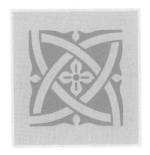

Physical Therapy Ethics

Donald L. Gabard, P.T., Ph.D.

Chair, Department of Physical Therapy
Chapman University
Orange, California

Mike W. Martin, Ph.D.

Professor, Department of Philosophy
Chapman University
Orange, California

F. A. Davis Company

Philadelphia

F. A. Davis Company
1915 Arch Street
Philadelphia, PA 19103
www.fadavis.com

Printed in the United States of America

Last digit indicates print number: 10 9 8 7 6 5 4 3 2 1

Acquisitions Editor: Margaret Biblis
Developmental Editor: Maureen R. Iannuzzi
Cover Designer: Louis J. Forgione

As new scientific information becomes available through basic and clinical research, recommended treatments and drug therapies undergo changes. The author(s) and publisher have done everything possible to make this book accurate, up to date, and in accord with accepted standards at the time of publication. The author(s), editors, and publisher are not responsible for errors or omissions or for consequences from application of the book, and make no warranty, expressed or implied, in regard to the contents of the book. Any practice described in this book should be applied by the reader in accordance with professional standards of care used in regard to the unique circumstances that may apply in each situation. The reader is advised always to check product information (package inserts) for changes and new information regarding dose and contraindications before administering any drug. Caution is especially urged when using new or infrequently ordered drugs.

Library of Congress Cataloging-in-Publication Data

Gabard, Donald L., 1946–
  Physical therapy ethics / Donald L. Gabard, Mike W. Martin.
      p. cm.
   ISBN 0-8036-1046-7
   1. Physical therapists—Professional ethics. 2. Physical
therapy—Moral and ethical aspects. I. Martin, Mike W., 1946– II.
Title.
   RM705.G334 2003
   174′. 2—dc21

2003043831

Permission to use information from Beauchamp T and Childress F: *Principles of Biomedical Ethics, 5e,* Oxford University Press, 2001, New York.

The following publisher has generously given permission to the authors to include in the case study and excerpts on pages 71–73 approximately 20 words; also a summary in their own words of Dr. Sacks's experience—which was submitted and approved by the author's agent. Excerpted with the permission of Simon & Schuster Adult Publishing Group from A LEG TO STAND ON by Oliver Sacks. Copyright © 1985 by Oliver Sacks.

For Clara and Clarence Gabard,
Lorraine Ogg, and Erasmo Borrego.
—Donald L. Gabard

For Shannon Snow Martin and Van L. Snow,
and in loving memory of Grace Snow.
—Mike W. Martin

About the Authors

DONALD L. GABARD, P.T., Ph.D., is associate professor of physical therapy at Chapman University. He earned his M.S. in physical therapy at the University of Southern California (USC), completed an additional two-year program in interdisciplinary medicine at its University Affiliated Program, and earned an M.P.A. and Ph.D. in Public Administration with a primary emphasis in administrative ethics. He also participated in seminars in medical ethics offered by the Hastings Center and by Georgetown University. Since 1978 Dr. Gabard has practiced pediatric physical therapy in a variety of settings, including in private practice and at Pacific State Hospital, the University Affiliated Program at Childrens Hospital of Los Angeles, Special Childrens Center in Pasadena, and California Children's Services. In addition to publishing a number of research articles, he has been a consultant to a variety of corporate and nonprofit organizations. Currently, Don Gabard is chair of the Department of Physical Therapy at Chapman University and teaches courses in physical therapy ethics, research design, and pediatric habilitation while maintaining clinical work and pursuing research in the distribution of health care to underserved populations.

MIKE W. MARTIN, Ph.D., is professor of philosophy at Chapman University, where he teaches medical ethics, business and professional ethics, and various other courses in applied ethics. He earned his B.S. (Phi Beta Kappa and Phi Kappa Phi) and M.A. at the University of Utah and his Ph.D. at the University of California, Irvine. He is author of many articles and nine books, most recently *Meaningful Work: Rethinking Professional Ethics* (Oxford University Press, 2000). His earlier book, *Ethics in Engineering* (with Roland Schinzinger), received the Award for Distinguished Literary Contributions Furthering Engineering Professionalism from the Institute of Electrical and Electronics Engineers, and his *Virtuous Giving: Philanthropy, Voluntary Service, and Caring* received the Staley/Robeson/Ryan/St. Lawrence Research Prize from the National Society of Fund-Raising Executives. In addition, he has received two fellowships from the National Endowment for the Humanities, two grants from the Association of American Colleges, the Arnold L. and Lois S. Graves Award for Teachers in the Humanities, and several awards for excellence in teaching.

Preface

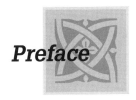

Ethics is the heart of professionalism. Just as much as technical skill, moral commitment enables physical therapists to provide quality services for patients, work effectively with colleagues, and maintain the trust of the public. At a more personal level, moral commitment motivates, guides, and gives meaning to work.

Physical therapists' special expertise and distinctive roles working closely and at length with patients allow them to bring a unique perspective to health-care ethics. Therapists also contribute to health-care ethics by participating in professional societies, serving on hospital ethics committees, revising health-care policies, and engaging in daily dialogue with other professionals. Hence, it is no surprise that the study of professional ethics now plays a prominent role in the curriculum and in professional settings.

Like health care itself, the exploration of physical therapy ethics is an inter-disciplinary effort. This book integrates the practical interests of physical thera-pists with philosophical ethics—a combination of disciplines that has similarly proved fruitful in the development of other branches of health-care ethics. Practical interests are engaged in many ways: by identifying and organizing a wide array of practitioners' concerns and debates within the profession, provid-ing numerous case studies of ethical dilemmas and responsible conduct, discussing relevant laws, and frequently referring to the *American Physical Therapy Association's Code of Ethics* and accompanying *Guide for Professional Conduct*. Philosophical approaches include attention to major ethical theories but primarily center around distinctions from and approaches to what philoso-phers call applied or practical ethics.

Our aim throughout this book is to provide tools for students and practi-tioners of physical therapy as they confront ethical dilemmas and moral contro-versy. Equally, our aim is to stimulate reflection on the moral significance of therapists' work, which remains a neglected area in the study of health care. Sometimes these aims are best served by withholding our views as authors, to provide balanced presentations of differing perspectives. Other times we present our position on issues, hoping thereby to provoke more discussion than would a mere summary of others' views.

Most of the chapters employ a dual organizing principle, as indicated by the chapter titles: a key value combined with a cluster of related topics in which that value plays a major role. For example, the key value in Chapter 7 is honesty, and the topics concern conflicts of interest. Usually the key value refers simultane-ously to a responsibility (an obligation) and a virtue (a good feature of charac-ter). Thus, honesty is owed as a duty to patients, and it is also a virtue of caregivers. Of course, no single value operates exclusively in any one domain of a profession, but we have found this approach contributes to thematic unity and pedagogical effectiveness.

Finally, we note that the *Guide to Physical Therapist Practice, Second Edition,* makes an important distinction between "patient" and "client":

> Physical therapist practice addresses the needs of both patients and clients through a continuum of service across all delivery settings—in critical and intensive care units, outpatient clinics, long-term care facilities, school systems, and the workplace—by identifying health improvement opportunities, providing interventions for existing and emerging problems, preventing or reducing the risk of additional complications, and promoting wellness and fitness to enhance human performance as it relates to movement and health. *Patients* are recipients of physical therapist examination, evaluation, diagnosis, prognosis and intervention and have a disease, disorder, condition, impairment, functional limitation, or disability; *clients* engage the services of a physical therapist and can benefit from the physical therapist's consultation, interventions, professional advice, prevention services, or services promoting health, wellness, and fitness.

For stylistic reasons, however, we have elected to most often use "patient," often the more vulnerable of the two categories, even though "patient/client" is in some cases most accurate.

Acknowledgments

We benefited from many insightful articles on ethics published in the journals *Physical Therapy* and *PT—Magazine of Physical Therapy*. Most of those articles are now available in a two-volume book, *Ethics in Physical Therapy*, published by the American Physical Therapy Association. Writers on physical therapy ethics and medical ethics who influenced our thinking are too numerous to list, but we wish to acknowledge Tom L. Beauchamp and James F. Childress, Robert M. Veatch and Harley E. Flack, Daniel Callahan, Laura Lee Swisher and Carol Krueger-Brophy, Janet Coy, Carol Davis, Amy Haddad, Ronald Munson, Ron Scott, and especially Ruth Purtilo, who has been a creatively commanding figure in the development of physical therapy ethics.

We thank our many students who over the years have challenged existing theory and offered their insights into ethical conduct. We also thank our colleagues and friends for their suggestions and support, including Gary Brahm, Deborah Diaz, Lauren Shepherd, Peggy Snow, and Virginia Warren. We are greatly indebted to Winkie Sonnefield, who read the entire manuscript and made many helpful suggestions. Don Gabard expresses gratitude to Terry Cooper for his generous mentoring in the study of ethics and management theory. Don Gabard's work on the book was partially supported by a sabbatical leave from Chapman University.

Margaret Biblis and Jean-François Vilain, our editors, along with Susan Rhyner, manager, creative development, and Maureen Iannuzzi, development editor, provided an ideal combination of encouragement, editorial advice, and creative freedom. We also wish to thank the reviewers for F. A. Davis who gave us helpful feedback as the project developed.

Oxford University Press granted permission to use our essay "Conflicts of Interest and Physical Therapy," from Michael Davis and Andrew Starks (eds.), *Conflict of Interest in the Professions* (Oxford University Press, 2001), as the basis for Chapter 7. The American Physical Therapy Association granted permission to print in the appendices its *Code of Ethics* and *Guide for Professional Conduct*. We note that these documents are periodically revised and made available at the Web site of the American Physical Therapy Association: www.apta.org/PT_Practice/ethics_pt.

Without the following support we would not have been able to incorporate some of this material into our book:

Case study adapted with permission of the American Physical Therapy Association from *Physical Therapy*, 1987(3):383–387, from Physical therapists as double agents: Ethical dilemmas of divided loyalties, by J Bruchner.

Excerpted with permission of the Americal Physical Therapy Association from *Physical Therapy*, 1989; 69(10):826-833, from Autonomy-based informed consent: Ethical implications for patient noncompliance, by JA Coy.

Case study adapted with permission of W.B. Saunders Company from *Ethical Dimensions in the Health Professions*, 2e, by Ruth Purtilo, 1993.

Excerpted with permission of the American Physical Therapy Association from *PT Magazine*, 1994; 2(10), from Culture and personal meanings, by K Parry

Excerpted with permission of the American Physical Therapy Association from *PT Magazine*, 1993(2):76-78, from An instrument of our own minds, by Ruth B. Purtilo.

Material excerpted with permission of the *Journal of the American Geriatric Society*, 1997;45(4):507, from Advance directives for seriously ill hospitalized patients: Effectiveness with the patient self-determination act and the SUPPORT intervention, by J Teno, J Lynn, N Wenger, et al.

Article reprinted with permission of the Los Angeles Times from "Agonizing Over Who Lives, Dies," by Marjorie Miller, Sept. 11, 2000.

Case Study adapted with permission of the American Physical Therapy Association from *PT Magazine*, 1996; 4(7):72-78, Modality utilization: Readers respond, by Ruth B. Purtilo, case study written by Ron Hruska.

Excerpted with permission of the American Physical Therapy Association from *PT Magazine*, 5(2):67-69, from Allocation of care: Readers respond, by JE Glenn, quoted by Ruth B. Purtilo.

Case study adapted with permission of Dr. Karen G. Gervais from *Ethical challenges in managed care: A case book* edited by KG Gervais, R Priester, DE Vawter, KK Otte and MM Solberg, 1999.

Case studies adapted with permission of Geri-Ann Galanti, from *Caring for patients from different cultures: Case studies from American hospitals*, pp. 19, 32, 40, 65, and 122-123 by Geri-Ann Galanti, University of Pennsylvania Press, 1997.

Appendices reprinted with permission of American Physical Therapy Association, from *Code of Ethics, Code of Ethics and Guide for Professional Conduct; Guide for Conduct of the Physical Therapist Assistant*.

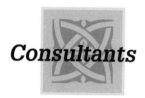

Consultants

Laurita Hack, P.T., M.B.A., Ph.D, FAPTA
Temple University
Philadelphia, PA

Z. Annette Iglarsh, P.T, Ph.D.
University of Sciences
Philadelphia, PA

Christine Kowalski, Ed.D., Ph.D.
Montana State University-Great Falls
Great Falls, MT

Cynthia Norkin, P.T., Ed.D.,
Ohio University (retired)
Athens, OH

Susan Roehrig, P.T., Ph.D.,
Hardin-Simmons University
Abilene, TX

Denise Wise, M.A., P.T.
College of Saint Scholastica
Duluth, MN

Jane Worley, M.S., P.T.
Lake Superior College
Duluth, MN

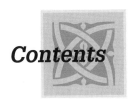

Contents

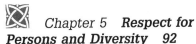

Professionalism and Ethics

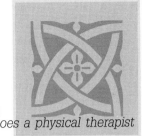

Does a physical therapist employed by a school district to attend to the needs of its student athletes owe primary loyalty to employer, students, or self?

Keywords

Professionalism	Physical therapy ethics	Ethical egoism
Compliance issues	Descriptive ethics	Psychological egoism
Moral disagreements	Normative ethics	Predominant egoism
Moral vagueness	Code of ethics	Mixed motive thesis
Ethical (moral) dilemmas	Ethical relativism	Moral development

Shirlaine

Shirlaine is a physical therapist working for a public school system.[1] Her duties consist primarily of screening high school athletes during the preseason and then treating injuries caused during practice or games. Currently she is treating Donald, the school's 11th-grade star wrestler and champion weight lifter, for a minor tear in his tendon at the biceps brachii muscle insertion. She notices excessive muscle hypertrophy as the tear heals. Because she knows that anabolic steroids are a common cause of such problems, and because she had previously suspected that Donald was using illegal drugs, she asks him whether he is using any steroids. At first he denies it, but eventually he confesses to using unprescribed methandrostenolone.

Shirlaine immediately urges him to stop using the drug and informs him of its potentially life-threatening side effects, including liver disease and cancer. He replies that he cares only about winning the state championship and begs her to keep the matter secret. He also says his competitors are using steroids, and it is unfair to deny him the opportunity to compete at their level. Moreover, he is confident he will not be caught. At one point he uses a threatening tone that makes Shirlaine feel her job might be in jeopardy if she divulges the information. In addition, Shirlaine knows the wrestling coach is an aggressive competitor who is lackadaisical about drug use.

Shirlaine faces an ethical dilemma, or, rather, several of them. In this chapter we discuss what ethical dilemmas are, how to identify them, and how to go about resolving them. After doing so, we define physical therapy ethics and discuss the connection between professionalism and ethics. We also discuss the specific contributions and limitations of ethical codes in resolving ethical dilemmas and, more generally, their role in professional ethics. We conclude by asking how morality and self-interest are related, particularly as they pertain to the goals of the study of professional ethics, a topic adumbrated in the example of Shirlaine. Throughout, we will understand **professionalism** as an umbrella value, one that encompasses the many more specific values professionals should commit themselves to.

 ## Ethical Dilemmas

Professionals encounter at least four types of ethical issues or problems: compliance, disagreement, vagueness, and dilemmas.

Compliance issues arise when it is clear what is morally right (or wrong) in a given situation and the only question is whether the professional will do it (or not do it). In general, knowing what is right is one thing, doing it is something else. For example, an individual who is in financial difficulty or angry at a supervisor might be tempted to steal from an employer, even though doing so is patently immoral. Living up to our moral responsibilities requires having integrity, self-discipline, and commitment, as well as avoiding apathy, weakness of will, and selfishness. In this book we sometimes discuss compliance issues, especially in chapter 8, "Integrity and Wrongdoing." The main emphasis, however, is on those issues for which a lack of clarity exists about what ought to be done because of disagreements, vagueness, or dilemmas.

Moral disagreements occur when individuals do not agree with each other about what is morally required in particular situations, or about which rules and policies are morally desirable, or even about which moral issues are important. Moral disagreements also play an important role in physical therapy, where therapists often share responsibility with others for an individual's health care. Physical therapists must work in unison with other health professionals who do not always agree on the best procedure or policy in specific situations. Physical therapists also work with their patients' family members, who sometimes disagree with each other. Thus, even when it seems completely clear to a therapist how best to resolve a moral difficulty, disagreements among colleagues who share responsibility for decision making can create new problems needing resolution, perhaps through reasonable adaptation and compromise. Also, as illustrated in the Shirlaine example, professionals and patients do not always see things the same way.

Moral vagueness means it is not clear what a specific moral value implies in a situation, what a particular moral idea means, or how best to structure (or "frame") a moral issue. For example, although it is clear that physical therapists are responsible for providing quality care to their patients, what exactly does that require in Shirlaine's situation? Also, therapists are expected to provide loyal service to their employers, but what is loyalty in Shirlaine's context?

Ethical dilemmas or **moral dilemmas** are situations in which two or more moral reasons come into conflict and it is not immediately obvious to the agent or to all rational persons what should be done. Ethical dilemmas also include situations in which one moral reason points in two opposing directions in a given situation. The moral reasons that enter into ethical dilemmas take different forms, such as moral duties, responsibilities, principles, rights, good consequences, ideals, or virtues.

Confronting moral dilemmas will occupy much of our time in this book because conflicting moral reasons are commonplace in the professions, as elsewhere. Why is that? Moral values are many and varied and enter into our lives in innumerable ways. Very often, multiple moral considerations apply to the same situation, as in the case of Shirlaine, and it is not immediately obvious which moral reasons have priority or even what the reasons require. Indeed, this complexity can even lead to alternative ways of formulating what the main dilemmas are in a situation. In part, these alternative ways of stating dilemmas reflect the central concepts in different moral traditions and ethical theories, such as those discussed in chapter 2. For example, dilemmas might be stated using the language of human rights ("rights ethics") or the language of utility, or producing the most good for the most people ("utilitarianism"). The way we identify ethical dilemmas reflects the values we find most important, both in general and in the situation.

Jan Bruckner, who developed the Shirlaine case study, suggests that Shirlaine faces a "double agent" or "dual loyalty" dilemma: "In this type of dilemma, physical therapists are forced to choose between loyalty to their employer and loyalty to their patients."[1(p383)]

> She must weigh her duty to her employer, the school system, and its interest, the team, against her duty to her patient, the athlete. The school system contracted with her to work with the coach and the team. The coach values the team's success over the welfare of the individual athletes. If Shirlaine chooses to act in loyalty to the team, she should act in a way to promote team success and probably ignore Donald's use of the contraband steroids.[1(p384)]

Certainly this is one plausible way to formulate the primary dilemma facing Shirlaine, but there are additional ways. On the one hand, it is not obvious that Shirlaine's duty to her employer unequivocally requires remaining silent. Suppose there is a "zero tolerance" state law requiring health professionals employed by the school district to report illegal drug use. Then, the loyalty to the school district might itself point in two different directions: loyalty to the school to maintain its zero tolerance policy by reporting Donald versus loyalty to the school to help its team win by not reporting Donald. On the other hand, it is not obvious what loyalty to Donald requires. Perhaps there is a duty of loyalty to turn him in, for the sake of his long-term physical health, but also a duty of loyalty not to turn him in, to respect his expressed desire to win the state championship.

At this point it might be objected that we have switched from (1) stating the dilemmas facing Shirlaine to (2) beginning to reason how to resolve the dilemmas, by reflecting on exactly what Shirlaine's responsibilities require in the situation. In fact, what we have discovered is that the very formulation of the pertinent dilemmas might involve discussing what one's responsibilities require in particular circumstances. In this way, the tasks of articulating ethical dilemmas and beginning to resolve them overlap. Stated another way, our moral perspective shapes what we see as dilemmas in the first place, as well as how we resolve them.

Bruckner points out that Shirlaine faces another ethical dilemma, this time concerning medical paternalism. Discussed in more detail in chapter 3, medical paternalism occurs when health professionals interfere with the autonomy (self-determination, freedom) of others with the aim of helping them. Shirlaine has a duty to promote the health of her patient; she also has a duty to respect his autonomy. Respect for Donald's autonomy seems to favor keeping his secret. In general, respect for autonomy also seems to imply maintaining strict confidentiality about patients, although there are exceptions, some required by law. In contrast, the duty to promote Donald's health suggests engaging in medical paternalism by overriding his autonomy in order to prevent him from risking his health. The issue might be complicated, however, by Donald's age. He is 17 and hence a minor in the eyes of the law. Does his age cancel out the duty to respect his autonomy, allowing Shirlaine to act directly in his self-interest, as she interprets that interest? Or, does she owe a duty to Donald's parents to inform them first, so that they, as legal guardians, can make decisions on behalf of Donald?

Shirlaine's choice might also be construed as a conflict between her self-interest and morality. Assuming that her primary moral duty is to help Donald, her patient, her self-interest, or personal well-being, might point in other directions. If she keeps quiet, most likely her job will not be affected. She would also avoid any wider repercussions for her career, such as difficulty getting another job if her contract is not renewed. Self-interest can itself be viewed as a moral consideration, however, in that we have moral rights to pursue our self-interest, within limits. We also have a duty to ourselves and to our families to pursue our self-interest, again within limits. Accordingly, Shirlaine's conflict can be viewed as an ethical dilemma that pits duty to others against duty to herself and to her family.

We will leave the resolution of these dilemmas to the Discussion Question section at the end of this chapter. As we proceed, however, we will return to the Shirlaine case study as a springboard for raising additional issues.

Resolution of Ethical Dilemmas

How, in general, should we resolve ethical dilemmas, arriving at a carefully considered conviction about what to do? There is no mechanical procedure, no moral algorithm. The following steps, however, are usually important in working out solutions in physical therapy, although not necessarily in this order.

1. Identify all the moral reasons that apply to the situation.

2. Consult the *American Physical Therapy Association* (APTA) *Code of Ethics* and *Guide for Professional Conduct*. (The current versions, dated January 2001, are reprinted in the Appendix, but periodically the documents are revised and posted on the Website for the APTA.) The code and guide state the professional requirements incumbent on all physical therapists, provide help in identifying the applicable moral reasons, and offer valuable guidance. Equivalent documents for the physical therapist assistant are the *APTA Standards of Ethical Conduct for the Physical Therapist Assistant* and the *Guide for Conduct of the Physical Therapist Assistant* (last amended in July 2001). These documents are available on the Website for the APTA and are also reprinted in the Appendix.

3. Gather factual information about the situation that is relevant in light of the moral reasons.

4. Identify applicable laws, if any. Laws function as legal constraints but also as moral reasons, given the general moral responsibility to obey the law.

5. Determine which moral reasons are most compelling in the situation. The ethical theories discussed in chapter 2 might be helpful in organizing, clarifying, and guiding one's thinking at this point.

6. Identify alternative practical responses to the dilemma that act on the moral reasons involved.

7. Weigh the reasons in light of the facts and with regard to the options: Which option best respects the most important moral reasons in the situation?

8. Talk with colleagues or others (without violating confidentiality) about how they see the dilemma. If one is in a situation of shared decision making in which there is disagreement, work out reasonable "compromises"—in the positive sense of a rational reconciliation of differences, not "compromises" in the pejorative sense of betraying one's integrity. In some cases realize that more than one reasonable solution is possible; in other cases the best solution might be to agree to disagree.[3]

Finally, we note in passing that some writers define ethical dilemmas in different ways than we have.[4] For example, Ruth Purtilo defines them as situations in which there are two correct but incompatible courses of action: "An ethical dilemma is a common type of problem that involves two (or more) morally correct courses of action *but you can't do both.* . . . As a result you (the agent, the responsible one) necessarily are doing something right *and also* wrong (by not doing the other thing that is also right)."[5] We find this definition misleading, at least as applied to most instances in which moral reasons conflict. In most ethical dilemmas, although admittedly not all, sound reflection and good reasoning lead to a verdict that one option is morally required, all things considered. Sometimes it becomes clear that one reason is most compelling in the circumstances and has priority over the others. Other times, reflection reveals that some of the responsibilities are limited and do not require as much as they initially seemed to require. Sometimes the right course of action causes some damage or harm, but it is still right. For example, the right thing to do might be to loyally support the interests of one's employer, even though it leads to putting a competitor out of business, thereby causing suffering to the competitor's employees.

Physical Therapy Ethics

Physical therapy ethics involves much more than the study of ethical dilemmas. In offering a fuller characterization of what it involves, we will distinguish two major meanings of the word "ethics" and two corresponding senses of "physical therapy ethics." Some are descriptive; others, the ones of primary interest in this book, are normative.

Descriptive Ethics

Descriptive ethics refers to what people actually believe in moral matters, or how they actually act, regardless of whether their beliefs and actions are justified. Thus, we speak of the ethics of Christians, Jews, Muslims, Hindus, Marxists, and members of the Ku Klux Klan. In a corresponding way, physical therapy ethics might refer to any or all of the following: (a) the conduct of physical therapists (as individuals or as groups), (b) the beliefs of physical therapists, and (c) the official views endorsed by the American Physical Therapy Association in its *Code of Ethics* and its *Guide for Professional Conduct*. Notice that each of these can be discovered by empirical inquiry, without evaluating the beliefs or conduct involved.

In a related sense, descriptive ethics can also refer to this empirical inquiry, in particular to scientific descriptions of people's beliefs and conduct in moral matters. Correspondingly, physical therapy ethics can mean the description and explanation of the beliefs and conduct of physical therapists concerning moral issues, without asking whether those beliefs and conduct are justified. These scientific studies might also seek to explain the origins of moral beliefs and behavior by identifying their causes. Generally, descriptive inquiries are conducted by psychologists, sociologists, anthropologists, and other social scientists. Also, biologists have created a new field called "sociobiology" that studies the genetic origins of morality.[6,7] The information gathered from these scientific inquiries is relevant in identifying areas needing moral critique and improvement. The information is also relevant in developing justified moral outlooks, for justified outlooks must be psychologically realistic—that is, attuned to what is possible for human beings.

As an example of descriptive inquiries relevant to physical therapy, we turn to the early days of the AIDS crisis. It was common knowledge that early on many physical therapists were reluctant to provide care to patients with AIDS. It was important to know if care was being compromised because of a fear of contagion, an avoidance of rendering what was perceived as futile treatment, or homophobia. If the answer had been contagion, then the profession should have dramatically increased its efforts and educational programs to explain the contagion risks. If it had turned out to be an aversion to treating persons with catastrophic illnesses or terminal illnesses, then treatment of patients with AIDS needed to be viewed in comparison with treatment of patients with cancer or other life-threatening diseases. If the results had been homophobia, then the profession would need to increase the educational effort around diversity and duty to treat. A scientific examination of the beliefs and values of physical therapists measuring fear of contagion, attitudes about terminal care, homophobia, and resulting behaviors would have been a timely and useful descriptive inquiry. Note that such a descriptive inquiry would not in itself make a moral judgment but would merely identify prevalent attitudes with relevant frequency, intensity, and a correlation with treatment variables.

Normative Ethics

In the main sense used in this book, "ethics" concerns justified or valid moral values. In one meaning, "ethics" refers to a normative study, an inquiry into what should be, not just what is commonly believed or usually done. **Normative ethics** means aimed at identifying, understanding, and applying justified moral values. Justified values are those values that stand up to full critical scrutiny in light of both broader normative perspectives and relevant facts about the world. This includes how those moral values are properly applied to issues, decisions, policies, organizational structures, laws, and questions of personal character. As such, ethics encompasses more than the study of ethical dilemmas. It includes, for example, appreciating justified moral values, understanding their meaning and importance in human life, developing sound moral policies, and fostering moral commitments and ideas.

Accordingly, as an area of study, *physical therapy ethics is the normative inquiry into the moral decisions and principles, ideals and virtues, and policies and laws concerning physical therapy.* This normative inquiry is an interdisciplinary study that draws on the insights of physical therapists, other health professionals, philosophers, religious thinkers, attorneys, administrators, and members of the public.

In a related sense, "ethics" is used as a synonym for morally desirable conduct, beliefs, and character. Using this sense, physical therapy ethics refers to the set of justified principles, policies, ideals, beliefs, attitudes, and conduct in physical therapy. And when we say that an act or a person is ethical (or moral), we are recommending or commending them.

In short, the word "ethics" has normative and descriptive meanings. In its descriptive sense, it refers to (1) scientific descriptions and explanations of what people believe and how they act concerning morality or (2) the actual beliefs and conduct of individuals and groups concerning morality. In its normative sense, it refers to (3) inquiry into identifying and applying justified moral values or (4) justified moral beliefs and conduct themselves, as well as morally desirable character. In this book, we will be interested primarily in the normative meanings, with the context making clear whether (3) or (4) is intended.

Morality

If ethics is the study of moral matters, what is morality? Some people use the words "moral" and "morality" narrowly, perhaps to suggest sexual attitudes, personal values, religious views, or other specific emphases within ethics. They distinguish moral reasons from the ethical reasons in professional life. In this book, however, we follow mainstream philosophical usage, according to which "moral reasons" include both professional and personal ethical values. What, then, are moral reasons?

To some extent, we all know what moral reasons are. They include honesty and integrity, justice and fairness, decency and compassion. A list of sample moral values, however, does not amount to a comprehensive definition. Nor does it explain why these items appear on the list—in other words, why are honesty and compassion moral values? It would be convenient to have a more comprehensive definition, yet providing such a definition is more difficult than it first appears.

Suppose we invoke a standard dictionary definition: Morality is about right and wrong, good and bad, what we ought and ought not to do. The difficulty is that all these terms have applications beyond moral matters, and hence they do not pinpoint our topic. For example, we speak of the right way to use a goniometer, the wrong way to interpret the developmental quotient for a premature child, the right way to turn on a computer, and the wrong way to test for a hip flexion contracture. There is a good and bad way to grow tomatoes and to mix paint. And when we say we ought to turn right at the signal in order to get to the restaurant, we are not issuing a moral prescription. The point is that distinctions of right-wrong, good-bad, and ought-and-ought-not are applied in numerous contexts having no special connection with morality.

As we try to be more specific, we become engaged in a normative inquiry, and the resulting definition is likely to be controversial. For example, if we say that morality is simply obeying the law and other dominant customs, we are embracing the controversial view called ethical relativism. Or, if we say morality is simply pursuing what is good for ourselves, we are embracing ethical egoism. If instead we say that morality is producing the most good for the most people, we are embracing the theory called utilitarianism. (These views are discussed later in this chapter.) Finally, if we say that morality is about human well-being, this characterization will strike some people as too narrow and others as too broad. It is too narrow because it excludes animals and the environment as having moral significance in their own right, independently of their uses for humans. It is too broad because it neglects how additional, nonmoral values also contribute to human well-being—for example, the values of art, recreation, and religion. In short, an informative and comprehensive characterization of morality requires sketching an ethical theory—a theory about morality—of the sort explored in chapter 2.

The expression "morally justified" is itself ambiguous. It might mean (a) morally obligatory (right, required), (b) morally permissible (all right, though perhaps not obligatory), or (c) morally good (desirable, even if not required). Obligatory principles are mandatory for all physical therapists, and failing to meet them makes therapists culpable. Yet ethics concerns more than duties and dilemmas, in physical therapy and elsewhere. Ethics also concerns personal ideals that individuals commit themselves to in their work, and some of these ideals are not mandatory for everyone. For example, some moral ideals are attached to religious commitments. Others are supererogatory ideals of caring and service that go beyond the minimum service required of all physical therapists. These personal ideals motivate, guide, and give meaning to the work of physical therapists (and other professionals), even when they are not incumbent on all of them.

Professions and Ethics

Physical therapy ethics is a branch of professional ethics, and more specifically a branch of ethics in the health-care professions. What is a profession? And what is the connection between professions and ethics (that is, "ethics" as morally desirable beliefs and conduct)?

In a loose sense, professions include all ways of making a living. Thus, we speak of professional athletes, truck drivers, spies, and even murderers. However, in the narrower sense used here, professions include only some forms of work—such as law, medicine, teaching, and physical therapy. Notice that very similar activities can be part of a profession or of work that is not yet a profession. For millennia engineers built roads and designed bridges, but engineering became a profession only in the late 19th century. Again, nursing, accounting, computer programming, and physical therapy became professions in the 20th century. What is this narrower sense of "profession"?

According to a standard definition, professions are those forms of work that meet at least four criteria: commitment to the public good, advanced expertise and education, independent judgment, and social organization and recognition.[8] Accordingly, physical therapy is a profession if it meets these criteria.

Commitment to the public good refers to a shared devotion to some aspect of the good of society. The specific aspect is part of the definition of particular professions. Thus, law is aimed at justice, engineering at efficient production of technological products, education at promulgating knowledge, and the health-care professions at promoting health. Physical therapy is a health-care profession distinguished by its focus on certain aspects of health as well as its distinctive social roles. Roughly, physical therapy focuses on functional movement, including preventing injury and reducing or relieving pain. The distinctive, if not altogether unique, ways these goals are pursued include rehabilitation and habilitation, which allows the person to enjoy a more functional, pain-free, and independent life that would not be possible without this specialized intervention.

Commitment to the public good provides the most obvious and direct tie to professional ethics. A profession's commitment to its distinctive public good is officially signaled in its **code of ethics** and related guidelines for professional conduct. Indeed, the drafting of a code of ethics and its promulgation within a profession are two of the earliest signs that a profession is emerging from what was previously a domain for technicians or craft persons. The American Physical Therapy Association's *Code of Ethics* and *Guide for Professional Conduct* were adopted in 1981 and have been revised several times since then.

Advanced expertise combines sophisticated practical skills with a strong grounding in sophisticated theory. Stated in another way, professional expertise combines practical *know-how* with *knowing-that* (numerous theory-based facts). The importance of practical know-how has always been clear enough in the case of physical therapy, which is quite literally a "hands-on" profession. The requirement of advanced theory-based knowledge has increased dramatically but still is in need of further refinement. The professionalization of physical therapy is manifested in the steady movement toward more advanced training in science and medicine and by the increased union between know-how and knowing-that, as exemplified in evidence-based practice.

Educationally, the profession started as certificate programs, many housed within hospitals or freestanding practices, apart from universities. Over time, most programs moved to or were developed in the university setting, and the professional training occurred simultaneously with acquisition of a bachelor's degree. At the present time most entry-level physical therapy programs are at the master's degree level.[9] The fairly recent emergence of the doctorate of physical therapy program as an entry-level degree extends the continuing educational evolution of the profession. The California Physical Therapy Association's goal is that, by the year 2004, half of the entry-level programs in physical therapy in California will award a master's degree and the other half will award a professional doctorate.[10] According to the California association's Vision Statement, the professional doctorate will be the only entry-level program acknowledged by the year 2010.

Still, while many feel that the theory-based aspect of the profession is adequate to consider it an advanced expertise, others regard physical therapy as still an emerging profession. The criticism has been expressed that some therapists fail to recognize that know-how is dependent on increasingly sophisticated forms of knowing-that. Know-how will not be recognized as a health-care contribution and thus be reimbursable by insurers as a medical expense until efficacy is demonstrated and supported within a theoretical framework.

Independent judgment implies the need for discretion—in contrast to mechanical or routine procedures—in making diagnoses of problems, considering alternative solutions, and reaching sound verdicts about how to proceed. Traditionally, so-called "true professionals" were said to act independently on their judgment, without supervision by others. That criterion has become somewhat unclear. While it is true that in more than half of the states in the United States physical therapists may evaluate and treat without a prescription, most still receive a prescription or diagnosis from a physician in order to receive reimbursement from insurance carriers. In many locations, that prescription is often open-ended and leaves the strategy for treatment up to the physical therapist.

Historically, the first physical therapists in this country were "reconstruction aides" who were employed by the government's Division of Special Hospitals and Physical Reconstruction during World War I and who had relatively little independence. The American Physical Therapy Association was founded in 1921.[11] In the aftermath of World War I, when physical therapy began to gain social recognition, physical therapists were regarded as technicians under the supervision of physicians, who were the true professionals.[12] As such, therapists' central responsibility seemed clear and simple: obey directives from supervisors. Physical therapists remained under the direct control of physicians into the 1950s, when private practice become a genuine possibility for significant numbers of therapists. California was the first state to legally allow direct access for physical therapy evaluation (1968), followed by 30 other states into the 1990s. Like those of other health professions, the standards of practice and education were continuously advanced as the profession became increasingly "professionalized." Today, most physical therapists again work in managed-care settings, but they have a professional identity grounded in wider responsibilities than simply obeying physicians' orders—especially responsibilities to provide quality care to patients.

How independent must practitioners be in order to qualify as "true professionals"? Nearly all professionals increasingly work in situations in which they share responsibility with others, and in which they are often accountable to managers and directors of organizations. Even physicians, traditionally the most independent of all professionals, now primarily work in managed-care facilities, where they are accountable to organizations. If anything, the "team" setting in which most physical therapists conduct their work has become the norm, in which the term "independent" judgment must be understood.

Social organization typically includes one national professional society—such as the American Medical Association, the American Bar Association, or the American Physical Therapy Association—together with organizations within each state. *Social recognition* means that the profession, through its professional organization, wins support from state and national governments to educate, license, discipline, and in other ways regulate their membership. In well-established professions, the profession wins not only the permission to engage in certain tasks but also a monopoly over services. Thus, only physicians can prescribe drugs. In the allied health fields, such as nursing and physical therapy, monopolies are less stringent and boundaries between professions can in some settings blur, as with occupational therapy and physical therapy for the pediatric developmentally delayed child. Even where there is not a vast, legally granted monopoly of services, however, the license that permits practitioners to write "P.T." after their name carries a public recognition that somewhat restricts unlicensed persons from engaging in certain public services.

⬡ Codes of Ethics

We have twice mentioned the APTA *Code of Ethics* and *Guide for Professional Conduct*, once in defining physical therapy as a profession and once as a resource in resolving ethical dilemmas. Throughout this book we will frequently cite these documents in connection with specific issues. It might be helpful at this point, therefore, to reflect on the contributions and limitations of the codes and guidelines promulgated within professions in general. What is the moral status of professional codes of ethics? Do they put into writing the standards that ought to govern the profession, or do they actually create at least some of the standards? In part, they do both.

Professional codes and guidelines are extremely important for at least five reasons.[13] First, as already emphasized, codes provide helpful guidance to professionals. Moral problems can be genuinely perplexing. Codes articulate, organize, and concisely present the backbone of moral understanding that informs the profession as it grapples with that perplexity. Moreover, within educational settings they also provide a useful tool in teaching professional ethics.

Second, codes represent a consensus within a profession that enables practitioners to work cooperatively and to compete fairly. Codes seek to establish a reasonable compromise and consensus about the restraints on self-interest in pursuing income within a competitive free-enterprise system. As such, they provide an essential understanding among professionals about what should and can be expected of each other, thereby establishing a field of fair play (work) that lessens cutthroat competition.

Third, codes give support to responsible professionals who are sometimes asked by their employers to cut (moral) corners in the name of profit. Under pressure, the isolated individual often has little recourse without the shared voice of the profession about responsible conduct.

Fourth, a code is the official statement by the profession that both individuals and the group of professionals are committed to promoting the public good and minimizing any harmful side effects. Professionals contribute to the fundamental public good—that is, good for the wider community—and are also capable of doing great harm to individuals and to the wider community. Because individuals differ considerably in their moral outlooks, a code expresses and establishes a consensus of shared standards in promoting public good, typically at a high level of excellence.

Fifth, and closely related, a code and its accompanying guidelines promote public trust. Codes function as a social contract between professionals and the public about what is to be expected of professionals. The code expresses a shared commitment to seek uniform ethical standards throughout the profession rather than a hit-and-miss approach that provides only occasional quality.

Having noted the great importance of codes, we can now question whether they are morally sufficient. Are they all that is needed to guide the professions? In our view, codes of ethics provide the backbone of professional ethics but not its full anatomy. Codes are generally the first word, but they are not a substitute for good moral judgment, much less for the deep personal commitments that individuals bring to their work.

For one thing, the principles articulated in codes are often too vague or incomplete to resolve ethical dilemmas. For example, Principle 9 of the APTA code says, "A physical therapist shall protect the public and the profession from unethical, incompetent, and illegal acts." Does that mean therapists should sometimes engage in whistle-blowing about their employer's or colleagues' unethical conduct? If so, exactly when is whistle-blowing justified? Of course, codes can always be rendered more precise, but there are limits. If they are to be useful as concise documents, they cannot possibly comment directly on every conceivable moral problem that might arise. Hence, with good reason, the APTA guide says that its ethical principles "should not be considered inclusive of all situations that could evolve."

Occasionally codes contain entries that do not belong there or that no longer apply. The code of the American Medical Association, as well as those in law, engineering, and other professions, once forbade advertising. The codes had to be rewritten in the late 1970s when the courts ruled that such codes were unconstitutional infringements of fair competition. Other entries in earlier codes forbade criticizing colleagues, which had the effect of silencing responsible free speech.[14]

In general, it is always intelligible to ask whether and why particular codes and their specific entries are justified. Codes are human documents, and they are only as sound as the judgment and foresight of the individuals and groups who write them. Suppose it were argued that a professional code is self-certifying, simply because it is written by the professional organization representing the group. Such a view presupposes that the group has final authority. In general terms, this view is called **ethical relativism**: Right action consists always and only in following the customs of the group or society to which one belongs.

There are many problems with ethical relativism. One problem is that one might be a member of many groups with conflicting standards. Thus, one might be a Catholic and an employee of Planned Parenthood, two groups that do not necessarily share the same view on abortion. Also, what constitutes the view of the group: complete consensus, a two-thirds majority, a simple majority, laws or other dictates of authorities within the group? The deepest problem, however, is that ethical relativism could be used to justify patent immorality. In an extreme case, it could be appealed to in justifying the treatment of Jews by Nazis during the Holocaust and any number of other horrors perpetrated by groups. In fact, scholarly reflections on the Holocaust, in addition to feminist objections to the treatment of women in certain societies, have prompted some anthropologists to question the extreme forms of ethical (or "cultural") relativism on which their discipline is founded.[15]

The central problem with ethical relativism, then, is that it makes nonsense of a fundamental aspect of moral reasoning: that sound moral reasons can be used to evaluate and sometimes reject particular laws and customs of groups. For example, human rights provide moral reasons that cut across national and even religious beliefs. The laws and customs of Nazi Germany patently violated human rights.

Moral reasoning can be used to evaluate the soundness of a professional code of ethics. A code of ethics that makes no mention of rights might well be flawed, and a valid code of ethics might make an appeal to human rights an important part of its outlook. We view it as a strength of the APTA code that its Principle 1 states, "A physical therapist shall respect the rights and dignity of all individuals and shall provide compassionate care."

At the same time, the customs of groups almost always have great moral importance. Although customs are not automatically the final word, they are typically morally *relevant* considerations in determining what ought to be done. Certainly that is true of the customs and standards expressed in professional codes. Indeed, professional codes have great moral significance even if they are not ideal documents, for they express the authoritative view of the entire profession as a basis for establishing public trust.

Codes are vitally significant for the five reasons we gave, but they do not replace the need for good moral judgment, perhaps guided in part by the study of ethical theory. Nor can they take account of the more personal commitments that individuals bring to their work, such as religious or humanitarian ideals that guide, motivate, and give meaning to their work. Finally, professional codes are human documents that from time to time need revision, and ethical theories can enter into discussions about how to make those improvements.

 ## Why Be Moral?

The study of professional ethics, then, involves much more than the study of codes and their applications to particular situations. It includes inquiry into broader moral concerns, such as ethical theories that might be used in grasping what kinds of entries should be in codes in the first place. It also involves reflecting on other basic moral matters as they pertain to the professions. It begins with this question: Why be moral, whether in one's profession or elsewhere?

The question can be taken two ways. On one hand, it might call for unfolding what is involved in the moral life, perhaps in a manner that elicits moral concern. Taken this way, it calls for invoking and elucidating moral values in some comprehensive way. For example, suppose the question is raised concerning why we should avoid cheating or paying bribes even when other people are doing so. The answer might be that participating in such practices would adversely affect our own character. It would make us persons whom we ought not to be: engaging in dishonest acts makes us dishonest persons, rather than persons of integrity. Thus, a question about why one should perform certain morally obligatory actions is answered by appealing to the virtues—that is, to the desirable features—of character that partly define who we are.

Again, suppose the question is why we should heed the standards of professional ethics in physical therapy. The answer might be that doing so would make us responsible professionals—and that says something important about the kinds of persons we are, the kinds of relationships we aspire to have, and the kinds of community we seek. In this regard, the primary reason for *doing* what is required as a morally responsible professional is that we will *be* responsible persons in our professions. We will be persons of integrity. We will be decent and compassionate healers.

On the other hand, the question "Why be moral?" might be presented as a challenge to justify the entire moral life itself—not just specific moral actions, but moral character and conduct in general. It might ask, Why should we care about any moral reasons? This question challenges the legitimacy of moral reasons and calls into question morality as a way of living. If morality is to matter, the question implies, it must have some nonmoral justification. Typically, that justification is understood to be self-interest. "Prove to me that morality pays," the question demands; "Prove to me that morality is worthwhile in terms of self-interest."

Many philosophers have attempted to respond to this challenge. Most notably, Plato, in his *Republic*, attempted to show that the moral person will be happier than the immoral person, and hence that morality pays.[16] He responds to the legend of the Ring of Gyges, in which a shepherd named Gyges finds a ring that allows him to become invisible—an idea two millennia older than H.G. Wells's science fiction tale of the invisible man. Using his magical powers, Gyges manages to gain control of the kingdom, placing all its riches under his complete control. Plato attempts to show that Gyges would of necessity be unhappy because his appetites would grow uncontrolled and overwhelm him. In contemporary terms, his mental health would be destroyed, and with it his well-being. Thus, Plato concludes, "virtue is, as it were, the health and comeliness and well-being of the soul, as wickedness is disease, deformity, and weakness."[16]

Other philosophers have argued that for the most part morality points in the same direction as an enlightened view of one's self-interest, or one's well-being.[17] For example, if we are selfish, we might have difficulty in love relationships; if we are callous and cruel, we will not have many friends; if we are dishonest, people will not be eager to engage in business with us; and so on. In short, moral endeavors and happiness-producing aspects of our lives largely overlap. If they did not, the moral life would be a nightmare of constant conflict between our natural desires to promote our well-being and our moral concerns. In fact, professional ethics and private interests generally overlap and mutually reinforce each other.

Even so, most contemporary philosophers reject the demand that morality must be justified entirely in terms of self-interest. Such a demand implies that only self-interested reasons are valid and that moral reasons must be validated in terms of them. To the contrary, as moral beings we affirm the validity of moral values themselves as ways to respect and care about persons (and other sentient animals). To adopt a moral point of view is to have such attitudes as respect and caring and to try to act on them. It is also to respond to other persons as having a moral worth that makes a claim on us and requires our attention. Indeed, it is to acknowledge moral values as especially important in how we live.

Or is it? There is one ethical theory that reduces morality to self-interest. **Ethical egoism** is the view that we ought always and only to care only about our own self-interest. This view suggests we ought to concentrate exclusively on our well-being and happiness rather than care about other people for their sake. The history of philosophy contains many attempts to refute ethical egoism. One attempt is to show it is logically inconsistent. For example, if I value myself as having inherent worth, mustn't I, to be consistent, value other people who, after all, are similar to me in relevant respects? The difficulty with this attempted refutation is that ethical egoists believe that each of us should have a singular moral concern for ourselves, and to that extent should view ourselves as morally singular. The charge of inconsistency is compelling only to people who have already abandoned ethical egoism.

Another attempt to refute ethical egoism is to appeal to moral principles about caring and respecting others for their sake. For example, the Golden Rule says we should do unto others as we would have them do unto us. Again, one might appeal to human rights, insisting that all humans have rights that make claims on us. The difficulty with all such strategies is that they assume the very thing that ethical egoists challenge—namely, that other people matter morally. Ethical egoists renounce such appeals to moral principles transcending self-interest precisely because they renounce moral reasoning as it is ordinarily understood. In this way, ethical egoism is a form of moral skepticism—skepticism about the validity of moral reasons.

Perhaps the most promising attempt to refute ethical egoism is to show that it is self-defeating. Its aim is to have us maximize our own long-term interests, well-being, and happiness. Yet, when we attempt to pursue our self-interest exclusively, we often fail. We become self-centered and selfish (excessively self-seeking) in ways that cut us off from the very things that promote our happiness: love, friendship, deep commitments in our professions, and additional commitments to humanitarian, environmental, spiritual, or other involvements. All these involvements presuppose that we cultivate caring for others for their sake.

The crux of the matter is the nature of the "self" whose self-interests are to be promoted. When the "self" is defined in terms of having caring relationships with others, self-interest and morality tend to converge.[18] Most ethical egoists, however, tend to resist such expanded conceptions of the self, and it proves difficult to shake them from their narrow conceptions of the self as preoccupied with good for themselves.

Instead of trying to refute ethical egoism directly, we might ask why some people find it an attractive doctrine, to see if there are any sound reasons for embracing it. An argument often set forth is that if we all look out for our own interests, then everyone will benefit. This is because we know best what is good for ourselves and are also in the best position to pursue that good. In reply, it is doubtful that these generalizations are true, since often we need others' help, especially when we are very young or very old. In addition, we sometimes fail to know what is good for ourselves. A more telling reply is that even if it were true that having everyone concentrate only on their own good would result in benefiting everyone, that would not provide an argument for ethical egoism. For such an argument presupposes that we should care about benefiting everyone, and that is exactly what the doctrine of ethical egoism denies.

Psychological Egoism

Perhaps the primary rationale for allegiance to ethical egoism is a particular view about human nature called **psychological egoism**, which says that all humans are always and only motivated by the desire to get what they believe are benefits for themselves. This is called "psychological" egoism because it is a doctrine about what actually motivates us, as distinct from "ethical" egoism, which is a doctrine about how we ought to act. If psychological egoism were true, then ethical egoism would be the only plausible ethical theory. All other ethical theories, as we will see in chapter 2, regard morality as placing restrictions on the pursuit of self-interest. But if all that humans are capable of caring about is good for themselves, the only plausible ethical theory is one that requires us to take a long-term view of our interests and to engage in prudent self-seeking.

Thus, it is no surprise that defenders of ethical egoism are invariably psychological egoists, including the 17th-century philosopher Thomas Hobbes and the 20th-century novelist Ayn Rand.[19,20] But a surprisingly large number of psychologists, economists, and political scientists have also embraced psychological egoism. Hence, it is worth asking what arguments support that view of human nature. Most of the arguments are simple, seductive, and specious.

The first argument states that people always act on their own desires. Therefore, people always and only seek something for themselves—namely, the satisfaction of their desires. Therefore, psychological egoism is true.

In reply, we can agree the premise is true: We do always act on our own desires. Even when we seek to please others we are acting on our desires to please them. And even when we do things we say we don't want or feel like doing (such as going to the dentist), we are actually acting on our desire (to maintain healthy teeth). Indeed it is true by definition that we always act on our own desires: by definition, my actions are based on my desires and my beliefs—that is simply what an action is, in contrast to involuntary reflexes or accidentally getting struck by lightning. Surely, however, this tautology cannot establish psychological egoism, which is a highly controversial view of human nature. In fact, the fallacy is easy to discern. "My desires" include desires for many different things: to get something for myself (self-seeking), to pursue my profession with excellence, and to help others who are in need of help. It is the object (target) of the desire that determines whether it is self-seeking, not the mere fact that it is my desire.

The remaining arguments for psychological egoism take this last point into account and focus on the objects of desires. Thus, a second argument asserts that people always seek to gain pleasure for themselves (from satisfying their desires) or to avoid their pain; therefore, psychological egoism is true. In reply, this time the premise is false. We seek many things that we value for themselves—love, friendship, creative expression, mountain climbing. We derive pleasure from these things because we value them in the first place. True, often we do seek pleasures, but the pleasures are attached to and derive from activities, relationships, and things that we value and desire. If we did not value these things in their own right, we could not derive enjoyment from gaining (and even pursuing) them.

A third argument asserts as a premise that we can always imagine an ulterior self-seeking motive for any human action. Even the most seemingly self-sacrificing action might be motivated by a concern for compensation of some kind, if only posthumous awards or divine salvation; therefore, people only seek something for themselves.

In reply, the premise is obviously true: we can always *imagine* a self-seeking motive for any human action. It does not follow, however, that the *actual* motive is self-seeking. For example, we can always imagine that soldiers who jump on grenades to save their comrades are only out to gain posthumous rewards or to escape depression. We can also imagine that the rescuers during the Holocaust who risked their lives and their families to save perfect strangers were only thinking about themselves. We can imagine these things, but that does not make them so.[21] One would have to be a cynic to believe that all forms of heroic and supererogatory conduct are mere variations on "looking out for number one."

A fourth argument says that when we examine closely any human action, we actually do find some element of self-seeking, some kind of benefit for the agent; therefore, psychological egoism is true.

In reply, this time the premise might well be true, but it does not establish the conclusion. That is, it might well be true that every human action is at least *partly* motivated by self-seeking, but that does not establish that the entire or sole motive is self-seeking. (It is a confusion to infer that because "one" motive for an action is self-seeking that the "only" motive is self-seeking.)

At this point, we leave to the Discussion Questions section a further analysis of whether psychological egoism can be supported by any better arguments. We conclude here with what we consider two important and plausible claims about human motivation.

It is probably true that most people, most of the time, are primarily motivated by a concern for their self-interest. This view has been called **predominant egoism**.[19(p444)] Predominant egoism differs from psychological egoism by acknowledging a significant, albeit limited, role for caring about other people. It leaves room for the possibility that responsible professionals genuinely can and do care about the people they seek to help. Specifically, physical therapists can and do care about their patients—for the sake of their patients and for their own personal benefit.

The second claim is that most human actions have multiple motives, often embedded within layers of motivation, and often combining legitimate self-seeking with concern for others. For example, taking a particular college class might be motivated partly by the enjoyment one derives from it and partly, perhaps primarily, by its contribution to a degree. In turn, the desire for the degree is motivated by multiple interests: earning a living, finding enjoyable and challenging work, and being able to help others. Call this the **mixed motive thesis**: Much human action is motivated by a mixture of motives, including elements of self-interest and altruism.

The motives of professionals might be sorted, very roughly, into three categories: craft, compensation, and moral concern.[22] *Craft motives* are desires to meet the standards of technical excellence as defined by state-of-the-art professionalism, as well as to seek creative solutions to technical problems. *Compensation motives* are desires to earn a living, have job stability, gain professional recognition, exercise power and authority, and other primarily self-oriented desires. *Moral concern* refers to motives specified in moral language, many of which fall into two overlapping categories: (1) integrity motives, which are desires to meet one's responsibilities and maintain one's moral integrity and (2) caring motives, which are desires to promote the good of others for their sake. Typically, all three types of motivation are interwoven in the life of the physical therapist. Moreover, it is generally good that this mixture is found, for the motives tend to reinforce and strengthen each other.

Why Study Ethics?

We are now in a position to examine the goals of the study of professional ethics. Why study professional ethics, and what can be gained from such a study? We will focus on the goals of physical therapy ethics courses required for earning a degree, but the same question arises in the study of professional ethics as part of continuing education, in ethics workshops within companies, and even in reflecting on one's own work as a practitioner.

A familiar objection to courses on ethics is that morality cannot be taught at the college level because moral values are already instilled, or not, in the early moral training of children. This objection contains an element of truth, but only an element. The essential foundation for moral decency must begin early in life. Without that foundation, little can be done at the college level. To cite an extreme example, there is no cure for those who are sociopaths—individuals said to have "antisocial personality disorders"—who enter adulthood without a moral conscience, without any sense of right or wrong.

Nevertheless, university courses can make a significant contribution to **moral development**.[23] The study of ethics is a lifelong process, and higher education provides an especially important opportunity for grappling with the complexity of moral issues in the professions. Courses on ethics strengthen capacities for dealing with moral vagueness (uncertainty, ambiguity), dilemmas, and disagreements. They do so by strengthening and refining such skills as:

- identifying and clarifying moral issues and moral reasons.
- weighing conflicting moral reasons.
- forming consistent and well-developed moral perspectives.
- maintaining imaginative awareness of alternative viewpoints, and integrating conflicting perspectives.
- using moral reasons and arguments with increased precision, both in writing and in dialogue with others.

Notice that this list centers on cognitive skills—skills of the intellect, such as perception, clarity, and argument. Presumably a thoroughly immoral person could possess these cognitive skills and yet lack moral concern and respect. The person could lack desirable moral attitudes and fail to act in morally desirable ways. In fact, such a person could abuse the skills by using them to rationalize immoral conduct. Consider, then, the following additional skill goals:

- The ability to argue in morally reasonable ways, toward beliefs that are justified (acknowledging wide room for legitimate differences among morally reasonable persons).
- Strengthening attitudes of care and respect for other persons, as well as for oneself.
- A developed and nuanced appreciation of diversity, as manifested in moral tolerance (noncoercive behavior toward people one disagrees with), open-minded (receptive to new ideas), and broad-minded (acknowledging a range of morally reasonable differences).
- Tendency to act in morally responsible ways as a professional.
- Ability to maintain integrity by integrating one's personal and professional life.

Should we add the last five goals to our list of aims for university courses on ethics? Our answer is yes, with a caveat. Without these goals, courses on ethics would have little *moral* point. Devoting classroom time to ethics should be done in the conviction, or at least with the reasonable hope, that such time will contribute to morally responsible conduct rather than mere cleverness in arguing that is aimed at rationalizing immoral behavior. Moreover, when teaching ethics is linked to clinical supervision, professors can and should assure that students are meeting appropriate standards of clinical practice.

The caveat: In our view, the direct emphasis in college courses should be on increasing cognitive skills, largely presupposing a foundation of moral concern—on the part of professors and students alike; teaching ethics is different from preaching. As for moral commitment, professors and students are in many respects moral equals. Professors have greater practical experience and theoretical expertise, but they cannot be presumed to "have the right answers" in resolving moral issues, nor even to be more deeply committed morally than students. Hence, in setting goals for courses on ethics, and especially in grading exams and papers, professors should reasonably focus on increasing skills of moral argument, including appreciation of alternative perspectives and awareness of the important variables involved in a decision.[24]

As stated in the Preface, the central aim of this book is to offer tools for students and practitioners of physical therapy to strengthen their capacities for responding to moral vagueness, ambiguity, conflicting reasons, and disagreements. We proceed in the conviction that such growth is both possible and commonplace. Although our focus is on increased cognitive skills, we address ourselves to morally concerned persons who will use these skills for ethical purposes.

Moral Development

The preceding discussion of classroom goals can be linked to controversies in the area of psychology that studies moral development—that is, the growth in moral understanding and character of individuals within their societies. Moral development theory has as many branches as does psychology in general. Thus, behaviorists, psychoanalysts, social psychologists, and others have all made contributions. Especially important work, however, has been done by the cognitive psychologist Lawrence Kohlberg (1927–1987) and his critics.

Kohlberg identified three levels of psychological development: preconventional, conventional, and postconventional.[25] Each level contains two stages, making a total of six stages. The stages are distinguished according to how individuals engage in moral reasoning and which motives or reasons they respond to.

At the preconventional level, typical for most children aged four to ten, individuals are narrowly egoistic in their reasoning and motivation. This level is akin to the outlook of ethical egoism, although children at this age are not yet able to envision their long-term good in the way required by the ethical egoist. At stage 1 they think in terms of avoiding punishment and deferring to physical power. At stage 2 they begin to pursue their desires by using stratagems to gain rewards, such as "You scratch my back and I'll scratch yours."

At the conventional level, the emphasis is on meeting the expectations of family, organizations, and wider society. This level encompasses stage 3, which accents stereotypes of "good boy" and "nice girl," and stage 4, which accents doing one's social duty so as to maintain the social order. The level is akin to ethical relativism. According to Kohlberg, many adults never grow beyond this level.

At the postconventional level, individuals move in the direction of autonomy, self-directing their lives in light of moral principles that are not reducible to customs of groups. Stage 5 is a social contract perspective in which principles are seen as justified when they represent agreements among rational participants in society. There is an emphasis on legal rules, but not an assumption that all actual legal rules are reasonable. Stage 6 is reasoning in terms of abstract principles that are comprehensive, universal, consistent, and ranked in a hierarchy of importance. The Golden Rule and general principles of justice and human rights are examples of fundamental principles.

Consistent with our earlier rejection of ethical egoism and ethical relativism, we agree with Kohlberg that moral development includes movement away from childlike narcissism and uncritical social conformity; it includes movement toward autonomous moral reasoning and conduct in terms of wider values. Yet, along with critics of Kohlberg, we challenge his assumption that the highest stages of moral reasoning are defined by using universal principles ranked in order of their general importance. To see what is at issue, consider Kohlberg's most famous example, the Heinz Dilemma.[25]

Heinz

Heinz is married to a woman who is dying of cancer but whom doctors believe might be saved by a very expensive radium-compound drug. A pharmacist in a European town where Heinz lives controls the drug and will make it available at a cost 10 times what it costs to make. Heinz cannot afford the drug, nor can he find friends who will loan him the money to buy it. After trying to convince the pharmacist to lower the price or to let him pay for it later, Heinz breaks into the pharmacy and steals the drug. The question is whether he was justified in doing so.

Kohlberg presented this and other dilemmas to people of many ages and studied how they reasoned about them. He concluded that those who said Heinz should worry about himself primarily were at the preconventional level. Those who argued that Heinz should not steal the drug because stealing is wrong (according to social conventions) were at the conventional stage. And those who reasoned that Heinz was justified (either permitted or obligated) in stealing the drug because the rule "Save lives" or "Help one's wife" overrides the rule "Do not steal" illustrated higher stages of moral development.

Suppose, however, that individuals argued that Heinz should keep talking to the pharmacist, trying to convince him to change his mind, and perhaps encouraging others to talk to the pharmacist as well? Kohlberg tended to interpret such respondents as being indecisive and wishy-washy rather than firmly principled. In contrast, Carol Gilligan, Kohlberg's most famous critic and his former research assistant, suggested that such dialogue-oriented and contextual approaches represent legitimate and perhaps even preferable responses to the dilemma.[26]

Gilligan drew a distinction between an "an ethics of care" and an "ethics of justice." She suggested that Kohlberg presupposed an ethics of justice in which moral growth meant moving toward reasoning using abstract, universal rules. In contrast, she reported that her studies of young girls revealed growth toward effective balancing of the needs of oneself and others. Gilligan adapted much of the basic structure of Kohlberg's levels of moral development, but she redescribed the three levels: Preconventional reasoning consists of exaggerated self-concern, conventional consists of reasoning based on what society demands, and postconventional implies being able to reasonably balance the legitimate needs of oneself with those of others. The latter is accomplished by paying close attention to context, maintaining personal relationships, sustaining communication, and making reasonable compromises. According to Gilligan, rather than a hierarchy of abstract rules of the sort Kohlberg emphasized, what matters is nuanced and responsible contextual reasoning.

We postpone to chapter 2 a discussion of moral rules and contextual reasoning. But here we ask: How can we tell whether Kohlberg, Gilligan, or some other developmental psychologist has accurately portrayed the highest stage of moral development? Clearly, "highest" means the most valid, justified, or insightful way of reasoning. Hence, to rank the stages requires defending a moral viewpoint. We should not assume that a particular psychologist is more adept than others in determining which moral viewpoint is most justified.

In general, we cannot rely on psychologists to tell us what is the best way of moral reasoning. Only a serious study of normative ethics can help us do that, and even then we might expect disagreement among reasonable persons. Each of us, as morally responsible and autonomous agents, must engage in that study for ourselves, gaining from the insights of others along the way. Thus, our view of the specific goals of courses of ethics cannot be uncritically imported from studies of moral development by psychologists. Those studies are valuable and enrich the study of ethics, but invariably they presuppose an ethical outlook that needs to be defended philosophically. Some of those insights can be gleaned from the moral theories we consider in chapter 2.

In concluding, we note that, ironically and regrettably, ethics, for some, has a bad name. For these people, it brings to mind negative things like blaming, self-righteous hypocrisy, and congressional ethics committees that themselves sometimes act in suspect ways. Or it elicits a groan by reminding us of the seemingly intractable disagreements involved in the "culture wars" over such issues as abortion, affirmative action, and the death penalty, if not more personal battles we have had with our parents and friends over other issues. Then, too, there is the humorous remark reportedly made by Nobel laureate Saul Bellow: "Socrates said, 'The unexamined life is not worth living.' My revision is, 'But the examined life makes you wish you were dead.' "[27]

Ethics does, of course, have a serious and complex side to it, and in this chapter we have highlighted its dimensions of vagueness, dilemma, and conflict. Yet ethics involves much more that is positive. Moral values permeate the daily practice of physical therapy as well as all other professions, even where no uncertainty or disagreement is present. All services to clients have a moral dimension, a dimension grounded in caring and respect. Professionalism implies a continual sensitivity to and mindfulness of these values in ways that contribute to meaningful, giving relationships with patients and other clients (such as family members, surrogate decision makers, or companies).

Discussion Questions

1. Present and defend your view concerning (a) how best to articulate the ethical dilemmas faced by Shirlaine, in the case study opening this chapter, and (b) how to resolve them. In developing your answer, consult the APTA's *Code of Ethics* and *Guide for Professional Conduct*. Which entries are directly applicable to the case, and do the entries provide the solution to any dilemmas involved? As you answer these questions and listen to others' points of view on the case, can you begin to characterize some of the values central to your view of ethics, both in personal and professional life?

2. Ethics includes moral inquiry into policies and laws, as well as individual conduct, and sometimes moral dilemmas can be resolved only by shifting attention to questions of policy. Which laws would help lessen the kinds of dilemmas faced by Shirlaine? Would the laws have any negative side effects?

3. What similarities and differences do you see in the professions of physical therapists, chiropractors, and physicians specializing in physical injuries? Do the differences imply any differences in ethical principles governing their work?

4. Some social critics believe that distinguishing certain forms of work as "professions" implies elitism and social superiority. Others share George Bernard Shaw's cynicism that professionalization is primarily a ruse designed to gain more money from clients, or, as he puts it in his 1913 play *The Doctor's Dilemma*, "All professions are conspiracies against the laity." Are these criticisms warranted, at least in part? If so, what remedies might be offered so as to strengthen public trust in professions and professionals?

5. Discuss the following questions:
   a. Is psychological egoism true?
   b. Is ethical egoism true?
   c. What is enlightened self-interest?
   d. If we understand the "self" (the person) as defined by its relationships with others, does the good of the self essentially become one with valuable relationships with others?

6. What limitations, if any, do you see in Lawrence Kohlberg's assumption that the highest (best) level of moral reasoning involves an emphasis on universal moral rules, ranked in order of importance? What dangers do you see in Carol Gilligan's emphasis on contextual reasoning aimed at maintaining personal

relationships rather than relying on general moral rules? Link your answers to your view concerning how Heinz should have acted and especially to the argument you would put forth to defend your view.

7. Ethics includes more than obligations. It also includes personal ideals of caring and service that transcend mandatory requirements, ideals that give meaning to one's career. To ask a highly personal but pertinent question, what ethical ideals do you bring to your profession? What prospects and obstacles do you anticipate in pursuing those ideals?

8. Roger Ortega is a physical therapist in a skilled nursing facility where many of the patients referred for physical therapy require modalities such as ultrasound and paraffin treatments as a part of the total physical therapy program. Roger discovers that the ultrasound machine is not functional but that the PT aides have continued to use it at the direction of the other physical therapist, Phyllis Smoyer. When Roger questions Phyllis about this practice, she acknowledges that the machine does not work but she argues that the primary benefit in most of these cases is the placebo effect and so no harm occurs. In fact, many do feel their pain is diminished. The only explanation offered to Roger for not having the equipment repaired is the cost of the repair. Is there an ethical problem here, and if so, what course(s) of action could Roger take?

9. Read through the APTA *Code of Ethics* and *Guide for Professional Conduct.* Do all the entries strike you as reasonable? Identify at least one possible conflict, and hence ethical dilemma, that might arise between two or more entries in the code—for example, between section 9 and section 11.3. (Check the APTA Website to see if the code and guide have been revised since January 2001, which is the version in the Appendix of this book.)

References

1. Bruckner J. Physical therapists as double agents: ethical dilemmas of divided loyalties. *Phys Ther.* 1987;67:383-387.
2. Benjamin M. *Splitting the Difference: Compromise and Integrity in Ethics and Politics.* Lawrence, KS: University of Kansas Press; 1990.
3. Moody-Adams MM. *Fieldwork in Familiar Places: Morality, Culture, and Philosophy.* Cambridge, MA: Harvard University Press, 1997;110-111, 182-183.
4. Sinnott-Armstrong W. Moral dilemmas. In Becker LC, Becker CB, eds. *Encyclopedia of Ethics.* 2nd ed. New York: Routledge; 2001:1125-1127.
5. Purtilo RB. *Ethical Dimensions in the Health Professions.* 2nd ed. Philadelphia, PA: W.B. Saunders; 1993:39-40.
6. Caplan AL, ed. *The Sociobiology Debate.* New York, NY: Harper and Row; 1978.
7. Thompson P, ed. *Issues in Evolutionary Ethics.* Buffalo, NY: State University of New York Press; 1995.
8. A related, but fuller, list of criteria is given by Bayles MD. *Professional Ethics,* 2nd ed. Belmont, CA: Wadsworth; 1989. Also see Callahan JC, ed. *Ethical Issues in Professional Life.* New York, NY: Oxford University Press; 1988:26-39.
9. American Physical Therapy Association. Accredited Educational Programs for the Physical Therapist. Available at: https://www.apta.org/Education/schoollistings/pt_schools/acd_edu_prg_pt. Accessed on March 16, 2001.
10. California Physical Therapy Association. 2010: California Vision Statement. Available at https://www.CCAPTA.org/PTVisionStatement2010.htm. Accessed on December 12, 2002.
11. American Physical Therapy Association. A Historical Perspective. Available at: https://www.apta.org/About/apta_history/history. Accessed on March 16, 2001.

12. Magistro CM. Twenty-second Mary McMillan lecture. *Phys Ther.* 1987;67:1726–1732.
13. Martin MW. *Meaningful Work: Rethinking Professional Ethics.* New York, NY: Oxford University Press; 2000:32-35. Michael Davis gives even greater importance to codes; see Thinking like an engineer: The place of a code of ethics in the practice of a profession. *Phil Pub Affairs.* 1991;20:150–167.
14. Unger SH. *Controlling Technology.* 2nd ed. New York, NY: John Wiley and Sons; 1994:124.
15. Fluehr-Lobban C. Cultural relativism and universal rights. In Sommers C, Sommers F, eds. *Vice and Virtue in Everyday Life.* 4th ed. Philadelphia: Harcourt Brace; 1997:220-225.
16. Plato. *The Republic*, trans. Cornford, FM. New York, NY: Oxford University Press; 1945:44.
17. Kavka GS. The reconciliation project. In Feinberg J, Shafer-Landau R, eds. *Reason and Responsibility.* 10th ed. Belmont, CA: Wadsworth Publishing; 1999:637-650.
18. Holley DM. *Self-Interest and Beyond.* St. Paul, MN: Paragon House; 1999. See also Paul EF, Miller FD, Paul J, eds. *Altruism.* New York: Cambridge University Press, 1993.
19. Kavka GS. *Hobbesian Moral and Political Theory.* Princeton, NJ: Princeton University Press, 1986.
20. Rand A. *The Virtue of Selfishness.* New York, NY: New American Library; 1964.
21. For a sampling of the vast literature on Holocaust rescuers, see Oliner PM, et al. eds. *Embracing the Other.* New York: New York University Press; 1992. See also Monroe KR. *The Heart of Altruism.* Princeton, NJ: Princeton University Press; 1996.
22. Martin MW. *Meaningful Work*, p21.
23. Callahan D, Bok S, eds. *Ethics Teaching in Higher Education.* New York: Plenum; 1980. See also Davis M. *Ethics and the University.* New York: Routledge; 1999.
24. Simon RL, ed. *Neutrality and the Academic Ethic.* Boston, MA: Rowman & Littlefield; 1994.
25. Kohlberg L. *The Philosophy of Moral Development.* Vol. I. New York, NY: Harper Collins; 1981.
26. Gilligan C. In *A Different Voice.* Cambridge, MA: Harvard University Press; 1982. Second edition, 1993. For an illustration of the influence of and controversies surrounding Gilligan's work, see Kittay EF, ed. *Women and Moral Theory.* Totowa, NJ: Rowman & Littlefield; 1987. See also Card C, ed. *Feminist Ethics.* Lawrence, KS: University of Kansas Press; 1991. Also, Tong, RP. *Feminist Thought.* 2nd ed. Boulder, CO: Westview Press; 1998.
27. Bellow S. Seeing the earth with fresh eyes. *New York Times.* May 26, 1977;13.

Good Judgment and Moral Reasoning

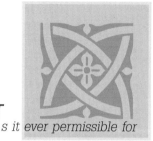

*I*s it ever permissible for
physical therapists to lie during the execution of
their professional responsibilities?

Keywords

Rights ethics
Human rights
Legal rights
Liberty rights
Welfare rights
Libertarians
Duty ethics
Autonomy
Rationality

Categorical imperative
Universalize
Absolute duties
Prima facie duties
Deontological ethical theories
Consequentialist (teleological)
   ethical theories
Utilitarianism
Intrinsic good/bad

Harm principle
Act utilitarianism
Rule utilitarianism
Virtue (character) ethics
Religious ethics
Divine command ethics
Pragmatism

Luis Alvarez

Luis Alvarez, a physical therapist working in a rehabilitation clinic, has a female patient who was injured in a domestic dispute. Luis was approaching the treatment area, where his patient was waiting, when her irate spouse approached him and asked if his wife was in "there," pointing to the treatment room. The man's demeanor suggested both anger and intoxication, and Luis feared his patient's spouse might complete the battering that led to her admission in the first place. Is it all right for Luis to lie and say that the patient has been discharged, thereby allowing himself time to call security and warn the proper authorities? Or should he pursue a different stratagem because lying is undesirable, especially in one's role as a professional?

Moral questions are answered by exercising good moral judgment. That means being sensitive to the full array of moral reasons applicable to particular situations. It also means integrating those reasons in morally reasonable ways in light of the relevant facts available. Given the complexity of the world and the multiplicity of moral values, moral judgment cannot be encapsulated in a simple algorithm. Even the most familiar acts, such as lying, have considerable complexity.[1] As the novelist George Eliot commented, "The mysterious complexity of our life is not to be embraced by maxims," and there is no substitute for the "growing insight and sympathy" earned "from a life vivid and intense enough to have created a wide, fellow feeling with all that is human."[2] Moreover, good judgment must often be exercised promptly, as in the situation faced by Luis Alvarez, with little time to ponder an ideal solution.

Regardless of the urgency of the situation, moral judgment is exercised against the background of moral understanding developed from childhood on, as suggested in the discussion in chapter 1 of Kohlberg and Gilligan's theories of moral development. Part of that development consists of learning an array of moral rules—such as tell the truth, keep your promises, do not cheat—and moral attitudes taught by parents and teachers using paradigms (clear-cut cases) of what is morally right and wrong. Ethical theories attempt to organize these rules and attitudes into systematic perspectives on morality. Although they cannot replace practical experience, ethical theories seek to provide helpful frameworks for approaching ethical dilemmas. They do so by pinpointing relevant moral reasons and by clarifying and ordering them in importance. They also help in justifying general moral principles. As such, they contribute to good moral judgment, even though they cannot replace the need for a continually "growing insight and sympathy."

Philosophers have not succeeded in formulating one ethical theory satisfactory to everyone. Indeed, today few philosophers believe that agreement on just one ethical theory will ever occur. Nevertheless, philosophers have developed several influential types of theories.[3] In this chapter we introduce six major types, each of which has many defenders, and each of which has greatly influenced thinking about health-care ethics; they include: rights ethics, duty ethics, utilitarianism, virtue ethics, religious ethics, and pragmatism. We will touch on additional theories in other parts of the book—for example, feminist theories are discussed in chapter 5—but the six theories discussed here represent a good sampling of major approaches in contemporary ethics, both in general and specifically within the field of health care. Because each of the theories developed over time and now has several variations, they all can also be regarded as *moral traditions* that remain vibrant today.

As we proceed, we will take note of the major variations within each theory. Doing so reveals that the details of a given theory, as well as its general direction, matter enormously. As we suggest later, often the differences between the versions of one type of theory are far greater than the differences among types of theories.[4] Also, given the complexity of these theories, it will be helpful to examine them in connection with the more familiar topics of lying (that is, knowingly stating falsehoods with the intent to deceive) and deception (intentionally misleading someone, whether by lying, pretense, or other means) and explore how each theory explains what is wrong with deception and also when deception is morally permissible (and occasionally obligatory).

Rights Ethics

The language of "rights" provides one way to formulate Luis Alvarez's dilemma. On the one hand, the battered wife has a right to life, as well as a right not to be assaulted by others, including her husband. On the other hand, the husband has a right not to be lied to. The dilemma consists of the clash of these rights, and the question is which right has priority in the situation. The dilemma is properly resolved by exercising good judgment in weighing these conflicting rights. It seems clear that the right to life is more important in this situation, as in nearly all situations, and hence we reasonably judge that the wife's right to life outweighs the husband's right not to be deceived.

But perhaps a lie is not the best solution. Another form of deception might be preferable, or perhaps the ideal solution is to avoid deception altogether, trying instead to calm the irate husband while withholding information. But sometimes the ideal is impracticable. If Luis's choice, because of the need for immediate action, is between lying and protecting his patient, we reasonably judge that lying is justified.

An ethical theory cannot be expected to make this particular judgment more certain, but it can place it within a broader moral framework. For example, an ethical theory might highlight the great importance of a person's right to life. It might also highlight that there is no general right to be told the truth in every situation, even though there is a presumption against lying—that is, lying must be justified by a stronger moral reason.

Rights ethics is the ethical theory that makes *human rights* morally paramount and fundamental. Whereas most ethical theories leave some room for employing the language of rights, only rights ethics views human rights as foundational—the moral bottom line. Accordingly, conduct is morally right (obligatory) when and because it respects human rights. The historical and contemporary power of this approach to morality is manifested in the names of important social movements, including the civil rights movement, the women's rights movement, the farm workers' movement, and the gay rights movement—not to mention the animal rights movement, which would extend rights to all sentient creatures. Most important for health-care ethics, the patients' rights movement has for several decades shifted the locus of moral decision making in health care to patients and away from physicians.

Rights ethics is probably the most familiar ethical theory, at least in the United States, for it is the theory on which the American political and legal system is founded. In the Declaration of Independence, Thomas Jefferson wrote, "We hold these truths to be self-evident; that all men are created equal; that they are endowed by their Creator with certain unalienable rights, that among these are Life, Liberty, and the pursuit of Happiness." The allusion to a Creator indicates how rights ethics might be connected with religious ethics, but here we consider rights ethics without assuming a tie to religion. Notice that Jefferson appealed to human rights as self-evident—that is, as intuitively obvious to a reasonable person. Ascribing human rights to each person is one way to express the dignity and the authority of individuals to be counted as moral equals with other individuals.

Exactly what are **human rights**? They are morally valid entitlements or claims on other persons, recognizing that others make similar claims on us. Mature and competent adults have the ability, as well as the moral authority, to assert these claims, but children and incapacitated adults need to rely on others to assert the claims on their behalf. Human rights, also called natural rights, are "unalienable" in that they cannot be abolished or taken away (made "alien" to us).

Of course, rights are sometimes violated. For example, the rights of enslaved persons are violated completely, but they still possess those rights. To complicate matters, we can voluntarily waive or exchange some of our rights in particular situations, as when we agree to undertake certain risks at the workplace in exchange for more desired benefits. We can also authorize others to exercise our rights on our behalf, as when we sign a durable power of attorney document, stipulating who has the right to make our health-care decisions should we be rendered unable to exercise our rights.

Human rights are distinct from legal rights, even though they overlap. **Legal rights** are simply the areas of freedom and benefits recognized in a particular legal system. In contrast, human rights are possessed by human beings whether or not the laws of their societies recognize them. The previous systems of apartheid in South Africa and slavery in the United States were systems of legal rights that violated human rights, and human rights are still violated by some legal systems of countries around the world. In the Declaration of Independence, are the rights to life, liberty, and the pursuit of happiness listed as legal rights or as human rights? The answer is both: they are human rights insofar as they are possessed by all humans, and they are legal rights insofar as that document, together with the U.S. Constitution and other laws, embeds human rights in the law.

Rights ethicists regard human rights as morally fundamental, but which are the most basic human rights? Different rights ethicists give different answers to this question. For example, in the 17th century, a hundred years before Thomas Jefferson drafted the Declaration of Independence, English philosopher John Locke formulated the first powerful rights ethic, listing the most basic rights as life, liberty, and property.[5] Jefferson simply changed Locke's British emphasis on property to the American emphasis on the pursuit of happiness. Closer to our time, A. I. Melden shortened the list of basic rights even further, to one: the right to pursue one's legitimate interests, essentially the right to liberty.[6] He suggested that the rights to property and the pursuit of happiness were implied by the right to pursue one's interests, and that even the right to life is implied by the right not to have one's liberty brought to an end. He also insisted that rights must be understood within moral communities based on mutual respect and goodwill, otherwise they easily degenerate into narrow self-seeking.

Another deep disagreement among rights ethicists concerns whether only liberty rights exist, or whether liberty rights also imply welfare rights. **Liberty rights** are rights not to be interfered with—for example, the rights not to be killed, not to be kidnapped, and not to have one's property stolen. (The "not" explains why they are also called "negative rights.") **Welfare rights** (also called "positive rights") are rights to receive essential goods when one is unable to earn those goods on one's own and when the community has the resources to provide them. An infant's right to receive care from its parents is an example. Other examples, recognized in American society beginning in the 1930s, include a disabled person's right to medical care, a fired worker's right to unemployment compensation, and the rights of senior citizens to social security.

Libertarians are those rights ethicists who believe that only liberty rights exist. They object to taxing people to support government welfare programs such as Medicare and unemployment compensation. Libertarian views have had increasing political influence in recent years, not only in dismantling parts of the welfare system but also in pushing for greater individual responsibility for financial matters. Yet these views remain a minority position among the general public, which continues to support Medicare, Medicaid, Social Security, and government support for education. Libertarians also represent a minority among rights ethicists, most of whom believe that human rights include both liberty and welfare rights.

Indeed, Melden is typical when he contends that liberty rights imply at least minimal welfare rights. What point would there be in ascribing liberty rights to severely handicapped children unless doing so placed a duty on communities to make available essential resources for enabling those children to develop their capacities for the appreciation of liberty? Thus, most rights ethicists support the allocation of public funds to provide physical and occupational therapy services to all disabled children. These services are provided regardless of the family's ability to pay through children's services agencies in each state, supported by local, state, and federal money.

It might seem that a wide gap separates respect for fundamental human rights and the mundane presumption against deception applicable in the example of Luis Alvarez. In fact, however, the connection is straightforward. The right to pursue our liberty (freedom, autonomy) is violated when others deceive us, thereby undermining the pursuit of our legitimate interests. Thus, lying to patients about matters related to their therapy undermines their exercise of liberty as they pursue the especially valuable goal of improving their health, as we discuss in chapter 3. The presumption against deception is frequently lessened when the interests being pursued are not legitimate, as in the case of the irate husband threatening violence. The presumption is also overridden by other competing rights that are more pressing, as with the wife's right not to be put at risk. The wife has this human right in general, but the right is bolstered by her special right to safety while under the care of the therapist.

This last point introduces a distinction between two types of moral rights: human and special. *Special moral rights* arise from contracts, promises, legislation, school membership, and relationships with professionals. Because special rights make reference to particular relationships and memberships, they are not human rights possessed by every person. Nevertheless, human rights enter into understanding special rights. For example, the special rights created by contracts should be respected because doing so respects the fundamental human right to liberty. Luis Alvarez's patient acquired special rights when she was accepted as a patient, under his care and that of his clinic. Yet those special rights are undergirded by her human rights to liberty and to not being assaulted.

In general, for rights ethicists, good moral judgment consists of identifying the full array of rights relevant to situations and finding the most reasonable way of balancing those rights. All rights have limits, and most have some permissible exceptions when they conflict with other rights. As with the other theories, balancing rights against each other can be complicated, and exactly what is required depends on how the theory is developed as well as on how rights apply to particular circumstances.

To sum up, the fundamental idea in rights ethics is that of human rights—a valid moral entitlement or claim on other persons because all humans have equal moral worth. Human rights are distinct from legal rights, which are entitlements or claims specified in a society's laws. Most rights ethicists believe there are two kinds of human rights: liberty rights not to be interfered with, and welfare rights to receive certain benefits from the community (when one cannot earn them and the community has them available). But libertarians deny that welfare rights exist as human rights, and they seek to dismantle legal welfare rights. There are also special moral rights—for example, those created by promises or contracts—that are justified by reference to human rights and to liberty. Taken together, these distinctions suggest how a major moral theory and tradition seeks to express the complexity of the moral life.

The next theory, duty ethics, is in many ways the mirror image of rights ethics. Rights ethics makes human rights fundamental and regards duties as derivative: Because you have a right to life, I have a duty not to kill you. Duty ethics inverts this approach. It begins with the idea of duties to respect persons and then regards rights as correlated with these duties.

Duty Ethics

A second way to formulate the ethical dilemma faced by Luis Alvarez is in terms of moral duties. Luis has a general moral duty to prevent harm to an innocent person, as well as specific duties to prevent harm to his patient while under his care. He also has a general duty not to lie. These duties clash, thereby creating an ethical dilemma. The dilemma can be resolved by understanding which duties have priority in the situation, presumably the duty to prevent harm to the patient.

Notice that this way of structuring the dilemma mirrors the earlier rights approach. Indeed, most rights and duties are correlated with each other: if you have a duty not to kill me, then I have a right not to be killed. Yet, whereas rights ethicists take human rights to be morally ultimate, duty ethicists regard duties as fundamental.

Immanuel Kant

Duty ethics is the view that actions are right when, and because, they are required by principles of duty that specify mandatory types of conduct.[7] German philosopher Immanuel Kant, who lived from 1724 to 1804, was the most influential duty ethicist. He attempted to articulate high-level principles that could identify our specific duties. One of these principles, the respect-for-persons principle, is among the most famous in the history of ethics: "Act so that you treat humanity, whether in your own person or in that of another, always as an end and never as a means only."[8] Roughly paraphrased, this means one should always show moral respect toward oneself and others—appreciating how persons place limits ("ends") on actions so that they are not merely means to gaining benefits for oneself. Paraphrased in another way: Always respect persons as having legitimate purposes ("ends") of their own that place limits on your own purposes, and also respect your own rational purposes as limiting how you act toward yourself.

Kant believed that all specific moral duties, including duties not to deceive, cheat, steal, and murder, are entailed by this principle as the varied dimensions of what it means to respect persons. In addition to duties to others, we have duties to ourselves, to respect our own rational nature as autonomous beings. Abusing drugs and alcohol, not developing one's talents, and committing suicide are some of his examples of damaging or destroying our autonomy. Kant calls these the duties of self-respect. This idea has been influential in ethics.[9,10]

What does it mean to treat humans as ends in themselves? Essentially it means respecting them as rational, autonomous beings who have their own rational purposes, their own "ends." If the word **autonomy** is omnipresent in medical ethics, it is because Kant made the word central to his moral perspective. Today, the word is often taken to mean self-determination. Insofar as Kant intended this meaning, his emphasis on respect for autonomy parallels the emphasis in rights ethics on respect for liberty. But Kant also built into his conception of autonomy the idea of **rationality**: having the capacity and disposition to act according to universally valid principles of action and on rational desires. Precisely what Kant meant by rational principles and desires was revealed in a piecemeal fashion, from his examples. Thus, in four famous examples, he argues that rational beings desire (1) to continue living; (2) to develop their talents and aptitudes; (3) to not have others make insincere promises to them; and (4) to receive necessary help when in severe hardship. As a result, suicide and neglecting our talents violate our duties of self-respect, and when we make false promises or fail to help others in severe hardship, we violate our duties to respect them.

Notice that Kant's respect-for-persons principle is formulated as a command: "Act always. . . ." Kant called this general principle of respect the **categorical imperative**, suggesting that it commands unconditionally. He also called specific duties, such as "Tell the truth" and "Keep your promises," categorical imperatives. By "categorical" he meant that there are no conditions or special goals attached, unlike the imperative, "If you want to be happy, be honest," or "If you want people to like you, keep your promises." These "iffy" commands are *hypothetical imperatives*—imperatives with a condition (or "hypothesis") attached.

Kant insisted that morality requires us to do certain things because they are our duties, not because these things contribute to our personal gain or self-interest. In this way, he made motives and intentions especially important in thinking about morality. We are to do our duty because it is our duty; we are to do what is right because it is right. Kant called this conscientious devotion to doing what is right the "good will," and he located our moral dignity in our capacity to exercise this moral goodwill. We have worth as moral agents because we are capable of caring about moral values as binding on us rather than acting solely out of ulterior motives of self-interest.

Kant set forth a second version of the categorical imperative: "Act only according to that maxim [motivating principle] by which you can at the same time will that it should become a universal law."[8(p340)] This idea of *universalizing* is familiar from the Golden Rule: Do unto others as you would have them do unto you. For Kant, the "others" are rational beings. He argued that moral duties are universal in that they apply to all persons who find themselves in morally similar situations. Thus, valid principles of duty are those we can—without self-contradiction or conflict in our rational will or intentions—conceive of every rational person acting on. For example, when we try to **universalize**—imagine everyone acting on—the rule "Lie when you can gain an advantage from doing so," or the rule "Make false promises when it benefits you," we become caught in a conflict with our rational will. As rational beings, we desire not to be deceived, and, in general, we want to live in a world where truthful communication is the norm. Hence our desire to deceive or to make a false promise conflicts with our rational nature, preventing us from endorsing these principles as universal principles. We can, however, conceive of all rational beings not lying and not making false promises, and so these are sound principles of duty.

Kant's universalization test expresses an important logical truth: Consistency requires that a moral judgment about a specific action extend to all relevantly similar actions. However, logical consistency is only a formal test; it is not a substantive way of identifying what our duty is. Stated in another way, it is a necessary but not sufficient condition for determining what our duties are. Thus, it is not a helpful guide in this respect unless we make a large number of assumptions about what all "rational beings" desire.

Despite Kant's enormous influence, nearly all ethicists agree that he made one monumental mistake. He believed that everyday moral principles, such as

"Tell the truth" and "Keep your promises," are **absolute**, with no permissible exceptions. In his view, we should never lie or make false promises—period. Yet, such an absolutistic view fails to help us when duties come into conflict and create ethical dilemmas. It provides no guidance when the duty not to lie conflicts with the duty to protect innocent life. Resolving an ethical dilemma often requires making an exception—a permissible exception—to a general principle of duty that clashes with another duty.

Conflicting duties are commonplace, and it is a puzzle why a thinker of Kant's stature could have failed to appreciate this familiar occurrence. Perhaps Kant was misled by confusing the ideas of absolute duties (duties having no permissible exceptions) and universal duties (duties applying to everyone placed in similar situations). Clearly, a rule could be universal while permitting some exceptions—for example, "Tell the truth except when doing so threatens a human life." Or, perhaps Kant was misled by failing to distinguish the idea of absolute duties from his notion of categorical imperatives (that moral duties must be heeded simply because they are our duties), a notion that carries a firm tone of "Do not deceive—period!" Or, as his harshest critics suggest, perhaps he was prone to *moralizing*, in the pejorative sense of being inflexible, dogmatic, parochial, lacking nuanced sensitivity to context, and being excessively judgmental or preachy.[11]

David Ross

Whatever the source of his glaring oversight about conflicting duties, Kant's ethics must be revised in order to be viable. British philosopher and scholar David Ross (1877–1971) made the needed revision by saying that everyday rules are **prima facie duties**: genuine duties that sometimes have exceptions when they conflict with other duties having greater importance in a given situation. Thus, there is a prima facie duty not to lie, but there is also a prima facie duty to protect innocent life, and a further duty to protect a patient under one's care. Lying to a criminal in order to protect one's family can be fully justified—not only permissible but even obligatory. One's *actual duty*, or "duty proper," in a situation—that is, one's duty, all things considered, in the particular circumstances—is to tell a lie in order to save a life. (The expression "prima facie" is now a standard term in ethics, and it is frequently applied beyond duty ethics. For example, rights ethics speaks of prima facie rights, meaning rights that have permissible exceptions when they conflict with other rights.)

How do we know that the duty to protect innocent life generally overrides the duty not to lie? Ross believed we can know our general, prima facie duties with certainty—that they are as self-evident as simple mathematical truths, and that we know this through immediate intuition, at least once we have reached moral maturity. In contrast, our actual duty in specific situations is frequently less certain. To Ross, we must simply think hard and sensitively:

> When I am in a situation, as perhaps I always am, in which more than one of these *prima facie* duties is incumbent on me, what I have to do is to study the situation as fully as I can until I form the considered opinion (it is never more) that in the circumstances one of them is more incumbent than any other; then I am bound to think that to do this *prima facie* duty is my duty *sans phrase* in the situation [i.e., my actual duty, all things considered].[12]

In emphasizing the need to reflect in this contextualized manner, Ross went beyond Kant, who thought our actual duties could be understood in the abstract, without attending to the complexities and nuances of specific situations. Yet Ross relied heavily on intuition in identifying prima facie duties. More recent duty ethicists have tried to go beyond intuition to formulate more general tests for identifying duties.

Basic Duties

Using Ross's version of duty ethics, good moral judgment consists of identifying the full range of duties relevant to a situation and reflecting carefully on how to balance those duties in light of the relevant facts about the situation. Doing all this can be complicated, and it gets more complicated as duty ethics is fleshed out. In particular, just as rights ethicists disagree on their lists of the most basic rights, duty ethicists differ in their lists of basic duties. Here is a list of four alternative lists of basic duties, set forth by some prominent 20th-century duty ethicists.

1. For his part, David Ross organized the most basic duties into six categories: (1) duties deriving from our own actions, either in making commitments (duties of fidelity) or in causing harm to others (duties of reparation); (2) duties deriving from other people's acts of service toward us (duties of gratitude and reciprocity); (3) duties to maintain fair distributions of benefits and burdens (duties of justice); (4) duties based on the sheer opportunity to help others (duties of beneficence); (5) duties linked to opportunities to develop our talents (duties of self-improvement); and (6) duties related to not injuring others (duties of nonmaleficence).[12(p21)]

2. William Frankena thought that all the more specific duties could be derived from two, which were based on: a principle of beneficence (concern for the good of others) and a principle of justice (treat people equally and fairly). His principle of beneficence was complex, however, and included four other principles, in descending order of stringency: do not inflict harm; prevent harm; remove harm; and promote good.[13]

3. In *Principles of Biomedical Ethics*, Tom L. Beauchamp and James F. Childress set forth a primarily duty-ethics approach inspired by David Ross and William Frankena and centered on four basic principles: (1) respect for autonomy, (2) nonmaleficence (do no harm), (3) beneficence (promote good), and (4) justice.[14] These four principles imply more specific "rules," such as professionals' obligation to maintain confidentiality and to obtain informed consent from patients. Beauchamp and Childress have been enormously influential in health-care ethics, to the point where some licensing exams take their four principles to be authoritative in the assessment of thinking about health-care ethics. However, in recent editions of their book, Beauchamp and Childress also incorporate virtue ethics (see page 37) to complement their primary emphasis on principles and rules.

4. In *A Theory of Justice*, John Rawls (1921–2002), the single most famous ethicist of our time, set forth a complex ethical theory centered around two principles of justice.[15] One is the obligation to maximize equal liberty, meaning that each person deserves the most extensive range of political liberties compatible with others having the same. The other is the obligation to abide by the "difference principle," which states that

inequalities in wealth and power are justified only insofar as they create a system beneficial to the most disadvantaged members of society. These principles have been especially influential in the current thinking about the distribution of scarce medical resources, as we will discuss more fully in chapter 9.

Rights Ethics vs. Duty Ethics

In summary, whereas rights ethics holds that duties are derived from human rights, duty ethicists make duties fundamental: your rights to liberty are correlated with my duty to respect your liberty. Kant thought that all specific duties are implied by a general duty to respect the autonomy (self-determination) of rational agents, agents who are capable of acting on universal principles and who possess rational desires, such as to respect themselves and to be respected by others. He also thought that moral duties are universal principles that we can envision all rational beings acting on without contradiction to or conflict with our own rational wills. Kant was an absolutist who believed that duties have no permissible exceptions. In contrast, most duty ethicists follow David Ross in acknowledging that duties are usually prima facie: they can have some legitimate exceptions when they are overridden by other duties. Determining priorities among duties requires exercising good judgment, although ethicists like John Rawls attempt to establish some general priorities among duties.

Both rights ethics and duty ethics hold that actions are right or wrong because of their inherent nature—for example, as acts of respecting liberty or being truthful—rather than solely because of their consequences. Stated another way, actions are right when they are required by principles of duty or rights. The overall consequences of actions are downplayed: rights are to be respected, and duties are to be met, even when doing so does not always promote the general good. In some versions of these theories, most notably Kant's, consequences are denied any importance at all, for only the motive (good will) and the nature of the act (required by duty) matter. (However, most duty ethicists and rights ethicists take consequences into account.) Because of this similarity, duty ethics and rights ethics are often lumped together and dubbed **deontological ethical theories.** As such, they are contrasted with **teleological** or, as it is more commonly termed, **consequentialist ethical theories** that determine right and wrong solely based on consequences.[16] Ethical egoism, discussed in chapter 1, is a consequentialist theory, in that it says we should maximize good consequences for ourselves. The most influential consequentialist theory is utilitarianism, which says we should maximize good consequences overall, taking into account everyone affected by our actions.

 ## Utilitarianism

Utilitarianism compresses all moral principles into one: Produce the most good for the most people, considering equally the interests of each person affected by our actions. This compression makes utilitarianism seem like a simple theory. It tells us to examine the facts, exercise our best judgment about the effects of our alternative choices, and make the choice that maximizes the good consequences overall. For example, lying is right when it promotes the most good, and it is wrong when it promotes more bad than good.

This appearance of simplicity quickly dissolves, however, as utilitarians unfold their theories in different directions. To begin with, what is the good that is to be maximized? It must be specified and tallied up without mentioning rights, duties, or other types of moral considerations—otherwise, the theory would bring in additional elements beyond good consequences. In particular, we must avoid assuming additional principles of justice about how goods are distributed. Utilitarians, then, set forth a theory of **intrinsic goods** (things worth seeking for their own sake) and intrinsic "bads" (things to be avoided, given their very nature) in nonmoral terms, without making additional moral assumptions.

Jeremy Bentham, an English jurist and philosopher writing in the late 18th century, held that the only intrinsic good is pleasure and the only intrinsically bad thing is pain (a view sometimes called *hedonism*).[17] Moreover, only the quantities of pleasures matter, so that equal amounts of the pleasures of love and wisdom are on a par with equal quantities of the pleasures of eating and sex. Bentham thought this approach would allow mathematical calculations of good, creating what he called a "hedonic calculus." Yet most utilitarians find this approach too simple. How do we measure the quantities of pleasures and pains—in love, friendship, or even sex—so as to be able to tally them up? Are all pleasures intrinsically good, including the pleasures of the rapist and sadistic murderer?

Perhaps most complex to answer is the question of whether pleasures are the only good things? Robert Nozick asks us to imagine an "experience machine," or what we might call a virtual reality machine:

> Suppose there were an experience machine that would give you any experience you desired. Superduper neuropsychologists could stimulate your brain so that you would think and feel you were writing a great novel, or making a friend, or reading an interesting book. All the time you would be floating in a tank, with electrodes attached to your brain. Should you plug into this machine for life, preprogramming your life's experiences?[18]

Few of us would plug into the machine for life (although we might for short periods of time). That is because we find intrinsic value in things beyond pleasures, and even beyond having experiences. We want to *do* things, including things we regard as intrinsically valuable, and we want to *be* persons who do things, rather than blobs floating in a tank of water.

John Stuart Mill, the greatest of the utilitarians, illustrates the complexity that emerges as a theory of intrinsic good is refined. Mill argued that the quality of pleasures, as well as their quantity, must be taken into account, saying that some pleasures are inherently better in kind than others. This sounds plausible. It allows us to count more heavily the pleasures of love and discount the pleasures of violence. Yet how in general are we to tell which pleasures are of higher quality? Mill suggested this test: "Of two pleasures, if there be one to which all or almost all who have experience of both give a decided preference, irrespective of a feeling of moral obligation to prefer it, that is the more desirable pleasure."[19] Restated, the relative quality of two pleasures is determined by a large majority vote of those who have experienced both.

However, can't a majority, even a large majority, be mistaken? Appealing to the widespread views of his time, Mill argued that the pleasures of love, friendship, intellectual endeavors—in general, those of the "higher faculties"—are inherently superior to the pleasures of the body. But Mill lived in the Victorian era, and today it is unlikely that most people would say that the pleasures of good sex or of athletic competition are of lower quality than the pleasures of, say, poetry.

Both Bentham and Mill confused pleasure with happiness, thinking that the injunctions "produce the most pleasure" and "produce the most happiness" were synonymous. In fact, pleasure is a relatively short-term conscious emotion or feeling, whereas happiness is a longer-term way of living that embodies many pleasures, some pains, and some unconsciousness—for example, one can be happy for an entire summer, during which one is asleep one-third of the time—in a pattern that one can affirm overall as enjoyable. Notice, too, that not all pleasures contribute to happiness: cocaine use might be pleasurable, but it can also destroy happiness.

Overall, Mill is best interpreted as saying that the intrinsic good is happiness or a happy life, not pleasure per se. He defined happiness as "not a life of rapture; but moments of such, in an existence made up of few and transitory pains, many and various pleasures, with a decided predominance of the active over the passive, and having as the foundation of the whole not to expect more from life than it is capable of bestowing."[19(p13)] Such a definition makes it clear that we have moved a long way from the initial air of simplicity surrounding the utilitarian view. And if grasping what happiness is, for ourselves and others, involves such complexity, the same is even more true in judging how happiness is to be promoted.

In *On Liberty*, Mill argued that each of us is best able to chart our path to happiness, and that we are helped in doing so by being allowed maximum personal freedom. To that end, he favored removing bans on illegal drugs, polygamy, and a host of other restrictions on how individuals shape their lives. Specifically, he argued for what is called the **harm principle**: "That the sole end for which mankind are warranted, individually or collectively, in interfering with the liberty of action of any of their number is self-protection. That the only purpose for which power can be rightfully exercised over any member of a civilized community, against his will, is to prevent harm to others."[20] In developing his thesis, Mill invoked rights language. Yet, unlike rights ethicists, he understood rights in terms of utility, that rights are those areas of liberty that tend to have especially beneficial consequences and hence deserve protection by laws and other social sanctions.

In both his language and his emphasis in *On Liberty*, Mill defended views very close to those of libertarians, and certainly his emphasis on respect for autonomy was as profound as Kant's. This overlap suggests an important truth: The details of an ethical theory matter enormously. Indeed, the details with which a type of ethical theory is developed can matter more than the general contrasts between different types of theories (such as utilitarianism versus rights ethics).

In the 20th century, utilitarians developed two alternative theories of intrinsic good. Troubled by the difficulty in quantifying pleasures and objectively measuring happiness, economists adopted a theory of goodness as *preference satisfaction*: Intrinsic good consists of satisfying human preferences as manifested in how individuals spend their money. Other utilitarians regard the economist's approach as too crude, and not only because satisfying preferences does not always contribute to pleasure or happiness. These more "ideal"-oriented utilitarians developed *pluralistic theories* that list many intrinsic goods, such as happiness, (most) pleasures, love, friendship, virtues, and appreciation of beauty.

Act Utilitarianism

In addition to disagreeing about what is intrinsically good, utilitarians disagree about whether good consequences should be measured against each action or instead against a set of rules. **Act utilitarianism** focuses on each action: an act is right when it maximizes good effects more than (or at least as well as) any other option available in a situation. According to act utilitarianism, moral decision making enjoins us to identify all the feasible options in each situation, to weigh up the likely good and bad consequences for each option, and then to select the option that maximizes good overall. In the case of Luis Alvarez, we look at the specific alternative actions available to him and select the one that maximizes the good in his situation.

Act utilitarians are generally critical of rights ethics and duty ethics because they view those theories as supporting dogmatism and rigid obeisance to rules. Yet, precisely because of their neglect of rules, act utilitarians often get into difficulties by allowing too many problematic loopholes that run counter to our most carefully considered moral convictions. For example, act utilitarianism would seem to justify dishonesty, such as cheating, lying, and stealing, in situations in which no one learns about the dishonesty and in which the benefit to the dishonest person is greater than the damage to others.

Consider this example. John, a physical therapist in the acute ward of a local hospital, neglects to deliver prescribed services to patient A in order to spend extra and nonreimbursed time with patient B, who is about to be discharged early and who desperately needs extra treatment. Nevertheless, to account for his time, John charts care for patient A. Subsequently, because of factors unrelated to physical therapy care, patient A dies. There is in fact virtually no way for John to get caught for his actions. According to the act utilitarian approach, John made the right decision because the measurable good outweighed any negative outcome. But perhaps because such conclusions seem mistaken, most contemporary utilitarians now focus on the consequences of rules rather than those of individual actions.

Rule Utilitarianism

Rule utilitarianism is the view that we should follow a particular set of rules that, were they adopted in a society, would maximize overall good.[21] Thus, actions are right when they conform to a set of rules that would maximize good (or at least promote as much good as any competing set of rules). Here the task is to compare sets of rules (presumably in some order of importance) against other sets of rules to determine which would be maximally beneficial to a society. For example, most lying to obtain benefits for oneself is wrong because if society adopted such a rule, havoc would ensue. People would be unable to trust one another and hence would be reticent to make agreements and form lasting personal relationships.

Of course, rules need to take into account general settings, but the benefits of avoiding lying would preclude far fewer objectionable loopholes than act utilitarianism permits. Moreover, because rules interact with rules, rule utilitarians usually think in terms of a set of interrelated rules—a code of conduct. They also allow that special sets of rules will have importance only in some settings—specifically, professional codes of conduct that apply to particular professions.

Summary

Utilitarianism says that right and wrong are exclusively a matter of maximizing good consequences (and minimizing bad consequences) overall, taking all persons affected into account equally. It has two major forms, depending on whether the consequences are measured with regard to each action (act utilitarianism) or with regard to sets of rules (rule utilitarianism). This distinction between act and rule utilitarianism was drawn in the 20th century, and scholars see elements of both forms of utilitarianism in the 19th-century writings of Bentham and Mill. There are also scholarly disputes about how far act and rule utilitarianism differ in practice. There is no doubt, however, that alternative theories of what is intrinsically good matter greatly. Most theories of intrinsic goodness fall into four categories: pleasure (hedonism), happiness, preference satisfaction, or a list of varied goods (pluralistic theory).

✵ Virtue Ethics

From the 18th-century Enlightenment until recently, ethical theories have emphasized right and wrong action (and rules about right and wrong acts). Certainly that is true of utilitarianism, duty ethics, and rights ethics. In contrast, the ethics of classical Greece and Rome emphasized what it means to be a good or bad person, together with related concerns about good lives, good relationships, and good communities. **Virtue ethics**, also called **character ethics**, shifts the focus to these latter concerns, especially to the kinds of persons we should aspire to be.[22–24] Virtue ethics has evoked renewed attention in recent decades, and it now plays a major role in health-care ethics.

Within the framework of virtue ethics, lying is objectionable when it manifests vices. Specifically, lying is wrong when it manifests the vice of dishonesty—both untruthfulness and untrustworthiness. Many lies are objectionable for additional reasons, such as when they enter into cruelty, corruption, and selfishness. Nevertheless, some lies are permissible and even admirable—for example, when they are necessary to protect our legitimate privacy (lies of self-respect) or to protect innocent lives (beneficent lies), as in the situation of Luis Alvarez. Because there are many virtues, resolving ethical dilemmas often requires balancing conflicting virtues within particular situations.

Virtues and vices have direct implications for conduct, although they highlight *habits* of conduct rather than individual actions or even rules of action. Equally importantly, virtues bear on all aspects of character: virtues are desirable patterns of desires, intentions, emotions, attitudes, and reasoning, as well as conduct. Vices are undesirable patterns of these things. A central challenge for virtue ethics is to establish the precise connection between conduct and virtues (and vices).

Plato left this connection as something of a mystery. In attempting to argue that morality is in our self-interest, as noted in chapter 1, he tried to show that the virtues provide an inner harmony that makes for mental health and well-being: "Virtue is as it were the health and comeliness and well-being of the soul, as wickedness is disease, deformity, and weakness."[25] This intriguing suggestion connects with modern emphases on holistic health and indeed with the World Health Organization's definition of health as complete physical, mental, and social well-being. Yet it led Plato to portray ethics (or justice, as he called it) as a matter of the inward self rather than of external behavior. More fully, Plato divided the soul or mind into three parts—Reason, Spirited Element (something like a sense of honor), and Appetites. Each part had its distinctive virtue—wisdom, courage, and moderation, respectively—that enabled it to perform its distinctive function with excellence. Thus, moral persons will have wisdom in guiding their reason, courage in exercising their spirited element, and moderation in governing the appetites, such as desires for food, sex, and earning money. Plato does not explain, however, how these virtues are identified in outward conduct. In practice, how do we tell what wisdom, courage, and moderation are?

Aristotle tried to answer this question by suggesting that proper conduct consists of exercising practical wisdom instilled through years of proper training in reasoning, perception, and emotion.[26] Given the complexity of the world, it is impossible to formulate the nuanced skills comprising good judgment in the form of simple rules. In practical situations, good judgment locates the "mean," or "golden mean," as it has since been called, between two extremes. The mean is the appropriate middle ground between two vices, deficiency (too little) and excess (too much). Aristotle thought that most virtues govern specific areas of our lives.

For example, temperance is the virtue governing our appetites, enabling us to locate the mean between hurtful self-denial (deficiency) and overindulgence (excess). Courage is the virtue in confronting danger by locating the mean between cowardice (deficiency) and foolhardiness (excess). Generosity is the virtue in giving whose mean lies between stinginess (deficiency) and wastefulness (excess). And truthfulness is the virtue in truth-telling that resides in the mean between lacking candor (deficiency) and revealing everything, even when it violates confidentiality or causes great harm to others (excess).

Aristotle's doctrine of the mean is interesting, but it does not provide sufficient guidance about what the virtues imply. Contemporary virtue ethicists are developing a variety of new approaches in clarifying the virtues. Yet the concern about specific guidance remains. Some virtue ethicists simply accept that a virtue ethics can provide only rough guidance in the form of highlighting key ideals of character and community. They see this not as a failing of their theory but simply as the nature of morality, which allows far less precision than mathematics. Perhaps most ethicists, however, believe that virtue ethics needs to be supplemented by some moral rules or principles that specify what comprises right action. Insofar as their theory warrants the label of virtue ethics, they continue to see the virtues as primary. Still other ethicists have come to believe that a complete ethical theory must integrate the virtues with moral rules of some kind.[27]

As with other theories, virtue ethicists debate which virtues are most fundamental. Aristotle, Plato, and the classical Greek civilization in general accented four cardinal virtues: wisdom (which is most important of all), courage, temperance, and justice. Alasdair MacIntyre, in *After Virtue*, an influential book that renewed interest in virtue ethics, reaffirmed these virtues and added honesty and integrity as especially important in contemporary society.[28] In the context of medical ethics, Edmund D. Pellegrino and David C. Thomasma's *The Virtues in Medical Practice* examines a longer list of virtues: practical wisdom, fidelity, justice, fortitude, temperance, integrity, and altruism.[29]

Virtue ethicists also disagree about whether the virtues must be all or nothing. Aristotle insisted that a virtue is a settled habit shown consistently. He even endorsed a doctrine of the unity of the virtues: to have one of the cardinal virtues—wisdom, courage, temperance, and justice—is to have them all. More recent virtue ethicists, however, understand the virtues to be more independent of each other, and sometimes at odds.[30] For example, to be fully honest may threaten being fully loving, and in making decisions about lying one might have to balance honesty against the virtue of friendship (which had great importance to Aristotle). Contemporary virtue ethicists also insist that persons can manifest a virtue to a certain extent but not fully, or within some contexts but not others. For example, a professional might maintain standards of integrity at work but in private life engage in spousal abuse.

In general, the resurgence of virtue ethics has broadly influenced thinking about morality in four directions. First, virtue ethics focuses greater attention on moral motivation and moral psychology—the psychology of the moral life. Kant highlighted motives, but he did so with a narrow emphasis on doing what is right because it is one's duty. Virtue ethicists, with their interest in how virtuous habits are taught, have led to a wide exploration of emotions, attitudes, and other areas of the inner life.

Second, virtue ethicists spur greater attention to personal relationships. Modern philosophy—especially rights ethics, duty ethics, and rule utilitarianism—has a distinctive bias in favoring abstract rules that require us to be impartial. Virtue ethics turns us toward communities and personal relationships that significantly define who we are as individuals. These ties make special moral demands on us that need to be balanced against general duties of justice. This theme resonates with the call for health-care ethicists to pay greater personal attention to their patients.

Third, virtue ethics highlights ideals of moral aspiration. Most virtues are connected with corresponding ideals—for example, compassion with ideals of compassionate devotion to others, and justice with ideals of a just society. Those ideals exist in degrees, ranging from a mandatory minimum to supererogatory levels far beyond that minimum. Professionals bring to their careers an array of ideals concerning caring for their patients, their profession, for society in general. In addition, virtue ethics highlights the importance of pro bono service—providing services to patients who are unable to pay the full cost for services.

Fourth, virtue ethics renews attention to communities, including to how communities instill values in children and in citizens. Virtues are not private merit badges. They specify desirable ways of relating to other people, to organizations, and to communities. Hence, virtue ethics can be developed in alternative directions using different social-political perspectives. The views of the ancient Greeks were aristocratic in emphasis, although it was an aristocracy based on talent rather than inheritance. Modern theories are democratic in spirit, although often critical of excessive individualism. In particular, MacIntyre's work is often interpreted as a version of communitarianism, the political theory that emphasizes the common good as being as important as individual rights.[31]

Religious Ethics

Religious ethics links moral virtues, ideals, and principles to their religious beliefs and ideals.[32] Thus, within religious ethics, lying might be condemned as betraying a religious covenant and as violating a divine commandment not to bear false witness against one's neighbor. At the same time, many religions promulgate the commandment to love one's fellow human beings, and that commandment seems to justify lying in order to protect them from serious harm. Once again, good moral judgment comes into play in determining when lies are permissible, but this time good judgment is understood and unfolded within a religion. We will focus our discussion around three possible ways of linking morality with religious belief: moral motivation, moral guidance, and moral justification.

Before turning to these topics, we should ask a preliminary question: What is a religion? In *The Varieties of Religious Experience*, William James suggested there is no essence to religion, in the form of a set of defining features that must be present ("necessary conditions") and suffice to specify it ("sufficient conditions"). Instead, as we examine paradigms of religions, "We may very likely find no one essence, but many characters [features] which may alternatively be equally important to religion."[33]

For example, we need to be skeptical of the familiar idea that religion, by definition, requires belief in God. It is true that belief in a single deity (monotheism) is central in most world religions, such as Judaism, Christianity, and Islam. But other religions believe in many gods (polytheism), most notably Hinduism, classical Greek religions, and the religions of some African tribes. Still other religions, like Zen Buddhism, do not believe in a supernatural deity at all, or, like Confucianism, downplay the importance of belief in a god.

Typically, however, a religion will have two general features connected with *moral motivation*: reinforcing moral motivation in everyday life and teaching morality and stimulating moral development. When these features are missing, individuals might say they have *spiritual* beliefs, even though they do not belong to a religion.

One feature is that religions typically provide a *world view*—some general perspective about the universe and the cosmic origins of humans—which they connect with morality. For example, theistic religions usually make central a deity (or deities) who created the universe with some plan for humanity. That plan includes rewarding moral conduct and discouraging immorality. In addition to these sources of self-interested motivation, the aim is to inspire emulation of the ideal moral goodness of God as well as the goodness found in moral paragons within the religious tradition.

As a second example, consider the doctrine of karma, prominent in Hinduism and Buddhism. It asserts that good deeds beget good fortune, and bad deeds bring bad consequences to the agent. The doctrine is not simply a social claim about reciprocity ("What goes around comes around"), nor simply a psychological claim about the effects of guilt feelings on future conduct. Instead, it is a metaphysical claim that morality is built into the very structure of the universe—a powerful source of moral motivation indeed.

Another typical feature of religions is that they are embedded in communities structured by shared beliefs, practices, rituals, scripture, and narratives. The rituals might be social, such as attending a church, synagogue, or mosque. Or they might be more private, such as prayer, meditation, and fasting. Either way, they provide a way to encourage moral accountability among believers and toward key authorities within the religion. They also seek to foster self-discipline and involvement in helping others.

In addition to strengthening moral motivation, religions typically seek to provide *moral guidance*. One way they do this is through promulgating specific principles. For example, the Golden Rule is found in all major world religions, either in its positive version ("Do unto others as you would have them do unto you") or in its more negative version, such as that which Confucius formulated in the 6th century B.C.E.: "Do not impose on others what you yourself do not desire."[34] Another way is to highlight selected virtues as especially central. For example, Christianity makes the virtue of love paramount, Buddhism emphasizes compassion, Judaism emphasizes *tsedakah* (righteousness, justice), Islam emphasizes *ihsan* (piety, pursuit of excellence), and Navaho ethics emphasizes *hozho* (harmony, peace of mind, health, well-being, beauty).

Religions often provide guidance in the form of parables and stories (narratives), such as the parable of the good Samaritan.[35] Whether through principles, virtues, or parables, most religions seek a higher standard of conduct or virtue than is common in society. To be sure, they can also have a lower standard—for example, the Aztecs' practice of human sacrifice and some contemporary religions' endorsement of female circumcision.

Distinct from moral motivation and moral guidance, religions make claims about *moral justification*, specifically that moral values are justified by appeal to commandments of a deity. This view is called **divine command ethics,** by which moral judgments are justified solely because they conform to God's commandments. This is a troubling view, and it is rejected by many theologians as well as most philosophers. Not only does it imply that if there were no God there could be no morality, but it also makes nonsense of the idea of God being morally perfect, for it suggests that moral reasons are created by God's commandments rather than being the basis for making those commandments in the first place. A morally perfect deity would command what is morally right on the basis of sound moral reasons. Those reasons provide a justification for those commandments just as they provide a justification for human actions of right and wrong. Divine command ethics essentially says that the commands create morality, literally by creating what counts as moral reasons. Hence, the reasons do not exist until after the commands are issued, thereby rendering God's commands arbitrary and lacking in any justification.

For example, according to divine command ethics, rape is neither right nor wrong until after God issues some command concerning it. Yet most religious people believe that God would forbid rape for good reasons, perhaps for the same moral reasons we condemn it: violation of autonomy, infliction of suffering, and so on. Rather than rape becoming wrong only after God condemns it, God sees that rape is wrong and for that reason condemns it.[36]

This brief discussion of religious ethics prompts the question, What relevance does religious ethics have to health-care ethics? For one thing, religious ethics enters into the reflection of professionals as they consider professional ethics, whether in the classroom or at work.[37] Catholic thinking has played a major role in the development of bioethics, and today health-care ethics has advanced to the point where entire books are written within the traditions of major world religions.[38] Ideally, religious and secular ethics can interact through mutually enriching dialogue, in the same ecumenical spirit that different religious traditions interact.

For another thing, patients' religious views frequently enter significantly into how they respond to their illnesses and the decisions they make about the direction of their health care. As we discuss in chapters 5 and 6, health professionals need to develop sensitivity to different cultural and religious traditions in order to properly care for their patients. In addition, respect for patients' autonomy, and more generally functioning as a professional, requires maintaining professional distance, an idea discussed in chapter 4, by not imposing one's own religious outlook on patients.

Finally, we must note that secular medical ethics arose out of a need to solve dilemmas for which most religious ethics offered little guidance. The rapid increase in technology over the past 50 years brought with it situations never before faced by humans in the delivery of care. An example is the proper determination of death when machines properly attached can create the semblance of life long after a cognitive or spiritual presence has been lost. It is essential to search for common, or at least overlapping, values in a pluralistic society. Such

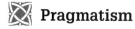

values make possible meaningful dialogue across multiple religions and diverse value systems.

Pragmatism

Pragmatism explores how we can exercise responsible moral judgment without resorting to a comprehensive theory such as rights ethics, duty ethics, utilitarianism, virtue ethics, or religious ethics. It elucidates how we exercise good moral judgment in balancing conflicting moral reasons and creatively extending them into new situations. These reasons include rights, responsibilities, and ideals of character, even though they cannot be encapsulated in comprehensive and systematic theories. **Pragmatism**, as an ethical outlook, does not mean that morality is reduced to expediency. Instead, it means that one pays close attention to the full range of moral values that enter into particular situations and tries to find the best way to give each its due—for example, when making decisions about whether to lie in Luis Alvarez's situation.

Broadly understood, then, pragmatism refers to a cluster of approaches to ethics that are wary of abstract rules and elaborate systems of principles. Pragmatists heavily emphasize the importance of context—of looking closely at the facts and values pertinent to particular situations. They also emphasize paradigms —clear-cut cases—as helpful guides in decision making, both in identifying routine cases and in understanding why moral dilemmas depart from routine cases to generate moral vagueness (lack of clarity about how to apply moral concepts and principles), moral ambiguity (more than one plausible moral interpretation of a situation), moral conflict (principles pointing in different directions), and moral disagreement (differing viewpoints among involved persons). In this sense, George Eliot was a pragmatist when she expressed doubts about the adequacy of universal principles and asserted that "the mysterious complexity of our life is not to be embraced by maxims."

If we insist that an ethical theory must be a search for systematization of the sort illustrated in utilitarianism, duty ethics, rights ethics, and virtue ethics, then pragmatism may seem to be an "antitheory" approach to moral reasoning, and indeed some of its defenders and critics portray it that way. In our view, however, pragmatism is an ethical theory, a theory about morality, because of the sophisticated development it received in the so-called classical era of American philosophy, represented especially by the work of William James (1842–1910) and John Dewey (1859–1952), and because of its refinements by contemporary pragmatists such as Richard Rorty, Hilary Putnam, and thinkers who adopt pragmatic approaches to health-care ethics.[39]

Both James and Dewey developed theories about moral decision making as an attempt to integrate the rich multitude of responsibilities, goods, social policies, and ideals of character that apply to particular situations. Dewey was especially concerned with making policy decisions, especially about approaches to public education, within democracies that embody an array of conflicting traditions and moral perspectives. In education, as elsewhere, morality calls for "creative intelligence" to find a practical solution that "coordinates, organizes and functions each factor of the situation which gave rise to conflict, suspense and deliberation."[40] More broadly, Dewey expanded Aristotle's emphasis on the importance of habits in shaping character and conduct. Habits acquire a power ("dynamic quality") of their own that propels actions, in good or bad directions—a fruitful idea in thinking about habits that maintain or harm health.[40(p37)]

That is not to say that moral principles are useless. Instead, it is to view principles more as general guides than as recipes for specific action. According to Dewey:

> A moral principle, such as that of chastity, of justice, of the Golden Rule, gives the agent a basis for looking at and examining a particular question that comes up. It holds before him certain possible aspects of the act; it warns him against taking a short or partial view of the act. It economizes his thinking by supplying him with the main heads by reference to which to consider the bearings of his desires and purposes; it guides him in his thinking by suggesting to him the important considerations for which he should be on the lookout.[41]

A recent variation of pragmatism can be found in Albert Jonsen and Stephen Toulmin's revival of casuistic thinking. In the relevant sense, casuistry is not sophistry—that is, hair-splitting rationalization—but instead careful attention to paradigm cases, models, analogies, and refined intuition. Jonsen and Toulmin were led to their approach during their participation in the work of the National Commission for the Protection of Human Subjects of Biomedical and Behavioral Research, from 1975 to 1978, whose charge was to develop national guidelines in the United States for protecting human research subjects in experiments. The commission was composed of people of widely differing cultural, religious, and political orientations, and as a result they failed to agree on many general ethical principles and priorities. Nevertheless, according to Jonsen and Toulmin, the group was able to reach substantial agreement at the level of specific cases:

> So long as the debate stayed on the level of particular judgments, the eleven commissioners saw things in much the same way. The moment it soared to the level of "principles," they went their separate ways. Instead of securely established universal principles, in which they had unqualified confidence, giving them intellectual grounding for particular judgments about specific kinds of cases, it was the other way around.[42]

Which Theory Is Best?

How do we assess ethical theories so as to determine which one is best? Showing that an action or rule is morally justified might involve appealing to an ethical theory, but what do we appeal to in deciding which ethical theory is most insightful and helpful?

The answer turns on what we seek from an ethical theory. We seek a moral perspective that is clear, consistent, and comprehensive by applying all moral issues of interest to us. It must be sufficiently simple and practical to provide useful guidance. Most important, it must be compatible with our most carefully considered moral convictions—that is, with the moral beliefs we have thought most insightfully about and are most certain of. To take an extreme example, if an ethical theory justified rape or torturing babies for fun, we would know the theory was false—and perverse. If act utilitarianism justified rampant cheating, then it should be rejected.

In this way, just as theories are used to justify actions and rules, our judgments about actions and rules provide a crucial touchstone for testing the adequacy of theories. To borrow an expression from John Rawls, this back-and-forth procedure seeks a "reflective equilibrium" between the ethical theory and a host of particular judgments. Rather than relying on isolated self-evident moral intuitions, as David Ross had us do, we regard the justification of both the theory and specific judgments as "a matter of the mutual support of many considerations, of everything fitting together into one coherent view."[43]

We believe the general type of ethical theory (utilitarianism, rights ethics, etc.) is not by itself crucial in deciding the usefulness of a theory. What matters is the detailed working out of the theory in a specific version. In the general sketches we have provided, rule utilitarianism, duty ethics, and rights ethics are all promising ethical theories. If they were not, they would not be as widely discussed as they have been (for centuries), nor would they continue to have many defenders. Notice that each of the ethical theories identifies the same basic moral principles, even though they each provide different moral languages in stating the principles and different ways of justifying them. For example, all of them agree there are prima facie obligations not to lie, steal, or cheat, whether because such principles have generally good consequences (rule utilitarianism), respect persons' autonomy (duty ethics), or respect persons' rights (rights ethics).

Virtue ethics is equally important and can be interpreted as complementing the rule-oriented theories. Essentially it sets forth a view of the kinds of persons we should aspire to be, as well as the kinds of relationships and societies we should live in. Such views complement rather than compete with theories of right action. In this spirit, the key values used to organize the remaining chapters in this book have dual dimensions, as responsibilities and as virtues. Good judgment, emphasized in this chapter, can itself be viewed as a virtue when it becomes a habitual tendency, or as an ability in meeting responsibilities, and the same is true of professionalism, the value highlighted in chapter 1.

Religious ethics, as already noted, will enter into an understanding of patients' views of their own well-being as well as into the moral ideals that many individual professionals bring to their work. In addition, occasionally we will take note of ideas from religious traditions, such as the Law of Double Effect discussed in chapter 6. Otherwise, given our pluralistic democracy, and especially the need for professional distance, religious discourse need not be prominent in public discourse about professional ethics.

Pragmatism has importance in responding to the many unprecedented situations with which contemporary societies confront us. It has special relevance to contexts of shared decision making, in the professions and elsewhere, in which individuals need to accommodate their moral convictions within groups without abandoning their most carefully considered principles. In our view, it is not an antitheory so much as a theory that can be developed with different emphases linking it with rights ethics or virtue ethics and so on. Or, if it is understood as an explicit rejection of systematic theories, it nevertheless remains an illuminating account of how most people engage in serious moral deliberation in practical situations.

In any case, all the theories seem to us worthy of consideration as ways of organizing moral reflection, stating and resolving ethical dilemmas, justifying principles of professional duty, and highlighting key moral ideas such as autonomy and respect for persons. Certainly all of them play prominent roles within health-care ethics. Even when we do not explicitly apply the ethical theories in the course of this book, they are offered as useful tools and illuminating perspectives for reflecting on all the issues raised here.

Discussion Questions

1. Monica Reid was angry and confused. After studying hard for the midterm exam in her neurophysiology course, hoping to get an A or at least a high B, she received a B–. She knew the professor graded on a scale and was one of toughest graders in the physical therapy program in which she was enrolled as a second-semester student. She also knew that at least three students who received higher grades than her had cheated on the exam. They had access to several pirated exams, kept in fraternity and sorority files, and one of them offered her access to the exams, which she refused. That student also informed her that the group was preparing crib sheets as backups and, if necessary, would excuse themselves to go to the restroom during the exam to consult notes in their pockets. Reid was in a quandary about whether to report the students to the professor. Was there any responsibility to report the cheaters, or would reporting them merely be a self-interested act of "ratting"? In answering this question, apply each of the ethical theories. What does each theory say about (a) what is wrong with cheating in general and (b) whether Monica Reid should report the cheating?

   Also, in deciding whether she should report the cheating, is it relevant how many students are cheating? What similarities and differences do you see between this issue and questions about whether physical therapists ought to report, to appropriate authorities, other health professionals who engage in wrongdoing? (You might revisit this issue in chapter 8 where whistle-blowing is discussed.)

2. Ethics includes moral inquiry into policies and laws as well as individual conduct, and sometimes moral dilemmas can be resolved only by shifting attention to questions of policy. Which university policies concerning plagiarism and other forms of cheating are morally justified? Is there a universal answer to this question, or does the answer depend in part on the nature of the university?

3. One objection to act utilitarianism is that it seems to justify some clear injustices.[44] For example, suppose we could kidnap a drunkard who is a nuisance in the local community, transplant his organs to save 10 other individuals who contribute greatly to the community but are now seriously ill, and do so without anyone finding out. The act utilitarian theory seems to permit or even require doing so. What would a duty ethicist and a rights ethicist say about such actions? How might utilitarians revise their theory, perhaps by shifting to rule utilitarianism, so as forbid such injustices?

4. Write down a list of absolute duties—that is, duties that never have a permissible exception under any circumstance. Is the list very long? Would you expect every reasonable person to agree with your list?

5. We said that, for the most part, rights and duties are correlated, so that if you have a right to life then I have a duty not to take your life. (There are some exceptions; for example, a newborn has rights but it is too young to have duties.) This suggests, as we also noted, that rights ethics and duty ethics can be viewed as mirror images of each other. Yet critics argue that rights talk tends to reinforce patterns of self-centeredness by leading to a preoccupation with one's own rights. In this connection, suppose that Thomas Jefferson had

written: "We hold these truths to be self-evident; that all people are created equal; that they owe duties of respect to all other rational beings, and are owed these duties in return." How might this difference in emphasis have affected Americans' view of community? For example, might it have helped create an atmosphere in which we would by now have a system of universal health coverage?

6. Plato believed that moral virtue and mental health substantially overlap. Assess this belief in light of what has been called a therapeutic trend: the tendency to approach moral matters using health-oriented perspectives.[45] In particular, consider the prevalent view that alcohol and drug dependency are diseases, either physical diseases or mental diseases, as listed in Diagnostic and Statistical Manual of Mental Disorders.[46] Is such a view compatible with holding individuals morally responsible for their conduct? Discuss, in this connection, the recent laws in Arizona and California to send nonviolent first-time drug offenders into therapy rather than to jail. Does responsibility for one's own health have any implications for how physical therapists respond to noncompliant patients—for example, those who fail to cooperate with the prescribed exercises? (Return to this question in chapter 4, on caring for patients, and in chapter 8, which touches on drug abuse by professionals.)

References

1. Bok S. *Lying: Moral Choice in Public and Private Life*. New York, NY: Vintage Books; 1999.
2. Eliot G. *The Mill on the Floss*. New York, NY: New American Library; 1965:521.
3. For a helpful historical overview, see Norman R. *The Moral Philosophers*. 2nd ed. New York: Oxford University Press; 1998.
4. Martin MW. *Everyday Morality*. 3rd ed. Belmont, CA: Wadsworth; 2001:39.
5. Locke J. *Two Treatises of Government*. Cambridge, England: Cambridge University Press; 1960.
6. Melden AI. *Rights and Persons*. Berkeley, CA: University of California Press; 1977.
7. Duty ethics is sometimes called "deontological ethics," from the Greek word *deon*, duty. Just as often, however, deontological ethics is understood as including both duty ethics and rights ethics.
8. Kant I. Foundations of the metaphysics of morals, trans. Beck, LW. In Melden AI, ed. *Ethical Theories: A Book of Readings*. 2nd ed. Englewood Cliffs, NJ: Prentice-Hall; 1967:345.
9. Hill TE. *Autonomy and Self-Respect*. Cambridge, England: Cambridge University Press; 1991.
10. Dillon RS, ed. *Dignity, Character, and Self-Respect*. New York, NY: Routledge; 1995.
11. Gordon L. Teenage pregnancy and out-of-wedlock birth: morals, moralism, experts. In Brandt AM, Rozin P, eds. *Morality and Health*. New York, NY: Routledge; 1997:253.
12. Ross D. *The Right and the Good*. New York, NY: Oxford University Press; 1930:19.
13. Frankena WK. *Ethics*. 2nd ed. Englewood Cliffs, NJ: Prentice-Hall; 1973:45-52.
14. Beauchamp TL, Childress JF. *Principles of Biomedical Ethics*. 5th ed. New York, NY: Oxford University Press; 2001.
15. Rawls J. *A Theory of Justice*, revised edition. Cambridge, MA: Harvard University Press; 1999:53. First published in 1971.

16. Purtilo R. *Ethical Dimensions in the Health Professions*. 2nd ed. Philadelphia: W.B. Saunders; 1993:10-11.

17. Bentham J. *The Principles of Morals and Legislation*. London, England; 1780. Relevant selections are widely anthologized—for example, in Pojman L, ed. *Moral Philosophy: A Reader*. 2nd ed. Indianapolis, IN: Hackett Publishing Company; 1998:113-115.

18. Nozick R. *Anarchy, State and Utopia*. Cambridge, MA: Harvard University Press; 1973:42.

19. Mill JS. *Utilitarianism*. Indianapolis, IN: Hackett Publishing Company; 1979:8. First published in 1861.

20. Mill JS. *On Liberty*. Indianapolis, IN: Hackett Publishing Company; 1978:9. First published in 1859.

21. Brandt RB. *A Theory of the Good and the Right*. Oxford, England: Clarendon Press; 1979.

22. Statman D, ed. *Virtue Ethics: A Critical Reader*. Washington, DC: Georgetown University Press; 1997.

23. McKinnon C. *Character, Virtue Theories, and the Vices*. Orchard Park, NY: Broadview Press; 1999.

24. Paul EF, Miller FD, Paul J, eds. *Virtue and Vice*. Cambridge, England: Cambridge University Press; 1998.

25. Plato. *The Republic*, trans. Cornford FM. New York, NY: Oxford University Press; 1945:444e.

26. Aristotle. *Nicomachean Ethics*, trans. Terence Irwin. Indianapolis, IN: Hackett Publishing Company; 1985.

27. Rachels J. *The Elements of Moral Philosophy*. 4th ed. New York: McGraw-Hill; 2003:173-190.

28. MacIntyre A. *After Virtue*. 2nd ed. Notre Dame, IN: University of Notre Dame Press; 1984.

29. Pellegrino ED, Thomasma DC. *The Virtues in Medical Practice*. New York: Oxford University Press; 1993.

30. Flanagan O. *Varieties of Moral Personality*. Cambridge, MA: Harvard University Press; 1991.

31. Avineri S, De-Shalit A., eds. *Communitarianism and Individualism*. Oxford, England: Oxford University Press; 1992.

32. Carmody DL, Carmody JT. *How to Live Well: Ethics in the World Religions*. Belmont, CA: Wadsworth Publishing; 1988.

33. James W. *The Varieties of Religious Experience*. New York, NY: Modern Library; 1902.

34. Confucius. *The Analects*, trans. Lau DC. Section 15:24. New York, NY: Penguin; 1979. For a general exploration of the Golden Rule, see Wattles, J. *The Golden Rule*. New York, NY: Oxford University Press; 1996.

35. Nelson HL, ed. *Stories and Their Limits*: *Narrative Approaches to Bioethics*. New York: Routledge; 1997.

36. Plato. *The Euthyphro*, trans Grube GMA. In Cooper JM, ed. *Plato: Complete Works*. Indianapolis, IN: Hackett Publishing Company; 1997:1-16. Also see Helm P, ed. *The Divine Command Theory of Ethics*. Oxford, England: Oxford University Press; 1979.

37. Lammers SE, Verhey A, eds. *On Moral Medicine: Theological Perspectives in Medical Ethics*. 2nd ed. Grand Rapids, MI: William B. Eerdmans Publishing; 1998.

38. For example, see Freedman B. *Duty and Healing: Foundations of a Jewish Bioethic*. New York, NY: Routledge; 1999.

39. Rorty R. *Consequences of Pragmatism*. Minneapolis: University of Minnesota Press; 1982. Also, McGee G, ed. *Pragmatic Bioethics*. Nashville, TN: Vanderbilt University Press; 1999; Stout J., *Ethics After Babel*. Princeton: Princeton University Press; 2001.

40. Dewey J. *Human Nature and Conduct*. New York, NY: Modern Library; 1957:183. First published in 1922.

41. Dewey J. *Theory of the Moral Life*. New York, NY: Holt, Rinehart and Winston; 1960:141. First published in 1908.

42. Jonsen AR, Toulmin S. *The Abuse of Casuistry: A History of Moral Reasoning*. Berkeley, CA: University of California Press; 1988:18.

43. Rawls J. *A Theory of Justice*, revised edition. Cambridge, MA: Harvard University Press; 1999:19.

44. Harwood S. Eleven objections to utiliarianism. In Pojman LP, ed. *Moral Philosophy: A Reader*. 2nd ed. Indianapolis: Hackett Publishing Company; 1998:181.

45. Martin MW. Alcoholism as sickness and wrongdoing. *J Theor Soc Behav*. 1999;29:109–131.

46. American Psychiatric Association, *Diagnostic and Statistical Manual of Mental Disorders*. 4th ed. Text revision. Washington, DC: American Psychiatric Association; 2000.

Respect for Autonomy and Information Control

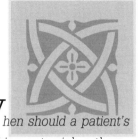

*W*hen should a patient's autonomous decision making outweigh a therapist's professional judgment?

Keywords

Veracity
Confidentiality
Autonomy
Substituted judgment
Best interest

Limited competency
Intermittent competency
Respect principle
Medical paternalism,
   weak and strong

Informed consent
Medical care standard
Reasonable person standard
Dialogic standard

The principle of autonomy asserts there is a responsibility to respect the autonomy (self-determination) of each person. No principle is more fundamental to health-care ethics, or indeed to all professional ethics. Despite its enormous importance, however, the responsibility to respect patients' autonomy is prima facie: it has limits, and there are justified exceptions in situations in which it conflicts with other, overriding moral principles. Controversy surrounds exactly what those limits and exceptions are.

This chapter focuses on three specific professional duties entailed by the principle of autonomy, each of which concerns the patient's control over treatment and control over personal information. These are the duties of informed consent, truth telling (**veracity**), and **confidentiality** (privacy). Our goal is to develop in the student a nuanced understanding of these duties, including their meaning, their moral foundations, and the moral dilemmas that arise when they conflict with other moral principles. We begin by commenting on the justification of the principle of autonomy and why respect for patients' autonomy has increased in importance in recent decades.

Respect for Autonomy

Autonomy has two aspects or senses: one moral and one psychological. In a moral sense, autonomy is the moral authority—or right, liberty, justification—to make our own decisions. To respect people's moral autonomy is to recognize their moral authority to form their own judgments about how to live and to act on those judgments. Respect for autonomy implies both an attitude and action, as ethicists Beauchamp and Childress explain:

> To respect an autonomous agent is, at a minimum, to acknowledge that person's right to hold views, to make choices, and to take actions based on personal values and beliefs. Such respect involves respectful *action*, not merely a respectful *attitude*. It also requires more than noninterference in others' personal affairs. It includes, at least in some contexts, obligations to build up or maintain others' capacities for autonomous choice while helping to allay fears and other conditions that destroy or disrupt their autonomous actions.[1]

Obviously, this moral authority to guide one's life has limits. In particular, it does not give one the right to violate others' rights. This consideration leads some ethicists to restate the principle of autonomy so that it includes exceptions. An example would be: We should respect others' autonomy except when they unjustifiably harm others. Yet, such built-in exceptions are already accounted for when we call this principle a prima facie principle.

Competency

In the psychological sense, autonomy refers to competency, in particular to having a certain minimum level of mental capacity and skill in reasoning and rational conduct. Autonomous persons must have the psychological capacity to guide their lives according to their own desires, beliefs, and intentions. They are rational agents in the minimal sense of being competent to make their own decisions, although "rational" does not mean they always act reasonably or with moral justification. Infants lack autonomy, in this sense, because they lack the minimal capacity and skill necessary to direct their lives in a way that protects and develops their potential (even though they have rights that surrogates exercise on their behalf). In time, normal infants gradually develop autonomy as they mature into adulthood. Adults also lack (psychological) autonomy when, for example, they are in a coma, or suffer from advanced Alzheimer's disease or other severe mental impairments, or in other ways lack the capacity to make choices.

The psychological capacities and abilities that define autonomy come in many different degrees. Nevertheless, one must attain some threshold of substantial decision-making capacity to be allowed to make health-care decisions. Adults, typically those aged 18 or older, are presumed legally competent until the courts declare otherwise. The threshold is specified by the law. However, as a rule of thumb, the need to ensure competence is proportional to the importance of the decision. We rarely assess competence when the decision is what the patient should order for dinner, but we require a diligent assessment of competence when the consequences of a voluntary decision are life threatening (as in undergoing some human experimentation) or irreversible (such as a request for a sex-change operation).

When a court decides that a patient is not competent, it appoints a guardian—usually a spouse, close relative, or someone the individual has specified in legal documents, especially in a durable power of attorney. Guardians then exercise autonomy, in the moral sense, on behalf of the noncompetent individual. Many troublesome issues concerning respect for autonomy involve such surrogate decision makers, as can be seen in the following discussion of the basic standards that should be used in making decisions.

There are two primary legal standards by which guardians might be asked by the government to render decisions on behalf of the patient. Under the first, guardians may be asked to render a **substituted judgment** for the patient. In this case, they use their knowledge of the patient and the patient's history of decision making to imagine what the patient would want under the circumstances. Of course, this requires that guardians have an intimate knowledge of the patient. Under the second primary standard, guardians base their decisions on what they think is in the **best interest** of the patient, regardless of what the patient might actually have chosen to do. The two standards can produce very different decisions.

Suppose that a woman never writes an advance directive—a "living will" specifying one's wishes for treatment under various conditions—but in conversation with her husband she has expressed strong feelings that she would not want to "linger" in life if there were any substantial pain involved. Using the substituted-judgment standard, the husband, as guardian, might refuse treatment on behalf of his wife if treatment would prolong life with the burden of appreciable pain. In contrast, using the best interest standard, the husband might decide that pain was natural and something to be endured in order to extend life, and order the treatment on behalf of his wife.

When advance directives are present, respect for autonomy should force us to regard a surrogate's "considered opinions," in the form of either a living will or a durable power of attorney, as having the same authority as if they were spoken in the present tense by a competent patient. There is an emerging argument that providers might be liable for a "wrongful life" if written directives are intentionally ignored.[2] Anyone with knowledge of these directives has a responsibility to make others on the health-care team aware of them, for both immediate and future decision making.

Children (under age 18) are not considered competent, and their health-care decisions must be made by their parents or guardians, although occasionally special state laws allow or require exceptions. Clearly, moral competency and autonomy do not magically emerge on the 18th birthday, and we have all probably known some 15-year-olds who were more competent than some persons at age 22. Legally, variations from the standard depend on the types of decisions in question. For example, some states have liberal laws about the legal age at which persons may obtain birth control and abortions, and rulings by judges can specify that minors are sufficiently "mature" to make their own decisions in these matters.

When profound consequences are involved, the state is especially protective of the emerging competency of the child, even if it means protecting the child from the parents. Parents may not refuse emergency or other essential medical treatments for a child if that refusal endangers the child's life. When parents refuse such treatments, often because of their religious beliefs, the courts will intervene and assume guardianship of the child and authorize treatment. Intervention of this sort is justified by respect for the (psychological) autonomy that the child will develop with time and the moral rights the child already has. As an adult, the former child can refuse the same kind of treatment that the court enforced, but because death cannot be reversed, those decisions must wait until children are old enough to make legally autonomous decisions.

In unusual situations, the courts might grant autonomous health-care decision-making rights to a person younger than 18 years old under the concept of the "emancipated minor." This award of rights usually goes to young adults whose parents refuse to act on their behalf, as is often the case with children who are "thrown away" rather than children who elect to "run away." There are also cases in which the courts have supported a minor's request to refuse medical treatment, as they did for Benito Agrelo, age 15. Agrelo was granted legal permission to discontinue the antirejection drugs given when he underwent a second liver transplant, even though it would mean his demise. The court accepted his desire to accept an early demise over a protracted state of discomfort caused by his reactions to the drugs.[3]

Even among autonomous adults, we should acknowledge "limited competency" and "intermittent competency." In our everyday lives we experience **limited competency**. For example, few of us have the training, even if we magically acquired the authority, to instruct the World Bank in the execution of its duties, yet most of us are competent to manage our own personal banking responsibilities. Similarly, patients might not have the capacity to make autonomous decisions in some areas of their lives even though they have adequate competency in other areas. For example, elderly patients with mild senility might not be competent to authorize participation in a research project that entails significant risk to the participants, but they can be adequately competent to select their meals from a menu.

Intermittent competency recognizes that there are times when otherwise autonomous individuals might be momentarily unable to deliberate thoughtfully and select a course of action. When we are under great psychological stress, we might easily be confused and unaware of the choices available to us, or we might be unable to make an appropriate choice. As an example, patients who have just learned that their diagnosis is life threatening might, for a period of time, be unable to assess their treatment options and make an informed decision. Parents who have just received word that their child was involved in a bicycle accident and suffered serious brain damage might not be able to give an autonomous directive to the health-care providers. In such cases, most experienced health-care providers know that they must preserve life or attend to all the patient's needs until decision makers have achieved a calmer state that allows them to understand medical information, assess their treatment options, and then make an informed decision.

Questions about autonomy and patient care have never been more relevant than in the managed care arena, as the following case study suggests.

Sam

Dr. Garcia is a well-known surgeon with an unparalleled success rate at hip replacements in Salem, a town of approximately 500,000 people. His surgical techniques are excellent, but he states openly that postsurgical rehabilitation is equally important. When his patients refuse therapy, he usually confronts them directly and rebukes them for having chosen him for the surgery in the first place if they were not willing to go all the way. He emphasizes that they will not reach their potential, and adds that they will damage his reputation and possibly make it necessary for him to fire their physical therapist. (He demands that his therapists, who are reserved exclusively for him by the physical therapy department of the hospital, work his patients for the full regimen each day.) He does not mention that at least daily one patient vomits from exhaustion or fear while in the gym.

Sam is new to Dr. Garcia's therapy team. As luck would have it, his first patient, Mrs. Samuels, refused to engage in strenuous exercise that made her nauseous. She tried to negotiate with Sam, stating that she still wanted to do therapy but not so aggressively. She reasoned that a slower pace would mean that she would need extra sessions but since she was willing to pay privately for the extra sessions, there was no reason not to take a less rigorous approach. When Sam presented Dr. Garcia with the proposal, the doctor exploded and threatened to terminate Sam if he did not get her out on time. He stated that every treatment session above and beyond his protocol robbed some new patient of time needed for rehabilitation and would mean that he would have to hire more therapists or reduce his surgical load. Instead, he would simply replace Sam. What is Sam to do?

We'll revisit this dilemma in the Discussion Question section at the end of this chapter.

Justifying the Respect Principle

It is worth exploring the more general questions about the principle of respect for autonomy, including its justification, its limits, and why it has become increasingly important. The **respect principle** can be formulated in various ways, most commonly in terms of correlated rights and duties: the rights of patients to exercise autonomy, and the duty of professionals to respect those rights. These formulations bring to mind, respectively, rights ethics and duty ethics. In practice, however, all ethical theories and moral traditions adapt these terms within their own framework.

Rights ethicists view patients' rights as directly implied by the basic human right to liberty. Duty ethicists derive patients' rights from the fundamental duty to respect persons who, as rational autonomous beings, have inherent dignity and worth. Virtue ethicists understand the virtue of respect as largely respect for persons as autonomous beings. Rule utilitarians understand patients' rights (and other rights) as those especially important areas of liberty whose protection tends to maximize overall good consequences. Although rights are not the most basic moral considerations for utilitarians, John Stuart Mill's utilitarian defense of liberty in *On Liberty* is in fact the most widely cited defense of people living their lives as they choose without interference and domination by others.

Although nearly all ethical theories justify a strong principle of respect for autonomy, they justify additional principles as well—in particular, beneficence (acting for the good of others) and benevolence (doing so motivated by a concern for their good). At least on the surface, beneficence and benevolence can conflict with the principle of respect for autonomy, thereby creating moral dilemmas. Throughout most of the history of medicine, these dilemmas were resolved by giving priority to benevolence, or, rather, the dilemmas were not even acknowledged because it was assumed that the benevolent physician had primary authority in making treatment decisions.[4] For 2500 years, the ethic of medicine was rooted in the Hippocratic Oath, which made paramount patients' health, not their autonomy. It was taken for granted that physicians knew better than patients what was good for them and that this knowledge gave physicians the authority to make decisions on behalf of their patients.

Stated another way, physicians embraced **medical paternalism**, or the view that physicians are justified in promoting the well-being of patients as defined by the physician, regardless of whether the patient gives prior consent. (Paternalism is sometimes called "parentalism," in order to avoid linguistic gender bias.) Paternalism takes various forms.[5] *Weak paternalism* is interfering with others' liberty to prevent them from harming themselves—for example, by forcibly stopping them from inadvertently walking into the path of an oncoming vehicle or requiring that motorcyclists wear protective helmets to prevent brain damage in motorcycle accidents. *Strong paternalism* is interfering with others' liberty to promote their good—for example, by using a placebo to help wean them from an addiction. The interference might mean promoting their good without their consent or even overriding their explicit choices, as when therapy is forced on someone against their will.

These forms of paternalism were once widely accepted in medicine and were reinforced by the Hippocratic Oath, which also forbids physicians from sharing their knowledge with laypersons, thereby further undermining patients' abilities to make decisions about their medical care.

Medical paternalism is declining dramatically. Even its defenders now argue for restricting its role in medicine. It is still accepted as a temporary measure, such as when health-care professionals entirely take over a patient's medical decisions during an emergency—when the patient is comatose or in shock—and relatives are not immediately available. But while the traditional rationale was that these were instances of justifiable paternalism, they are now reconstrued as signifying an implicit respect for autonomy, based on the assumption that rational individuals would choose this care if they could.

What led to this dramatic shift away from medical paternalism and toward an emphasis on respect for autonomy? Rights ethics, duty ethics, utilitarianism, and other ethical theories developed since the 18th-century Enlightenment played a role, although these theories generally reflected and systematized deeper movements in the direction of individualism. These movements were intensified by several events during the second half of the 20th century. The Nuremberg Code of 1946, drafted in the aftermath of the Holocaust, made central a principle of informed consent to ensure patients' ability to make their own decisions when confronted with powerful social institutions.

Other key forces included the social movements of the 1960s and 1970s, which accented individualism and gave rise to the patients' rights movement. During this period, several additional influences coalesced to prompt concern about risks to patients' autonomy: the increasing vulnerability of patients within modern health-care institutions; dramatic technologic changes that extend life and make possible an ever-increasing variety of treatment options; the widening gap of understanding between patients and professionals; and the augmented power of professionals. These issues began to be widely explored in the 1970s when medical ethics emerged as a discipline involving extensive interdisciplinary collaboration among health-care professionals, philosophers, attorneys, and social scientists.

In more recent years, both feminist ethics and the ethics of care have challenged how autonomy is defined. According to many feminist ethicists (about whom we say more in chapter 5), the problem is not that the principle of autonomy is incorrect, but that it instead does not capture the full scope of the moral life, including the role of decision making in governing one's life. In particular, the principle does not recognize that self-governance has different meanings for people, and that people define the "self" in different ways. Carol Gilligan, author of *In a Different Voice*, felt that most women and many men defined their "self" not as an isolated decision maker who should be considered competent only in the absence of the influence of others, but rather as a center of relationships and responsibilities that included many other significant persons. Therefore, persons who solicit the opinions of important people in their lives on crucial medical decisions are no less autonomous than those who make their decisions alone.

Most important, feminist ethicists have raised profound questions about the impact on autonomy of the uneven distribution of power, and they question whether women and minorities have the freedom to truly act autonomously when others are in positions of power. They also question if it is possible for those in power to treat those with lesser status as equals and to respect their choices with the same commitment as they would the choices of a peer. Although the concept of true autonomy is still a work in progress, Virginia Warren offers the following perspective, which addresses both power and respect for autonomy:

> On a larger scale, I believe that the feminist goal of eliminating conflicts over power can be permanently attained only by solving this problem: How can people be helped to develop a sense of self and of self-worth (identity) that is not based on putting down or controlling someone else (power over others)?... To eliminate discrimination across the board, a radical strategy is needed: educating people to value themselves in a way that does not depend on branding anyone else inferior.[6]

In light of these general considerations, we turn to the first and most important implication of respect for autonomy in health care: the duty of informed consent.

 ## Informed Consent

The duty of **informed consent** requires health professionals to respect the informed consent (and refusal) of their patients concerning the course of therapy. For patients to make informed decisions, three conditions must be met. The first is *competence*: patients must be sufficiently rational or competent to understand and make health-care decisions. In practice, requisite competence is defined legally, usually as the age of legal adulthood (18, for most purposes) unless the individual has a legal guardian because of a severe mental impairment or has authorized another person to make decisions. In the latter case, competent, autonomous adults can authorize someone to make decisions for them while they are still competent. However, the person who delegates the authority, not the surrogate decision maker, remains responsible for the outcomes of those decisions. For example, when competent patients authorize a physician or minister to make health-care decisions for them, the responsibility for the outcome rests with the patients, even though they did not directly make the decisions that produced the outcome. In such cases there is clearly the potential for abuse, but until that abuse is observed, one should respect the surrogate's decisions.

The second condition that must be met is *information*: patients must be given relevant information concerning their condition and treatment in a manner that they can understand so that they can make an informed decision. "Relevant information" includes facts about what is involved in the proposed therapy and alternative therapies, risks and benefits of the proposed therapy and of alternative therapies, financial costs, and additional information the patient requests concerning therapy. Precisely how much information is required is sometimes difficult to identify. In a practical sense, patients cannot be given all information concerning medical procedures, nor could most understand that information anyway (without a relevant health-care degree).

The difficulty comes in defining which information is relevant. At the time of this writing, there are two legally recognized standards that define which information must be given to the patient. The **medical care standard,** which is recognized in some states, defines it as the information that providers in a region agree is important for the patient to know. Other states recognize the **reasonable person standard,** which says that relevant information is that which any reasonable person would want before making a decision. A more recently proposed **dialogic standard,** which emerged from feminist ethics, would require that providers and patients have a dialogue in which patients define what they uniquely need to know so that the decision is their own individualized decision. This differs from the reasonable person standard in that it takes into account factors that might not be shared with "any reasonable person" but that are nonetheless important and reasonable to a particular patient. For example, a mother with terminal breast cancer wants to prolong her life in a pain-free environment until after the marriage of her daughter, which takes place in eight weeks. A generic reasonable person might not need or want such time-specific information or medical treatments that would help achieve a "success" that is unlike the success desired by others.

The information condition places requirements on how information is given as well as on what the information is. Disclosure of information in English to a person who speaks only Arabic does not constitute informed consent! And patients in emotional distress might need help in grasping even simple facts about their situation. Conveying the information requires skillful communication, rather than merely passing on a list of facts. It must be relayed in terms that the patient can understand, free of professional jargon and assumptions about what the patient ought to understand.

The tone of voice and the structure of the presentation are just two of the many subtle ways a provider may bias a patient toward one treatment or another. That is not to say that health-care providers should not express their opinions when asked. They should, however, express those opinions directly and overtly rather than covertly through a biased presentation of the relevant information. Moreover, professionals should be careful to give only information within their domain of practice. Out of respect for the autonomy of other providers, and in wise recognition of the limits of their own understanding, health-care professionals should not interpret the recommendations of other disciplines unless their help has been specifically requested in informing the patient. There is, however, a responsibility to make sure that corrections are made when a patient has received mistaken information because of either provider error or patient misunderstanding, which can often be discovered by asking patients to repeat or explain the information.

What if patients state that they do not want certain information, or perhaps any information, about their medical condition? For example, suppose they say their destiny is not in their hands and that additional information will be a burden, or that they prefer to follow their instincts. Does the right to informed consent include, paradoxically, a right *not* to be informed? Ultimately, patients should be free to use whatever decision matrix they prefer, be it sound reasoning, intuition, or magic. The right to self-governance implies a right to informed consent and, if one so chooses, a right not to be given certain information.

In fact, sometimes there are cogent, though unstated, reasons for refusing information. When researchers offered free counseling, educational programs, and genetic testing for a specific type of cancer to a group of high-risk individuals, only 43 percent elected to take the test, even though there was an 80 percent to 90 percent lifetime risk. The researchers in this particular study found that the most significant deterrent to the testing was potential discrimination by healthcare insurers once the results became known.[7]

One of the most important considerations for patients in refusing information has little to do with insurance. Ethnic background can affect how much information is desired by the patient, and belief systems can influence how information should be distributed and acted upon. One study found that Korean-Americans and Mexican-Americans were significantly less likely to believe that a diagnosis such as metastatic cancer should be given to the patient than were African-Americans or European-Americans. They were more likely to hold the belief that a patient should not be told of a terminal prognosis or asked about the use of life support by technology. Rather, those informational elements and decisions were most appropriately handled by the family.

The researchers concluded that the Korean-American and Mexican-American cultures used a family-centered method of making medical decisions as compared to the individual patient autonomy model used by European- and African-Americans. In family-centered cultures, it is the responsibility of the family to make the difficult decisions and the patient is protected from bad news. This practice is based on the belief that the information is an unnecessary burden to the patient and likely to lower the patient's morale, hindering recovery or a sense of well being. The researchers pointed out that this is also the predominant model in Italy and Greece. They report that in Italy, "autonomy is not viewed as empowering. Rather, it is seen as isolating and burdensome to patients who are too sick and too ignorant about their condition to be able to make meaningful choices."[8] These cultural differences do not undermine the concept of autonomy; instead, they expand it. A thorough understanding of autonomy allows others to work from the model that best suits their patients' individual and cultural needs.

When patients request that they not be told their diagnosis, forcing this information on them can be callous. In cases in which patients indicate an unwillingness to make their own decisions, the provider should ask what information they want, which decisions they would like to make, and who they will designate to make all other decisions. In medicine, respect for autonomy locates control with the patient or their designate rather than with the provider.

The third condition defining informed consent is *voluntariness*: patients should not be coerced or otherwise manipulated. Physically forcing therapy on patients against their explicit desires is the most flagrant violation of this condition. A more common violation is the use of subtle threats or other forms of emotional manipulation. Most common of all is the use of deception to "guide" a patient to making a particular decision.

Deception is the intentional misleading of a person, either by lying (intentionally stating a falsehood designed to create a false belief), withholding important information, exaggerating, understating, or using pretense. Deception typically violates both the information and voluntariness conditions, and to that extent those conditions can be viewed as overlapping.

All the conditions are sometimes challenged as changes in health-care practices and institutions occur. For example, many HMOs imposed "gag orders" on physicians and other providers, forbidding them to inform patients of alternative (usually more costly) approaches to their care or to refer them to sources outside the HMO for care— such as additional sessions with a physical therapist—which would increase their maximum benefit and the HMO's expenses. Medical ethicists and the courts condemned the gag orders, but the episode reminds us that patient rights remain vulnerable.

Let us illustrate the last two conditions, information and voluntariness, by adapting three examples from therapist Janet A. Coy. Each example involves patient noncompliance with a recommended course of therapy.

Physical Coercion

Mrs. S

Mrs. S, a 54-year-old woman, has received two and a half weeks of physical therapy during recovery from a right cerebrovascular accident. The muscle tone in her left upper extremity is improving, but the gain has brought with it increasing pain during range-of-motion (ROM) exercises. On her next visit she refuses treatment because of the pain, and she continues to refuse even after the therapist carefully explains the importance of treatment to improve arm movement and to prevent contractures. Convinced that she "cannot really appreciate the long-term implications of her refusal . . . the therapist performs the ROM exercises against Mrs. S's wishes. Meanwhile Mrs. S cries throughout the treatment session and at one point tries to gently push the therapist's hand away."[9]

Only a few decades ago the therapist's behavior might have been condoned, or at least tolerated, but today it is understood as unethical coercion. In legal terms, it constitutes battery: an unlawful attack; touching done without the consent of a person. While the presence of good intentions and a genuine desire to help Mrs. S makes the behavior paternalistic rather than a malevolent assault, immoral and illegal coercion are involved nonetheless.

There can be many variations in the details of this case. For example, Mrs. S might not express her refusal until after a therapy session is underway. Thus, by arriving for her appointment, she indicates a tacit consent to proceed with the routine exercises, but she exclaims "Please stop!" when the pain catches her by surprise during therapy. Or, in pain, she indicates refusal by shaking her head as she grimaces, a response calling for the therapist to pause and talk with her. Thus, in general, consent is not something always settled at the outset of either a discussion about a course of therapy or a particular therapy session. Instead, consent is part of an ongoing interaction with the therapist.

Deception and Threats

Mr. J

Mr. J, age 38, was in an accident that caused third-degree burns over his face, upper extremities, and back.[9(p46)] His skin grafts are healing successfully, and he has been cooperative during his three months of physical therapy. He starts refusing to wear his counterpressure garments, however, because he finds them uncomfortable. The therapist insists on the importance of the garments in improving his long-term appearance, but Mr. J replies that appearance is not important to him. The therapist is aware that there is considerable debate about the efficacy of the garments, but she remains convinced that they are an essential part of responsible care. Convinced that Mr. J will later deeply regret his decision, and knowing that Mr. J is strongly motivated to return to his job, she tells him that not wearing the garments might prevent sufficient recovery to return to his job as a mechanic and even jeopardize his insurance coverage. These are lies, because the garments will not affect function and, because Mr. J is compliant overall, his insurance coverage is not at risk. ▨

As in the first example, this case involves paternalism based on a sincere belief that the patient will benefit from the therapy being declined. Unlike the first case, the therapist manipulates Mr. J into making a particular decision by using deception. This violates the information condition for informed consent, but it also violates the voluntariness condition. Mr. J quite plausibly hears the therapist's remarks as a threat—the threat that health-care coverage will be revoked (regardless of whether the therapist is directly part of that revocation). Threats undermine voluntariness by creating fears or otherwise pressuring individuals to make decisions they otherwise would not want to make. Even without threats, deception itself interferes with voluntary choices when the deception manipulates a patient's decisions.

Manipulation

Mr. B ▨

Mr. B, age 68, has chronic obstructive pulmonary disease. Unable to care for himself, he enters a long-term nursing facility where he is mobile only with the help of a wheelchair and portable oxygen. He declines physical therapy, declaring he had had it before and it did not help. The therapist, however, believes that he would function more comfortably with the help of physical therapy and tries to convince him to at least undergo an evaluation to establish baseline information. "When Mr. B continues to refuse, the therapist begins to discuss her 'genuine desire' to help him be more comfortable, the importance of following a physician's order, and the 'terrible' consequences of not participating in physical therapy and of not being as active as possible. After 20 minutes of 'discussion,' during which both Mr. B and the therapist become increasingly agitated, Mr. B finally says, 'O.K., I give up. If I let you do the evaluation, will you leave me alone?' "[9(p46)]

There can be a fine line between assertively promoting understanding and encouraging patients to make reasonable decisions versus pressuring and harassing them. Obtaining informed consent requires more than dryly reciting facts, and a responsible therapist would undertake rational persuasion designed to convince Mr. B that it is in his interests to undergo the baseline tests. Yet getting patients to "appreciate" the importance of therapy easily shades into badgering them to make decisions through emotional agitation rather than calm deliberation. Even a tone of voice can increase or decrease rational deliberation by patients.

The last case involves a nursing facility where, as with many health-care institutions, special attention needs to be paid to subtle pressures. The courts have seen difficulties in the use of informed consent within "total institutions" (such as prisons and mental hospitals) that shape all areas of life. Nursing facilities are not generally thought of as total institutions, and yet some of them share striking similarities, ranging from a lack of privacy to the uniforms and hierarchy of the personnel. One could even argue that the ailments and limited fiscal resources of many elderly take away even their voluntariness (ability to choose) concerning placement in a skilled nursing organization. Living with a chronic ailment in a health-care institution for a long period of time can subtly affect an individual's overall sense of autonomy, leading to even more psychological dependence and vulnerability.

Especially in caring for patients who are elderly and enfeebled in long-term care facilities, providers may be tempted to confuse consent with simple compliance, and to interpret the lack of compliance with mental incompetence. As A. A. Guccione writes, elderly patients "who refuse to accept professional recommendations will often have their mental competency challenged."[10] The assumption is that any rational person would accept a certain course of therapy, and hence refusing it is a sign of irrationality so extreme as to call into question their general psychological capacities to be self-determining. In fact, sometimes this assumption is accurate. More often, however, health professionals fail to appreciate the right of patients to make their decisions in light of their moral values and intellectual outlook.

Martha Sullivan

Martha Sullivan is an 83-year-old widow who was admitted to a skilled nursing facility because of a broken hip, secondary to a fall. The hip had mended well and now the physical therapist is working on balance skills. This was not the first fall for Ms. Sullivan, and in fact she had been having increasing difficulty in caring for herself since her husband's death. Her children are worried that she might be injured in her home with no one available to help her. Both her children live out of state, and since her husband's death, Ms. Sullivan has lost interest in maintaining the friendships she previously had found rewarding.

Anna is Ms. Sullivan's physical therapist, and the two have developed an excellent rapport. Ms. Sullivan has been the ideal patient, doing all her home exercises. But Anna was caught by surprise when she went to Ms. Sullivan's room 15 minutes early to find her with her face in her pillow to hush the sounds of her crying. Anna put her arm around her patient and asked why she was so upset. Ms. Sullivan responded that she found therapy scary because she was afraid she would fall again and she was sure she would not live through another convalescent period. All she really wanted to do was to use a walker in her room and use a wheelchair when she went outside. Anna asked her why she had not mentioned this before. With great clarity, Ms. Sullivan explained that she was afraid that if she refused anything, the nursing facility would either have her declared incompetent or would put her out. If they declared her incompetent, she could be sent to a far worse location and would lose control of what little money she had left. She also stated that neither of her children wanted her with them and that she had no place else to go.

Anna feels sure she can coax Ms. Sullivan into continuing therapy, but she also feels unsure about whether she should attempt to change Ms. Sullivan's mind or merely stop by for social calls until Ms. Sullivan requests more therapy.

You will revisit Anna's dilemma in the Discussion Questions section at the end of this chapter.

Truth Telling

The duty to tell the truth to patients is also called the principle of veracity, honesty, or truthfulness. Negatively stated, it forbids deception, or intentionally misleading someone. As in everyday life, deception is objectionable for many reasons, including reasons reflected in the language of the various ethical theories we have discussed. Thus, deception undermines autonomy (duty ethics), violates the right to the truth (rights ethics), tends to generate a host of bad consequences (utilitarianism), and manifests the vice of dishonesty (virtue ethics). In addition, professionals enter into fiduciary relationships—special relationships of trust—in which strong requirements of truth are expected. In fact, receiving medical information can be thought of as one of the services that patients pay for as part of their health care.

Obviously, the duty of truth telling largely overlaps the duty of informed consent, but nevertheless it is distinct. It is rooted in a general duty of truthfulness (veracity, honesty) and as such applies to all information rather than only to information about health-care procedures. In practice, however, within therapeutic contexts, the relevant application of the duty concerns health-care information.

Moral dilemmas can arise when a physician asks a physical therapist not to convey to the patient certain information about the patient's health, particularly information that normally the therapist would not be required to divulge in obtaining informed consent about physical therapy procedures, but that has implications for the therapist-patient relationship. Ruth Purtilo presents the following case.

Andrew Gordon

Andrew Gordon is a 43-year-old contractor who fractured his right tibia in a fall from a scaffold. Mr. Gordon has been hospitalized for three weeks because the fracture is not healing quickly. A fever prompts tests that reveal lymphosarcoma, a cancer likely to be fatal within a year. His physician, Dr. Hammill, calls Kim Segard, the physical therapist, to say that he has talked with Mrs. Gordon and they have agreed that Mr. Gordon would not want to know the truth. The physician does, however, ask Kim whether Mr. Gordon has said anything suggesting he would want to know the truth. Kim reports that he had not. But 10 days later Mr. Gordon does say to Kim, "I have come to trust your judgment. . . . I've tried to cooperate with the doctors and everyone, but I have a feeling that something funny is going on that I can't get at. My wife and Dr. Hammill are acting strange and that is scaring me. . . . Do I have cancer or some fatal illness?"[11]

A direct lie, "No, you do not have cancer," would violate the relationship of trust between Kim and Mr. Gordon. Saying "I'm a physical therapist, not a doctor," would avoid a lie but perhaps constitute deception in the form of withholding information. Saying "You need to talk to Dr. Hammill about that part of your health care" might cause Mr. Gordon to feel additional anxiety that people are not being fully honest with him about something fearful. One way to preserve trust would be for Kim to offer to call Dr. Hammill and then get back to Mr Gordon within a day or so. This would provide the opportunity to convince Dr. Hammill that his patient wants the truth. But suppose Dr. Hammill still refuses, perhaps after talking again to Mrs. Gordon?

The case illustrates the moral complexities of working as part of a health-care team. A physician's choice to lie or otherwise deceive a patient can implicate coworkers in a web of deception. Fortunately, there is an increasing consensus that respect for autonomy creates a strong moral presumption to tell the truth, except in highly unusual circumstances. Today, the consensus would probably be that Dr. Hammill is at fault for failing to inform Mr. Gordon about his cancer. As a competent adult, Mr. Gordon has the right to be told the truth. And much is at stake: he should have the opportunity to choose how he wants to spend the remainder of his life in light of the truth. Perhaps he would want to prepare a will or take his family on a final vacation to some destination they had planned on visiting for years.

Dr. Hammill reflects the traditional medical paternalism that is now in decline. The change is relatively recent. A 1961 poll of American physicians revealed that 88 percent of them would routinely withhold from patients a diagnosis of their terminal cancer. By 1979 a poll revealed a dramatic change: 98 percent of physicians polled said they would reveal that diagnosis to their patients.[12,13]

Is this shift in attitudes morally appropriate? Sissela Bok offers one of the strongest arguments in its favor.[14] Many of her reasons are utilitarian arguments that highlight the good consequences of truth telling. She cites polls showing that people usually want to know the truth, even about terminal diseases. Moreover, they need to know the truth so they can set their affairs in order, make peace with their loved ones, and seek a meaningful way to live their last months or years.

The reason that health-care professionals often find it difficult to inform their patients of bad news is a fear of unpleasantness, and perhaps their own fear of death. As for the objection that telling a patient about a terminal illness could precipitate suicide, Bok emphasizes the importance of providing support services for patients. Nevertheless, she feels that patients have a right to the truth if they so desire. In some cases it could be argued that suicide can be a rational choice, especially when the option is uncontrolled pain followed by certain death (a topic we return to in chapter 6).

John Borrego

John Borrego is a physical therapist at a university teaching hospital. He was assigned a patient, Raymond Sinclair, who has low-back pain of unknown origin but progressive in nature. Mr. Sinclair works for the U.S. Postal Service, which ships large packages, and he attributes his pain to job-related back strains. He has filed a worker compensation claim. John initiates a treatment plan that consists of mild stretching, abdominal strengthening, and modified positions for sleep, lifting, and activities of daily living (ADL). A week following implementation of the program, John drafts a recommendation to the physician that they add ultrasound as a preliminary treatment to stretching, to create a faster and less painful course of treatment. He notifies the patient that he is making this request and will begin as soon as approval is received.

After several days of no response from the physician, John calls his office. The physician says that he wishes John had not told the patient of this proposal because he is afraid to authorize it, fearing that the back pain is caused by a malignancy that has migrated into the vertebra. He is in the process of evaluating current test results and ordering additional tests, but he does not want to alarm Mr. Sinclair if his clinical judgment should prove to be incorrect. To prevent Mr. Sinclair from suspecting anything, the physician tells John to give Mr. Sinclair the usual ultrasound treatment but without turning on the switch that delivers the impulse to the application head. That way, the physician reasons, Mr. Sinclair will not notice anything out of order. Perhaps he might even be one of those patients who will experience improvement because of the placebo effect, with no harmful side effects. John immediately understands that he is being asked to be untruthful by withholding information from the patient. He is also being asked to risk the trust of a patient who has grown to respect his recommendations.

Situations will always arise in which physicians feel justified in withholding some relevant information, at least for a certain period of time, thereby creating dilemmas for therapists.

Confidentiality

The duty of confidentiality is the duty to maintain privacy of information concerning patients by not divulging it to unauthorized persons. In principle, the scope of the duty is broad and includes *all* information about patients obtained during professional interactions with them. In practice, this consists of any intimate and potentially sensitive information, including that concerning the immediate care provided, additional health-related information, financial information, and other potentially sensitive information (though not, say, the color of clothing they wear on a particular day, or their hobbies).

During the past decade, the most frequently discussed example of confidentiality in health-care ethics has concerned patients with HIV/AIDS. Swisher and Krueger-Brophy offer this situation:

Larry Dulles

According to Swisher and Krueger-Brophy, "Larry Dulles is a 26-year-old man being treated in physical therapy for generalized weakness and neurological problems associated with acquired immunodeficiency syndrome (AIDS). One day his mother took him to therapy. After his treatment session, she remarked to his therapist that he did not seem to be improving. The therapist said, 'Well, we don't always see dramatic changes with AIDS patients.' Larry's mother was previously unaware of his diagnosis."[15]

The therapist's error was a casual lapse in judgment and probably well-intended, since the therapist was responding to the mother as a key family member whose involvement was both appropriate and valuable in contributing to the care of Mr. Dulles. Nevertheless, regardless of how understandable or well-intended, the therapist's error constituted a serious violation of confidentiality.

How serious is it? Swisher and Krueger-Brophy point out that in some states the lapse would violate the laws protecting patient confidentiality and in addition violate laws specifically passed to protect HIV information. In addition, both the therapist and his or her organization would be open to major civil lawsuits for invading privacy and causing emotional distress. The therapist's license could be at risk as well.

Suppose the therapist had inadvertently disclosed the information to Larry Dulles's wife or life partner? Or suppose the therapist happened to learn from Mr. Dulles that he is engaged in unprotected sex with several partners? Confidentiality does have justifiable exceptions. Most of them are specified within the law. In particular, health-care professionals must report child abuse, elder abuse, gunshot wounds, and some contagious diseases.

Confidentiality may be legally compromised when medical records are ordered by the courts in criminal investigations. But are there justifiable exceptions beyond what the law requires or permits? And which exceptions ought to be established by law in the first place? Answers to the last two questions have always been controversial. Extreme and even unforeseeable situations can arise that make it difficult to apply moral principles. In our view, the exceptions should be few, and confidentiality needs increasing safeguards.

To begin with, there is wide consensus that the duty of confidentiality is extremely important for at least four reasons. First, control over sensitive information is required by the principle of respect for autonomy. Maintaining control over sensitive information about us—"sensitive" as defined both subjectively, by each of us, and objectively in terms of risk of harm—is part of controlling our lives. The example of Larry Dulles illustrates how one fact about us can influence our entire self-image and the image that others have of us.

Second, professionals create a shared understanding with the public that they will take special care in maintaining confidential information. They do so, as a group, by promising the public (through their codes of ethics and other official documents) to maintain confidentiality. Like all promises, this commitment generates an obligation.

Third, in light of this shared understanding, a relationship of trust is created with each patient. Violating this fiduciary relationship is a breach of trust.

Fourth, and underlying all the previous reasons, confidentiality promotes health care (and other professional services). One reason why the fiduciary relationship is created in the first place is to ensure that patients will feel free to divulge sensitive information to health-care professionals in order to receive the health care they seek and need. Many patients already have a general reluctance to discuss intimate details about their bodies and lives. They must be encouraged to maintain frank and honest dialogue throughout the therapeutic process in which that information is relevant to the diagnosis or treatment at hand.

Despite the philosophical need for strict confidentiality, a hierarchy of legal entitlements to types of information does exist among health-care providers, based on the "need to know." Psychiatry and psychology have the greatest legal protection for the most intimate personal information about a person, because it is this type of information that is most important for successful diagnosis and treatment in these professions. Physical therapists, in contrast, have very limited legal entitlement to protect personal information in a court of law, aside from medical and physiologic information. This is because information about a patient's personal life is usually not an essential element for creating a treatment plan and intervention. Physical therapists should restrict their inquiries into the personal lives of their patients to the information relevant to their care. They should also avoid leading patients to believe that their deepest secrets are legally protected in a court of law, unlike the situation of psychological therapists.

Confidentiality is increasingly at risk in health-care settings. In 1982, physician Mark Siegler had already called confidentiality a "decrepit concept" because modern hospitals had ended the Hippocratic tradition of strict doctor-patient confidentiality. At the behest of one of his patients who was especially concerned about his privacy, Dr. Siegler investigated how many people had access to his patient's medical record. He discovered that at least 75 people had access, including physicians, nurses, pharmacists, nutritionists, therapists, students, financial officers, secretaries, and auditors. The access was a result not of carelessness but of caring for patients in light of the contemporary forces within health care: "the rise of health-care teams, the existence of third-party insurance programs, and the expanding limits of medicine."[16] Having sounded the alarm, Siegler recommended that access to sensitive information be limited to a "need to know" basis. He also called for informing patients about what "medical confidentiality" now means, and allowing patients to review their records and to indicate their wishes about restricting especially sensitive information in the records.

Since the time Siegler made these recommendations, far greater concerns have arisen concerning computer data banks that contain medical information— leading to both unauthorized uses and authorized abuses.[17] On the one hand, alarming examples of *unauthorized use* of medical information have been widely publicized. For example, some government employees in Maryland sold confidential medical information from the state data bank used for cost-containment purposes. The information was purchased by health maintenance organizations and later accessed and used by a banker to call in loans on cancer patients.[18] In 1994, an HMO discovered that over one hundred employees had accessed the medical records of a famous figure skater Tonya Harding after a visit for a sprained wrist. Most of these employees had no involvement in the case.

On the other hand, *authorized abuses* are institutionalized and legally permissible arrangements that channel information acquired in health-care settings to non–health-care parties, such as employers and businesses marketing products. Employers motivated to reduce health-care costs for themselves and their employees, or simply to ensure a healthy workforce, often use such information in making hiring and firing decisions, unless laws specifically prohibit doing so. Pharmaceutical and health-care-equipment manufacturers use the information to target audiences in selling their products. Recently, the popular press has been releasing investigative reports alerting the public to current databases that include medical histories and future possible links through the Internet that threaten to destroy privacy.[19]

A. Etzioni calls upon health-care professionals to reshape their institutions with an eye to counterbalancing corporate abuses to ensure that sensitive information is used to provide cost-efficient health care to patients. In tune with Siegler's emphasis on "need to know" access, he distinguishes three groups: the inner circle directly involved in providing health care, the intermediate circle of health insurance and managed-care corporations, and the outer circle of employers, marketers, and insurers. The primary goal should be to prevent the outer circle from gaining sensitive information that the inner and intermediate circles must have to provide good health care. This can be accomplished by establishing "layered records and graduated release" of information to appropriate groups. In some countries, such as France, genetic information is considered so confidential that it is maintained in a separate chart and is strictly maintained by the primary-care physician.

To conclude, we began this chapter with the theme that respect for autonomy has replaced medical paternalism as a dominant theme in medical ethics, especially concerning the control of information. The traditional case for medical paternalism was an appeal to beneficence or benevolence. Properly conceived, however, respect for autonomy and beneficence are not inherently opposed. As Edmund D. Pellegrino and David C. Thomasma suggest,

> Paternalism, whether benignly intended or not, cannot be beneficent in any true sense of that word. Beneficence and its corollary, nonmaleficence, require acting to advance the patient's interests, or at least not harming them. It is difficult to see how violating the patient's own perception of his [or her] welfare can be a beneficent act. Paternalism is obviously in a polar relationship with autonomy, but it is diametrically opposed to beneficence and nonmaleficence as well.[20]

Principle 1 of the APTA *Code of Ethics* expresses this basic unity of respect and caring: "A physical therapist shall respect the rights and dignity of all individuals and shall provide compassionate care." In the next chapter we turn to a discussion of caring for patients within a framework of respect for their autonomy.

Discussion Questions

1. Using the example discussed in the opening section of this chapter, discuss what Sam should have done in response to Dr. Garcia. Are there several morally permissible responses, or is one option most desirable or even obligatory?

2. Muriel Thomas is a 76-year-old widow who, as a consequence of a fall, had a hip replacement. Her only living relative is a son who shows little interest in her. Almost everyone in the rehab unit recognizes that most of Muriel's complaints are not related to the replacement but instead are thinly veiled attempts to get attention. She complains of various pains that change location and have no obvious connection to her injury, surgery, or therapy. Her functional status with a walker is nearly where it was prior to the accident. Although the physician and the therapist agree that therapy goals have almost been achieved and should be discontinued in a week or so, the physician asks the therapist to make up some kind of treatment to appease her complaints. The physician states that the attention will probably make the pains go away, at least until she is discharged. The physician also states that she will enter a diagnosis that will allow insurance to cover the therapist so that no revenue will be lost to the department. The therapist complied and started administering low levels of ultrasound to Muriel's forearm, the site of her most recent "pain." Much to the therapist's surprise, Muriel asked her directly how this therapy was supposed to help.

   What are the moral issues in this case, and how do you think they should have been handled?

3. Review the sections on confidentiality, truthfulness, and respect for patient autonomy in the APTA *Guide for Professional Conduct*. What does the guide require concerning the three examples from Janet A. Coy and the example of Ms. Sullivan discussed in the section on "Informed Consent"? In general, does the guide provide adequate guidance in these areas?

4. Paternalism (or "parentalism") is now widely suspect, both because of past abuses and because of the contemporary emphasis on respect for patient autonomy. Yet Gerald Dworkin argues that, ironically, some paternalism can be justified by appealing to respect of autonomy.[21] According to Dworkin, autonomy is lessened when persons become seriously ill, and it is ended when they die. Conversely, individuals' autonomy is broadened and protected by many laws that interfere with individuals' liberty for their own good, especially by encouraging them to be more prudent in basic matters of health and safety. Examples of such laws include: (a) requiring motorcyclists to wear safety helmets, (b) requiring drivers to wear seat belts, (c) forbidding swimming at beaches when no lifeguard is on duty, (d) prohibiting use of dangerous drugs such as heroin and cocaine, (e) compelling participation in Social Security or other retirement plans, (f) prohibiting dueling, (g) putting fluoride in public drinking water, and (h) requiring professionals (such as physical therapists) to be licensed. Dworkin adds that the burden of proof should be on the government to justify each of these interferences with liberty, and that the restrictions should be minimally restrictive. Do you agree or disagree with him, both about these examples and about his appeal to respect for autonomy as a justification for them? Would you favor further laws, such as those banning advertising of cigarettes, alcohol, and firearms?

5. Discuss how each of the major ethical theories discussed in chapter 2—utilitarianism, duty ethics, rights ethics, virtue ethics, religious ethics, and pragmatism—would justify the duty of confidentiality. In doing so, link to each theory the four reasons why confidentiality is important: respect for autonomy, professional obligation, trust, and promotion of health.

References

1. Beauchamp TL, Childress JF. *Principles of Biomedical Ethics*. 5th ed. New York, NY: Oxford University Press; 2001:63.
2. Stolberg S. Kept alive, but to live what kind of life? *Los Angeles Times*. October 22, 1996:A1, A10.
3. Associated Press. Teen-age patient gets ok to stop transplant drug. *Los Angeles Times*. June 12, 1994:A19.
4. Veatch RM. *The Basics of Bioethics*. Upper Saddle River, NJ: Prentice Hall; 2000:2-10.
5. Sartorius R, ed. *Paternalism*. Minneapolis, MN: University of Minnesota Press; 1983.
6. Warren VL. Feminist directions in medical ethics. In Holmes HB, Purdy LM, eds. *Feminist Perspectives in Medical Ethics*. Bloomington: Indiana University Press; 1992:38-39.
7. Lerman C, Narod S, Schulman K, et al. BRCA1 testing in families with hereditary breast-ovarian cancer. *JAMA*. 1996;275:1885-1892.
8. Blackhall LJ, Murphy ST, Frank G, et al. Ethnicity and attitudes toward patient autonomy. *JAMA*. 1995;275(10):824.
9. Coy JA. Autonomy-based informed consent: ethical implications for patient noncompliance. *Phys Ther*. 1989;69(10):45. Coy's excellent essay guides our discussion in this section.

10. Guccione AA. Compliance and patient autonomy: ethical and legal limits to professional dominance. *Top Geriatr Rehabil.* 1988;3(3):72.

11. Purtilo RB. *Ethical Dimensions in the Health Professions.* 2nd ed. Philadelphia: W.B. Saunders; 1993:109.

12. Oken D. What to tell cancer patients: a study of medical attitudes. *JAMA.* 1961;175:1120-1128.

13. Novack DH, et al. Changes in physicians' attitudes toward telling the cancer patient. *JAMA.* 1979;241:897-900.

14. Bok S. *Lying: Moral Choice in Public and Private Life.* New York, NY: Vintage; 1999.

15. Swisher LL, Krueger-Brophy C. *Legal and Ethical Issues in Physical Therapy.* Boston: Butterworth-Heinemann; 1998:151.

16. Siegler M. Confidentiality in medicine—a decrepit concept. *N Engl J Med.* 1982;307:518-521.

17. Etzioni A. Medical records: enhancing privacy, preserving the common good. *Hastings Cent Rep.* 1999;29. For an expanded discussion, see Etzioni A. *The Limits of Privacy.* New York: Basic Books; 1999.

18. Gunter B. It's no secret: what you tell your doctor—and what medical documents reveal about you—may be open to the scrutiny of insurers, employers, lenders, credit bureaus, and others. *Tampa Tribune.* October 6, 1996.

19. Consumers Union. Who knows your medical secrets? *Consumers Report.* August 2000:22-26.

20. Pellegrino ED, Thomasma DC. *The Virtues In Medical Practice.* New York, NY: Oxford University Press; 1993:58.

21. Dworkin G. Paternalism. *Monist.* 1972;56.

Caring for Patients

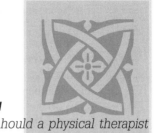

*S*hould a physical therapist
report suspected familial abuse of a patient if the
report is likely to cause therapy to be discontinued
without remedying the abuse?

Keywords

Principle of beneficence	Medical good	Emotional neglect
Malady	Total good	Sexual abuse
Illness	Professional distance	Emotional abuse
Illness narrative	Pity	Domestic elder abuse
Empathy	Physical abuse	Institutional abuse
Sympathy	Child neglect	Abandonment
Compassion	Physical neglect	Financial exploitation
Profession-specific good	Education neglect	Self-neglect

Like other health-care professions, physical therapy exists as a caring response to human maladies—suffering, disease, injury, and disability. Accordingly, the central norm for health-care professionals is caring, or what is called the **principle of beneficence**: the moral requirement to promote the well-being of patients. Caring for patients implies and is limited by respect for autonomy and also by professional standards of "due care," as discussed in Chapter 3. Here we take up several additional aspects of caring for patients: patients' experience of illness; the interaction between patients' medical good and their total good; and dealing with family violence and other forms of child and elder abuse. We will also discuss the issues of professional distance and character, and the role of caring motives in promoting health care.

"Caring" has several relevant meanings. Health-care professionals are *caregivers* (service providers) who have responsibilities to *take care of* patients (provide appropriate services) according to contractual obligations, state-of-the-art standards of competency in the profession, and respect for patients' autonomy. In meeting their responsibilities, therapists must be *careful* (cautious) in dealing with risks, *take care* (be conscientious) in meeting responsibilities, and exercise *due care* (reasonable caution) to meet standards of professional competence. Their work requires developing a good "bedside manner" in *showing care* (presenting themselves as concerned and considerate).

Professionals can "show care," however, without genuinely *caring about* (being benevolent regarding) their patients—in other words, without having a positive attitude toward them. A show of care might only be an elaborate game of appearances and pretense aimed at maintaining a profitable practice. That is, professionals could engage in helping actions (beneficence) without having caring motives and character (benevolence). Should therapists aspire to be *caring persons* (benevolent) who are genuinely concerned about helping patients for the sake of the patients and not simply to earn a living? Does such caring interfere with the professional distance needed for objective judgment and successful coping with the stresses of work, causing professionals to become *care-ridden* (burdened with anxiety), debilitated by "compassion fatigue," and even involved inappropriately (either emotionally or sexually) with patients? We will work toward answers to these questions in this chapter.

Experiences of Illness

It will be helpful here to distinguish between a malady and an illness.[1,2] A **malady** is a negative medical condition such as pain, disability, injury, disorder, loss of freedom, loss of pleasure, even the process of dying, or an elevated risk of suffering such harms. An **illness**—or feeling ill—is how a malady (or what one believes is a malady) is experienced by an individual. Accordingly, persons might be diseased or injured but not ill. For example, a person may have degenerative lumbar disk disease but not experience low back pain or other symptoms of illness, and a person might have hypertension without conscious symptoms of the disease. Conversely, persons can be ill but not diseased, which is the case with hypochondriacs, who genuinely suffer distress even though they have no actual physical malady.

The distinction between maladies and illnesses is blurred, and some maladies are partly defined by experiences of illness. Thus, many mental disorders are defined by experiences such as chronic depression, paranoia, or phobia. Severe physical pain can be both a symptom of a disease and a critical component of the illness experienced. In theory, however, there is a difference between disease or injury (which are objectively defined) and experiences of illness (which are subjectively defined). Of special interest is the fact that individuals might experience essentially the same malady differently. The same physical injury might be experienced in strikingly different ways, depending on individual attitudes, emotions, and beliefs.

Pain is one of the most important determinants in a therapist's decision about both intensity and duration of treatment, making the understanding of a patient's perception of pain an important factor for the clinician to consider. Sometimes, for example, chronic-pain sufferers have an elevated pain threshold, resulting in the underreporting of pain. This, in turn, misleads therapists to believing they are operating within normal physiological limits when in fact they are overtreating. Conversely, there are patients with such a low threshold for pain that the equivalent of a needle prick prompts undertreatment or may cause them to discontinue therapy. Thus, understanding pain is critical to appropriate healthcare delivery.

It is important to distinguish suffering from physical pain. Just as illness is the way in which a malady is experienced, suffering is one way an illness is interpreted by individuals. While physical pain can be explained by neurology, suffering is the interpretation of physical pain by the individual, and hence is better illuminated by the psychologist. Suffering, Cassell suggests, is "the severe distress associated with events that threaten the intactness of person."[3] More fully,

> . . . suffering occurs when an impending destruction of the person is perceived; it continues until the threat of disintegration has passed or until the integrity of the person can be restored in some other manner. It follows, then, that although it often occurs in the presence of acute pain, shortness of breath or other bodily symptoms, suffering extends beyond the physical. Most generally, suffering can be defined as the state of severe distress associated with events that threaten the intactness of person.[3]

In our view, Cassell's definition focuses on the most severe forms of suffering, but there are many milder forms as well. His definition does, however, help us clarify a phenomenon often seen in patients following a severe trauma. The idea of suffering as a threat to the entire person applies to many patients treated by the physical therapist, for patients often feel threatened by a change in their physical functioning. When they are without the core of their familiar self, which can be drastically changed by pain or disability, they are confused and disorganized, and experience what Cassell calls a "loss of central purpose." They are unable to focus on creating a revised (long- or short-term) self-definition until the suffering is relieved or diminished.

The first step in reducing suffering and pain is to acknowledge their presence. In doing so, we need an awareness of the patient as a total person, insofar as we can develop such an awareness without violating the patient's privacy. We also need to offer a simple expression of concern for patients' suffering. Even when we cannot fully understand another person's suffering, we can be respectful of it and offer hope through both our compassion and the application of our professional skills. Once suffering is reduced to a manageable level, the patient can effectively undertake the rehabilitation process.

The way to initiate an assessment of pain and suffering is through an **illness narrative**—a verbal account, brief or extended, written or spoken, of an illness.[4-7] Narratives, in general, are the stories (interpretations) we tell ourselves about events and relationships, challenges and achievements, and other aspects of our lives. Meaning (or significance) is a combination of intelligibility and value; it is a making sense of our lives in light of our values. Illness narratives, then, are interpretations of experiences of health problems (our own or others). An illness narrative typically makes sense of those experiences by placing them within the wider narrative of our lives. As an illustration of the manner in which caring for patients involves sensitivity to their experiences of illness and suffering, consider Oliver Sacks's illness narrative, A Leg to Stand On, aspects of which are described in the following case study:

Dr. Oliver Sacks

Dr. Sacks, a distinguished neurologist, underwent his first major experience as a patient when he severely injured his left leg, tearing the quadriceps from the patella, ripping the cruciate ligaments, and causing major nerve damage that paralyzed the entire leg with the exception of some motion in the toes. The accident occurred during a solitary hike on a mountain in Norway. Upon encountering an enormous bull, he ran in panic and was injured falling from a cliff. He managed to drag himself for hours until he was rescued by some other hikers. Airlifted to England, he underwent a major operation.

For a frightening two weeks he was left without any sensation in the injured leg, although he could wiggle his toes. Indeed, he experienced the leg as an alien appendage, something attached to his body but not part of it. This strange experience had a deeper impact on his general self-conception, dislocating his sense of who he was. These odd and alarming feelings were compounded by being thrust for the first time into the passive role of a hospital patient governed by prison-like requirements of impersonal clothing, identification bracelets, and strict structuring of his time. Fortunately, sensation in the leg gradually returned, followed by quick flashes of extreme pain. At that time he began a course of physical therapy that would eventually restore normal function. The experience of recovery would transform both him and his understanding of the role of health professionals.

Despite his years of experience in medicine, he was shocked to encounter in his surgeon a brusque "mechanic" who had no interest in him as an individual. When Sacks tried to convey his alarming sense of alienation, both from the leg and from his sense of self-identity, the surgeon "didn't even listen to me. He showed no concern. He doesn't listen to his patients—he doesn't give a damn."[8] In the few and brief times the surgeon visited, he dismissed Sacks's attempts to communicate his fears and uncanny feelings, bluntly saying he was a busy and a practical man, then walking out of the room. In retrospect, Sacks felt that he might have been somewhat unfair to the surgeon and that perhaps their formal roles were preventing both of them from making human contact. ◈

We do not know how Sacks's physician would respond to this assessment, but we can imagine that he might have responded that he did indeed care about Sacks; it was just that he had many additional patients who also needed his time. If he engaged with patients and spent more time with each, fewer patients would be seen. Although those fewer patients might feel better about him, his surgical performance probably would not be enhanced by the exchange. He might contend that he should consciously focus his time only on that which is relative to his task—surgery—which is based in anatomy and physiology. Certainly in the current managed-care environment, with its high demands on productivity, professional detachment might serve to achieve the completion of some tasks most efficiently, as we discuss more fully later in this chapter.

Patients generally expect, or at least hope for, personal concern from healthcare professionals. That concern might mean empathy, sympathy, compassion, and caring. **Empathy** is sympathetic identification with others. It combines cognitive understanding of what others are feeling with at least some tendency to respond with interest rather than indifference. As one writer states, "Empathy means 'I *could* be you,' " but it also implies something more than indifference.[9] In some contexts empathy involves vicariously experiencing what others are feeling and thinking, but it need not always mean having emotions paralleling what they are feeling. (In a weaker sense, empathy is simply understanding what others are feeling, without any sympathetic response to them. In this sense, sadists might have empathy for their victims.)

Sympathy is an emotion of concern for others' difficulties and especially a sharing of their sorrows or suffering. **Compassion** is deep caring in response specifically to suffering. Empathy, sympathy, and compassion are all manifestations of caring, an emotion of direct concern for others' well-being, with an active disposition to contribute to their well-being.

All these forms of personal concern were manifested by the physical therapists who worked with Sacks. For example, when the day came for him to attempt his first walk, the therapists gently urged him to stand, encouraging him with both practical advice and good humor suitable to the occasion and to the particular patient: "Come on, Dr. Sacks! You can't stand there like that—like a stork on one leg. You've got to use the other one, put weight on it too!"[8(p138)] When he was seized by terror as he began to fall, he cried out to the therapists, "Hold me, you must hold me—I'm utterly helpless." The therapists calmed him: "Now steady yourself—keep your eyes up." Sacks replied that he was unable to move the leg and, to his astonishment, he had utterly forgotten how one walks. In response, one therapist "wordlessly moved my left leg with her leg, pushing it to a new position, so that it made, or was made to make, a sort of step. Once this was done, I saw how to do it. I could not be told, but could instantly be shown."[8(p143)] Throughout the process, the therapists were gentle but persistent, conveying a firm sense that "one must 'get on with it,' one must proceed, one must take the first step."[8(p142)]

When Sacks finally managed to take that first step, motion returned rapidly. Full convalescence, however, took many weeks of gradually strengthening both muscles and physical self-control. It also required grappling with emotional disturbances that for Sacks were out of character. As his earlier terror diminished, he felt venomous spite, bouts of anger and irritation, and resentment at the more healthy patients in the convalescent center. Here again he credits a physical therapist with helping him: "When I started on the physiotherapy program, and the therapist was affirmative and profoundly encouraging, giving me the feeling that I might hope for a virtually complete recovery, I discovered that the hateful feeling was gone."[8(p178)]

Sacks concludes his illness narrative by reflecting on how modern medicine, with its fixation on physiological processes, has lost contact with "the experiencing, suffering patient."[8(p205)] Poetically, he calls for something like a "neurology of the soul" to restore an appreciation of listening to patients, of engaging their experiences as part of the therapeutic encounter. For the patient, convalescence is more than a matter of improving muscle tone and range of movement; it is also a matter of confronting fear, suffering, and vulnerability, and of needing help in summoning realistic hope.

Physical therapists are not trained as psychotherapists. It would be presumptuous for them to take on the role of "neurologists of the soul," although they should have an awareness of when patients might need help from a professional psychotherapist. Yet, like all health professionals, physical therapists treat their patients as persons when they are sensitive to the emotional aspects of suffering in addition to physical pain. A comprehensive ethical framework requires that we attend to the whole person, not just body parts or systems in need of repair. From this perspective, caring is not a "bonus" of good health care but instead is an essential, for two reasons. First, caring makes us attentive to patient needs and alerts us to subtle individualized feedback that is essential for personalized and effective treatment. Secondly, caring enhances us as therapists by continually expanding our ability to feel a connectedness with patients—and indeed with our profession.

Medical Good and Total Good

One important dimension of caring is sensitivity to how patients' medical good relates to their total good. For each profession, we can identity a **profession-specific good** defined by the relevant professional service—for example, in law, it is a client's share of legal justice; in education, it is a student's growth in understanding and skills; and in investment professions, it is a client's growth in income.[10] Patients' **medical good**, then, is their well-being measured in terms of health. In contrast, patients' **total good** is their overall, unified well-being. It includes health but also involves many more elements, such as happiness, valuable personal relationships, meaningful work, financial security, enjoyment of beauty, and, for many, religious or spiritual involvements.

Clearly, the contrast between medical and total good depends upon what is meant by "health." Conceptions of health differ, in both general outline and specific detail, and these differences reflect one's understanding of the appropriate scope of health care. At one extreme is the World Health Organization (WHO), which defines health as complete physical, mental, and social well-being. This definition would essentially collapse the distinction between one's medical and total good. At the other extreme is the concept of health as simply the absence of organic maladies. In between are many variations, such as Daniel Callahan's definition of health as "adequate physical well-being."[11]

We will not attempt a precise definition of health, leaving that as a discussion topic. We endorse, however, a holistic conception of health as biopsychosocial and as involving more than the mere absence of disease and injury. Nevertheless, health does not encompass the entirety of well-being, contrary to the WHO definition, for health does not include all aspects of such things as financial well-being or happiness in relationships.

Allan H. Macurdy's illness narrative will help clarify the distinction between medical and overall good as well as raise questions about how they are related.

Allan H. Macurdy

At age eight, Allan Macurdy was diagnosed with Duchenne's muscular dystrophy. His parents were told that the deterioration of his muscles would likely cause his death by age 15. His childhood remained relatively normal, punctuated by monthly visits to a physical therapist and an orthopedist. By adolescence, however, the normal challenges of becoming independent were compounded by frustration when Allan would fall down while climbing stairs and need help in order to regain his stability. For a while he was consumed with rage and bitterness, believing he had only a few years to live. Gradually these feelings subsided, and by the end of junior high school he was learning to cope with his disability. The early death sentence turned out to be mistaken. He completed college, earned a law degree, and became a practicing attorney.

Macurdy reports that one experience in particular became a parable for him about how health professionals often fail "to consider the person behind the symptoms."[12] Two days before he was scheduled to take the bar exam, he had extreme difficulty breathing and was diagnosed with pneumonia. Antibiotics and chest physical therapy proved insufficient to restore breathing. Given the complications caused by the muscular dystrophy, the doctor decided to place him in an iron lung. Already frightened, Macurdy became terrified and claustrophobic. The physicians who might have alleviated his fear failed to offer even minimal words of comfort. Instead they "trivialized and excluded" him with, at most, perfunctory remarks and "chattered on among themselves with great enthusiasm about arterial blood gas levels, titer volumes, and the comparative advantages of negative versus positive pressure ventilation."[12] Only one nurse intervened to talk with him and try to lower his anxiety, responding to him as a person rather than as merely an interesting medical problem. ◪

Macurdy's narrative reminds us that to provide health care for patients requires listening to them, engaging them as participants in a healing process, and respecting their autonomy in making decisions about the course of their therapy. It also reminds us that listening to patients can be integral to treating their medical conditions. Macurdy's terror when he was placed in the iron lung compounded his difficulty in breathing, and his convalescence depended in part on helping him manage his anxiety and strengthen his capacity to exercise self-determination. The narrative also introduces the distinction between a patient's medical good and total good. Good health tends to promote one's total good (in addition to being part of it), but it does not always do so. Unless one elevates health to a supreme value that overrides all other values—a morally dubious gambit—maintaining health must sometimes be weighed and balanced against other goods. Macurdy writes, "Health care is a means to a full and meaningful life; it is not an end in itself. But because the professionals deal only with the medical aspects of my life, they often lose sight of the impact of their recommendations on my career, home life, and relationships."[12(p14)]

In particular, his care providers continually urged him to exercise greater caution and take lower risks. For example, because he had a tracheostomy, Macurdy was especially susceptible to infections, and because his chest muscles had deteriorated, infections easily developed into pneumonia. But carried to its logical extreme, the attempt to eliminate all risk would lead to life in a bubble: "I would not be able to teach, represent clients, see friends, have an intimate life with my wife, play with my nephews and godchildren, or hug my dog. In other words, all those things that give my life value, purpose, and meaning would be sacrificed in order to protect me from infections that might kill me."[12(p15)]

Should the goal of health-care professionals, then, be to promote patients' total good or simply their medical good? Robert Veatch suggests that both goals are problematic in some respects: "If the goal is total well-being, no physician can be expected to be able to be skilled in all aspects of living well. But if the goal . . . is medical well-being, one has to recognize that no rational patient wants to maximize his or her medical well-being at least if it comes at the expense of other goods in life."[13] That is, on the one hand, health professionals are not trained to promote patients' overall good, for that good involves all major aspects of life, from finances and law to family and friendship. On the other hand, solely to maximize medical well-being would constitute a kind of fanaticism regarding only one aspect of life, however important that aspect is.

The resolution of the conundrum, as we see it, is that patients have the right and the responsibility to balance medical good against other goods in forming their autonomous views about what is reasonable for them. For their part, health professionals must respect the autonomy of patients. Thus, a physical therapist should encourage patients to sustain a rigorous regimen to restore maximum function of an injured limb, just as the physician should urge patients to stop smoking and exercise more. But therapists and doctors alike must accept the patient's right to weigh these medical goods against other important demands, such as earning a living. We cannot, however, expect patients to make the cognitive leap from selected treatments to functional outcomes. Care for our patients involves explaining the relationships between what we do and the patient's defined total good.

Professional Distance

Not all forms of caring are desirable within professional relationships; some forms are inimical to those relationships and undermine professional distance. **Professional distance** is the idea of not becoming inappropriately involved, emotionally or behaviorally, with patients and others involved in one's work. It does not mean emotional uninvolvement and indifference. Instead, it is what Aristotle called a mean between extremes: neither excessive or inappropriate involvement with patients (underdistancing) nor absence of caring engagement (overdistancing).[14,15] Professional distance is both a moral concept that refers to heeding professional responsibilities and a psychological concept that alludes to managing emotions and attitudes.

Oliver Sacks's surgeon illustrates overdistancing. The surgeon had difficulty relating to his patients as persons; perhaps he treated them as little more than interesting technical problems to challenge his medical skills. In any case, he didn't listen with sympathy. A more subtle example of overdistancing is the expression of pity, which should not be confused with compassion and sympathy. Compassion and sympathy are caring responses to other human beings as our moral equals. They are based on a sense of human solidarity, a sense that the patient is in an unfortunate situation that might befall us too, and a concern for the patient's well-being as a fellow human. In contrast, **pity** is a distorted form of caring that involves looking down on patients, often as a way of (over-) distancing ourselves from their plight.

Underdistancing can cause equally severe problems as professionals become emotionally enmeshed in their patients' suffering. Health professionals often deal with patients who suffer great pain, are disfigured, or are severely disabled. These problems are often compounded by personal crises involving finances, personal relationships, and psychological traumas. Caring professionals may be drawn too deeply into these problems in ways that can harm professionals and patients alike. Patients might be harmed by professionals' loss of objectivity in making therapeutic judgments, and professionals might inadvertently foster harmful forms of patient dependency rather than encouraging independence. In turn, professionals might be harmed by becoming so preoccupied with their patients that they take their work home with them in ways that undermine a healthy personal life. "Compassion fatigue" is a familiar consequence of excessive emotional involvement with patients.

As an example of just how subtle the loss of professional distance can be, consider the following case.

Karen Jarvis

Karen Jarvis is a 78-year-old woman who has spent the last two years in a nursing home.[16] During the past two months, following a stroke, she has received physical therapy for gait training with a walker and for acquiring more functional activities of daily living. Her physical therapist, Steve Clayton, knows that Mrs. Jarvis has reached a plateau stage in which continued physical therapy is unlikely to have any physical benefits, and he informs Mrs. Jarvis of his assessment. Mrs. Jarvis protests, insisting that she feels much improved after each therapy session and implores Steve to continue working with her. Steve is willing, indeed eager, to do so. He knows that Mrs. Jarvis has no family or other visitors, and that the therapy he offers undoubtedly has a positive impact on Mrs. Jarvis's overall health. He also looks forward to working with her, simply because he enjoys doing so. Medicare will continue paying the bills for physical improvements but not for mere psychological reassurance. At the same time, Steve believes he is working in the gray area in which a patient's positive attitude and sense of well-being can themselves bring physical improvements, or at least slow down physical deterioration. ◪

As this case suggests, the skills of physical therapists include more than applying medical knowledge. They include constructive personal responses to patients in establishing, modifying, and ending clinical encounters. Competence is central in providing services for patients, but such competence involves both knowing and caring. As the example also suggests, caring is a complex idea that can point in conflicting directions. Would the caring response be to focus on therapies directly linked to physical benefits, or is it permissible to consider the psychological benefits of therapeutic procedures?

Concerned that health-care professionals will lose objectivity, Howard J. Curzer argues that they "should be no more emotionally attached to their own patients than to someone else's patients or to the proverbial man on the street."[17] To foster a good bedside manner, they should learn to pretend to care for their patients without actually caring: they "should act *as if* they are significantly emotionally attached [to their patients], but in fact should involve their feelings relatively little. . . . They should hug patients who need to be hugged. But they should not really care."[17(p62)]

Curzer directs his arguments to physicians in hospitals, but they pertain to many additional health-care contexts. He argues that caring generates problems in at least six ways. We believe he identifies genuine dangers, but in each case we find his conclusions inconclusive.

First, Curzer argues that forming emotional attachments, unwanted by patients, invades patients' privacy.[17(p56)] In reply, we agree that respect for patients' autonomy includes respect for their desires not to have emotional expressions and demands forced on them. But that merely reminds us that some *expressions* of emotion are inappropriate, not that the emotions themselves are undesirable. Imposing emotional involvement against a patient's desires shows insensitivity and an absence of the virtue of caring.

Second, Curzer argues that caring threatens patient autonomy. On the one hand, he believes caring tends to make some people think they can control the lives of others in order to help them, thereby increasing the frequency of inappropriate paternalistic deception as well as making it hard for the professional to convey bad news about medical conditions. On the other hand, he says, caring can foster undesirable dependency of patients on the caregiver. In reply, we agree that the emotions of caring can be hurtful in the absence of respect for autonomy, including awareness that some forms of dependency undermine patient autonomy. But the virtue of caring is manifested in attitudes of respect for persons, including respect for their autonomy. Power, not caring, is the primary motive (usually a disguised one) that generates objectionable instances of paternalism. As a virtue, caring opposes that power impulse and respects patient autonomy.

Third, Curzer contends that health-care professionals "ought to be as impartial as possible toward patients" because emotional investment invites bias and favoritism, and even discrimination based on sex, race, age, or religion.[17(p58)] We agree that professionals should be impartial in the sense of not allowing their emotions to bias and distort medical treatment, and that bigoted attitudes should be rooted out. Impartiality, however, does not require emotional indifference. Teachers often like some students more than others, but professionalism requires setting these attitudes aside when grading. Similarly, professionalism in providing health care requires discipline but not total lack of emotion.

Fourth, since caring about patients leads one to seek the best treatment for them, Curzer claims this can cause inefficiency and injustice both through indifference to other patients and through driving up the cost of health care as one goes all out for unnecessary and perhaps even inappropriate services for one's patients, thereby skewing the distribution of limited health-care supplies within one's hospital. In reply, we agree that *excessive* emotional attachment to patients does distort good medicine. Any time professionals have reason to believe that their judgment is compromised, they should seek the medical opinions of other colleagues; in extreme cases, they should withdraw from a case. However, if one believed that emotional attachment generally destroyed the capacity for good judgment, then friends and family would never help each other.

Fifth, Curzer states that "emotional ties to patients tend to compromise the objectivity of professionals" in ways that threaten accurate diagnosis and treatment decisions.[17(p60)] In reply, we believe that insofar as caring leads to trying to get the best for one's patients, it is desirable. In rare instances in which caring for particular patients threatens another role one may have, perhaps as a hospital administrator, then one should be self-critical about conflicts of interest and take appropriate action to meet one's wider responsibility to the public.

Finally, according to Curzer, since it is difficult to leave emotions behind at the end of the workday, emotional involvements with patients carry into one's personal life in disruptive ways and use up limited emotional resources. Emotional investments are especially harmful in health-care careers because of the frustrations felt by clinicians when patients suffer, die, and foolishly ignore medical advice. Even the ideal of caring can generate guilt when one is unable to live up to it. In reply, we agree that caring health professionals are indeed at special risk for burnout, but burnout is not solely or primarily related to patient contact; it comes largely from organizational structures and managements that strip providers of a sense of control and purpose. It can also come from systematically stifling emotional responsiveness to patients who are the focus of one's professional life.

In the helping professions, a sense of meaning in one's work is sustained through at least some direct caring relationship with the people we help. As one nurse reports, "The people I've cared about, felt something for, become close to, the people I've invested a certain amount of myself in—these are the people I've learned something from. They are the reason I stay in nursing."[18] It is only in being whole, being genuine, that we can fully experience the intrinsic rewards of our profession, rather than spending most days just pretending to care. In addition, systematic emotional indifference to patients can easily become an emotional habit and carry over to relationships with other health professionals, with patients' family members, and even with one's own family.

In short, although Curzer identifies genuine dangers about how inappropriate caring can distort judgment, his arguments do not warrant abandoning ideals of caring in the health professions. Too much would be lost in doing so. In Chapter 8 we will extend this discussion of professional distance by focusing on one area of special concern: inappropriate sexual behavior, a topic that pertains to relationships among colleagues as well as professional-patient relationships.

 ## Family Violence

Understanding patients' family situations can be essential to caring for them as persons. In the next chapter we will discuss this theme in connection with multiculturalism and respect for diversity. Here, we explore it in connection with family violence.

Family violence takes many forms, including emotional abuse, but we will focus on physical violence. Moreover, although all members of families can be at risk of domestic violence, including adult males, we focus on the groups which are most vulnerable and hence most at risk: children, women, the elderly, and the disabled. Violence against members of these groups is all too common, and most physical therapists will encounter it. A therapist who sees a patient and family three or five times per week for one-half to one hour is usually the health-care professional most consistently involved with the family and hence uniquely placed to identify family violence. Indeed, a therapist can unwittingly become part of a dysfunctional family.

In a study by T. Clark, L. McKenna, and M. Jewell conducted in 1994 and published in 1996, 43 percent of physical therapists surveyed said they had treated a patient whom they knew or suspected had been physically abused by their spouse or partner, and 71 percent of these therapists said they had treated at least one battered patient during the previous year.[19] The number of battered women encountered by therapists might be even higher; only 5 percent of the therapists surveyed make routine inquiries about patients' relationships with their partners, 1 percent asked routinely about patients being battered, and 58 percent had never asked patients whether they were battered. Moreover, the study suggested that many physical therapists are not well informed about physical abuse. For example, fewer than half of the therapists were aware that the most common battery injuries occur in a central pattern around the head, neck, chest, and abdomen.

According to this study, therapists who did identify battered patients rarely informed the police. Indeed, only one therapist had done so, even though the study was conducted in California, which had, during the previous year (1993), passed a law requiring all health professionals working in health facilities to telephone the local law-enforcement agency when partner abuse is reasonably suspected. Over half the therapists provided battered women with information about shelters or counseling services. One in three notified a supervisor, and one in five contacted the patient's physician. Only 20 percent documented the injury by taking a photo or gathering other evidence, a step which is especially important when cases enter the legal system. Our further examination of these issues will begin with a case involving a child:

Trevor

Trevor, a three-year-old child with a diagnosis of cerebral palsy, presented himself as compliant and willing to follow requests, but for some reason he appeared to be very sad. He rarely spoke of happy events and was always worried about meeting expectations. His mother and father seemed devoted to the child. A speech therapist who was involved in the child's care suspected child abuse, but she had little evidence. She also feared that a less-than-convincing report to authorities would only result in the parents pulling him out of the center and keeping him at home, precluding outsiders from knowing what was going on. The physical therapist noticed some bruises that might be consistent with falls, which are common in patients who, like this child, wore bilateral long leg braces. When the physical therapist asked the mother about the child's facial bruises, she replied that he had fallen.

As time went on, the child became more comfortable with the therapist and in one session cried when he could not perform a requested exercise. The therapist reassured the child that they would do another activity instead, but the child kept weeping. When asked what was wrong, the child explained that his mother would "whip him when he did not do good." The pieces began to fit together and were confirmed the following week when the therapist saw the mother pull her son from the car by one hand with a force that nearly dislocated his arm.

What should the therapist have done? If the setting had been a hospital, a committee would have been available to take over the case once abuse was reported. In this case the therapist worked in a small private clinic where no such committee existed. The therapist doubted whether there was sufficient evidence to make a convincing case to the police, and he knew the parents could easily explain the bruises as resulting from the child's coordination and balance problems. The therapist also feared that the child would be severely beaten when he returned home and would not be brought to therapy again, anywhere. Even asking too many questions of the parents might simply alert them and lead them to cancel appointments. The health-care team decided to suggest to the mother that she join a "mothers' group" so that she might get some support and perhaps some better parenting skills. The speech therapist, however, became concerned about both the clinic's and her own legal liability and reported the family to the authorities. Within 12 hours the child was removed from the home by the sheriff at the direction of Child Protection Services. The clinicians never heard from the family again.

Tammy and Frank

Next consider Tammy, a 43-year-old female who was referred to physical therapy for an evaluation of vestibular, balance, and equilibrium functions, as well as for gait training with crutches. When her therapist, Frank, reviewed the emergency room chart, he noticed that the referring physician had cast her broken femur and treated her for lacerations and multiple bruises. The physician reported that Tammy had said her injuries were caused by a fall down a flight of steps in the home she shared with her husband and four-month-old daughter. Everything seemed routine to Frank except the requested evaluations. Upon further examination of the chart he realized that Tammy had been admitted on several other occasions for various injuries resulting from accidents. The occasion prior to this event was only six months earlier, while she was pregnant with her daughter. In that accident, which she attributed to slipping on a spill on the kitchen floor, she sustained a concussion along with multiple bruises, many of which were documented to be on the dorsal surface of her hands and arms.

When Frank met Tammy, she pointed to her bruised face and laughed about how clumsy she was. She was charming and tried with diligence to learn crutch walking. Frank suggested she go home and try out her new skills and return in three days to start the testing. At that time they could remedy any problems she was having with the crutches.

At Tammy's next appointment she had some problems with the crutches, but they were minor and quickly solved, allowing Frank to start the testing. Her balance reflexes, equilibrium, and vestibular functions were normal in every way that could be tested at that time. In reporting the results to her, he casually stated that he did not understand how someone could have so many accidents and have such good reflexes. Tammy confided that she had not fallen; her husband had lost his temper and hit her. She quickly attempted to clarify her response by saying that it was her fault because she knew what things set him off and yet she still had done something stupid that deserved to be punished. Frank asked her what had caused this last episode. She replied that she had overcooked the meat for dinner and knew how much her husband hated a ruined meal after he had worked hard all day. Tammy looked Frank straight in the face and said, "This is between you and me; if you ever tell anyone, I will deny it."

Frank wondered what he should do with this information. He could pretend Tammy never said anything to him. He could record the conversation and her history of suspicious injuries in her medical record, then report the abuse to the authorities, who would launch an investigation and subpoena the records. He could go to the physician and discuss the conversation and the history. He could schedule her for one more visit and try to convince her to seek help, although he sensed she would not listen.

At first Frank decided to do nothing, but he grew concerned that if she were seriously injured or killed the next time, he would be partly responsible for failing to provide the kind of preventive care she needed. He reasoned that since all the care was delivered through the emergency room, a conversation with the doctor would be futile, since neither of them was likely to see her again if another attack occurred. He would most certainly have gone to a committee designated specifically for investigating and reporting all types of abuse if he had worked at Forsythe Memorial, where such a team existed. But at his current place of employment, no such committee had been established.

After lengthy agonizing, he reported his suspicions and the conversation to the authorities. Tammy denied ever having had the conversation with Frank. She called him at the office to plead with him to tell the police that he had made a terrible mistake. When Frank refused, Tammy told him how hurt she was that he had breached the confidentiality she expected. Besides, her husband was now so angry that she was afraid that he would kill her.

Frank began to wonder if he had indeed had made a mistake. As it turned out, the investigation discovered neighbors who had seen physical abuse, and, even without Tammy's cooperation, the prosecutor tried the case and the jury found her husband guilty of assault and battery. After his release and their reunion, there were multiple violent events that increased in frequency and intensity. After several trial separations, Tammy finally went to a shelter and, with the help of authorities there, filed for divorce. On the last violent occasion, her husband had beat not only her but also their child. ❖

This case raises several general ethical conflicts for therapists. Exactly when does concern for patients' safety, as well as respect for reporting laws, override respect for patient autonomy and confidentiality? Why does the law intervene even when the victim might lie to protect the attacker and frequently reunites with the abuser? Ethically, we are justified in intervening because the victim is psychologically dependent on the aggressor and cannot act autonomously. When and how to proceed can be a difficult matter—one calling for good moral judgment and sometimes good luck.

Domestic violence is a complex and not yet fully explained pattern of behaviors used to oppress and exploit, and all too often results in death.[20,21] Generally, the victim progressively loses self-governance through a series of stereotypic behaviors by the aggressor that reduce the victim's self-esteem. Typically the family unit is isolated, with few if any social connections, thereby enabling the aggressor to go undetected by outsiders, the isolation limiting the resources available to help the victim. In an effort to save the relationship, the victim may temporarily leave the relationship an average of four to five times before actually dissolving the relationship.[22] Fears of retaliation are well founded: women are more at risk of being killed by a male partner than by anyone in or out of the family.[21(p115)] To compound matters, domestic violence does not begin and end with a single family unit. Scholars refer to the "social heredity of family violence" to remind us that these patterns of behavior are passed from parents to children.[20(p281)] To help break this intergenerational cycle, some cities, such as Los Angeles, provide a witness protection program for women who will testify against their abusers, so that they can be secretly relocated and given a new identity that will make it impossible for their abusers to find them.

Reporting Child Abuse

Abuse of children and the elderly is now a matter extensively circumscribed by law. In addition, public interest groups have developed more explicit definitions of these abuses. We discuss these matters in this and the next section. We also comment on the responsibilities of supervisors within organizations related to reporting incidences of abuse. Although reporting child abuse is the direct responsibility of the person who witnesses the actual signs and symptoms, the supervising therapist is often consulted because the symptoms and the laws are themselves frequently ambiguous. State and federal laws are generally very clear that supervisors may not inhibit or obstruct the reporting of abuse by the therapists they supervise. There are further positive roles for supervisors beyond advising and facilitating reports of abuse.

S. Kalichman identifies four clusters of factors that influence whether a professional reports abuse: situational, professional, legal, and organizational.[23] Situational factors, such as type and severity of abuse, and professional factors, such as number of years of professional experience, influence the treating therapist's decision to report. Legal factors, most notably knowledge of the law and the wording in the law, also influence the decision. Awareness of legal factors can certainly be enhanced if the supervisor posts the laws in the therapy office and discusses them at staff meetings or in-service training sessions led by speakers from the local protective agency. Finally, organizational factors are especially important in influencing reporting. These factors include the institution's own reporting policies, the degree of readily available support for reporting, and the organization's ethics policies and guidelines as well as its professional guidelines. It is the responsibility of the supervisor to determine that all of these guidelines are readily available to the staff.

Child abuse is so prevalent that it is unlikely that any center treating children will not at some point be faced with contacting child protective services. Based on 1998 state statistics from the National Child Abuse and Neglect Reporting System (NCANRS), there were an estimated 2,806,000 referrals, of which 66 percent were transferred for investigation and 34 percent were screened out. Over half (53.1 percent) were referrals from professionals.[24]

Federal legislation sets forth minimum standards for identifying child abuse and neglect and for sexual abuse through the Child Abuse Prevention and Treatment Act (CAPTA), as amended and renewed in October 1996.[25] Each state then enhances these definitions as it deems worthy, thus creating variations in regulations among the states. CAPTA stipulates that a child, in the case of abuse and neglect, is any youth under the age of 18, but in cases of suspected sexual abuse, the states must specify the age for their state. At a minimum, according to CAPTA, child abuse and neglect is "any recent act or failure to act on the part of a parent or caretaker which results in death, serious physical or emotional harm, sexual abuse or exploitation." Construed more broadly, it is "an act or failure to act which presents an imminent risk of serious harm."[26]

The National Clearinghouse on Child Abuse and Neglect Information, along with the American Prosecutors Research Institute, has summarized nearly 40 state statutes, both civil and criminal, resulting in the following descriptions:[26]

> **Physical abuse** is characterized by the infliction of physical injury as a result of punching, beating, kicking, biting, burning, shaking, or otherwise harming a child. The parent or caretaker may not have intended to hurt the child; rather the injury may have resulted from overdiscipline or physical punishment.
>
> **Child neglect** is characterized by failure to provide for the child's basic needs. Neglect can be physical, educational, or emotional.
>
> **Physical neglect** includes refusal of or delay in seeking health care, abandonment, expulsion from the home or refusal to allow a runaway to return home, and inadequate supervision.
>
> **Educational neglect** includes the allowance of chronic truancy, failing to enroll a child of mandatory school age in school, and failing to attend to a special educational need.
>
> **Emotional neglect** includes such actions as marked inattention to the child's needs for affection, refusal of or failure to provide needed psychological care, spouse abuse in the child's presence, and permission of drug or alcohol use by the child. The assessment of child neglect requires the consideration of cultural values and standards of care as well as recognition that the failure to provide the necessities of life may be related to poverty.

Sexual abuse includes fondling a child's genitals, intercourse, incest, rape, sodomy, exhibitionism, and commercial exploitation through prostitution or the production of pornographic materials. Many experts believe that sexual abuse is the most underreported of child maltreatments because of the secrecy or "conspiracy of silence" that so often characterizes these cases.

Emotional abuse (psychological/verbal abuse, mental injury) includes acts or omissions by the parents or other caregivers that have caused, or could cause, serious behavioral, cognitive, emotional, or mental disorders. In some cases of emotional abuse, the acts of parents or other caregivers alone, without any harm evident in the child's behavior or condition, are sufficient to warrant child protective services (CPS) intervention. For example, the parents/caregivers may use extreme or bizarre forms of punishment, such as confinement of a child in a dark closet. Less severe acts, such as habitual scapegoating, belittling, or rejecting treatment, are often difficult to prove and, therefore, CPS may not be able to intervene without evidence of harm to the child.

This brief summary cannot pinpoint all instances that may be relevant to therapists. For example, laws governing citizens in the state of Texas include in their definition of child abuse any child born addicted to alcohol or illegally acquired controlled substances.[27] The laws describe signs and symptoms of abuse as well as the presence of any of the substances in the child's bodily fluids. In several states, the laws provide permission for parents to reject nonemergency and non–life-threatening health care if such care is against their religious beliefs.

State definitions must be consulted and shared with every therapist, not only those treating children. This is because any therapist may come in contact with the children of patients they treat, or their patients might confess elements of abuse to therapists in the context of the professional relationship.

All states specify the persons who are mandated by law to report abuse. Some states, such as Alaska, Connecticut, and Wisconsin, specifically name physical therapists. Other states use broad categories such as "licensed professionals" or "practitioners of the healing arts." In most cases, all professionals who work with children are mandated to report.[28] Eighteen states make any citizen a mandatory reporter.[29] Failure to do so results in variable consequences, according to different state sanctions. In 45 states and the District of Columbia, penalties in the form of fines or imprisonment or both exist when someone fails to report what was known or should have been known.[29] In Mississippi the penalty is a fine of up to $5,000 and jail time of up to one year, or both, and in Montana the nonreporter is liable for civil damages and is guilty of a misdemeanor.[29] All states include a statement regarding issues of confidentiality, and no health-care professional is allowed to honor their perceived confidential patient relationship in child abuse cases. Some states, such as Wyoming, allow no confidential relationships whatsoever to inhibit or prevent the reporting of child abuse, but most states provide sweeping protection of confidential relationships between attorneys and clients, and between clergy and penitents.[29] In exchange, CAPTA mandates that if states are to receive federal grants, they must provide immunity to those who report abuse from prosecution under any state law (civil or criminal) and local regulations for making a good faith report. Of course, if a false report is made knowingly for malicious reasons, then that immunity does not apply.

The standard for reporting child abuse is reasonable suspicion, not certainty. Since all states allow anyone to report child abuse, the system is geared to screen out cases that are not likely child abuse and to investigate the balance to determine if child abuse has taken place. California's definition of reasonable suspicion is: "It is objectively reasonable for a person to entertain a suspicion, based upon facts that could cause a reasonable person in a like position, drawing when appropriate, on his or her training and experience, to suspect child abuse."[30] Kalichman states that "professionals who have reached a level of reasonable suspicion but not reported because they have not backed up their suspicion with evidence are in noncompliance with reporting laws. Thus, gathering evidence of abuse is not among the expected roles of mental health professionals. . . . Because most practitioners have not acquired adequate skills to investigate the occurrence of abuse, they may be overstepping their boundaries by doing so."[23(p55)] Institutions, however, often have procedures designed to facilitate protective services' investigation, such as taking photographs of injuries, being certain to have the face of the child in the picture, or even taking x-rays and providing temporary care for the child. Various states explicitly give permission for these types of policies without the consent of the parents.

Since there are no validated assessment tools to detect abuse, therapists must rely on their professional judgment. In the case of suspected physical abuse, there may be symptoms which promote a low level of suspicion, such as emotional distress. Suspicions may be greater if the therapist encounters a patient with unexplained bruises, welts, imprints of ropes, and burn impressions of irons.[23(p67)] In cases of suspected sexual abuse, the continuum may run from emotional distress (low suspicion) to verbal disclosure (high suspicion). Somewhere between the extremes the therapist has to determine a reasonable level of suspicion.

When it is determined that a suspicion is reasonable, state laws are in general agreement that an oral report must be made, immediately followed by a written report. The time frames for the written report have great variability among states. Colorado requires the written report to be filed within 48 hours, California requires it within 36 hours, and Arizona requires it within 72 hours. In each state the child protective agency will instruct the caller on the content of the written report.

For the oral report, most states require the name of the child, the child's current location, the parent's or caretaker's address and telephone number, the child's age, and the extent of the injuries. The person reporting must then request instructions on whether to tell the caretaker, whether to retain the child to await the child protective agency, or whether to pursue other options depending on state law. Although the report is usually made to the child protective agency in the state, it may also be made to the local police, depending on state requirements. In either event, child agencies typically report the incident to all other relevant agencies and departments. Some states, such as Maine, allow one report from a team, such as a multidisciplinary team, instead of separate reports from all who have a reasonable suspicion.[31] In those cases, however, personal liability for the therapist who has a reasonable suspicion is not excused if the team fails to file a report.

Reporting Elder Abuse

The results of the National Elder Abuse Incidence Study, requested by Congress and prepared for the federal Administration on Aging and the Administration for Children and Families, were released in 1998. The study used a stratified, multistage sample drawn from 20 counties in the nation that were believed to be representative of the country.[32] Researchers found that, if self-neglect was not considered, an estimated 449,924 elders over the age of 60 had been subjected to abuse or neglect. However, only 236,322 cases were reported to adult protective services, and of those, only 48.7 percent were substantiated. The balance either did not reach their state's level of proof or were still under investigation at the end of the study.

Among those cases that were substantiated, 75 percent of elders who were abused were physically frail, most were women, and most were clustered in the yearly income range of $5,000–$9,999. Cultural patterns also emerged, with extremely low percentages among all minorities except African-Americans. Whites generally committed between 79 percent and 86 percent of offenses in the categories of abuse and 41.3 percent of cases of abandonment. For African-Americans, figures ranged from 9 percent to 17 percent for the categories of abuse, with a 57.3 percent rate of abandonment. Of all abusers, nearly two-thirds were either a spouse or an adult child. T. Hickey and R. Douglass stated that 62 percent of professionals who deal with the elderly had seen indications of physical abuse.[33] In nursing homes, researchers found that within the last year of the study, 36 percent of workers had seen at least one act of physical abuse and 81 percent had seen psychological abuse. Among the workers themselves, 10 percent admitted that they had committed physical abuse, and 40 percent admitted to committing psychological abuse.[34]

Compared to child abuse, however, elder abuse receives significantly less attention. In a review of the literature in *Index Medicus*, only 26 articles on elder abuse appeared in a five-year time frame, compared with 248 on child abuse. Only 4 of the 26 had primary data.[35]

Unlike that for child abuse, no overarching federal act or regulation with a minimum standard makes federal money contingent on state compliance and funds services and shelters for elders. In 1975 the Older Americans Act created an ombudsperson program in all states to investigate and resolve nursing-home complaints.[36] There are also adult protective services (APS) in most states to investigate reported cases, and some provide the victims and families with protective services or treatment. Even where there are few, if any, laws specifically targeted for elder abuse, local and state laws exist to cover theft, assault, and other common forms of elder abuse. Amendments to the Older Americans Act passed in 1987 did provide relevant definitions to help states identify the problems, but they were not for enforcement purposes. As a consequence, states vary greatly in how they define elder abuse. In general, elder abuse is most often described as follows:[38]

> **Domestic elder abuse** generally refers to any of several forms of maltreatment of an older person by someone who has a special relationship with the elder (e.g., a spouse, a sibling, a child, a friend, or a caregiver in the older person's own home or in the home of the caregiver).
>
> **Institutional abuse**, on the other hand, generally refers to any abuse that occurs in residential facilities for older persons (e.g., nursing homes, foster homes, group homes, board and care facilities). Perpetrators of institutional abuse usually are persons who have a legal or contractual obligation to provide elder victims with care and protection (e.g., paid caregivers, staff, professionals).
>
> **Physical abuse** is defined as the use of physical force that may result in bodily injury, physical pain, or impairment. Physical abuse may include but is not

limited to such acts of violence as striking (with or without an object), hitting, beating, pushing, shoving, shaking, slapping, kicking, pinching, and burning. In addition, the inappropriate use of drugs and physical restraints, force-feeding, and physical punishment of any kind are also examples of physical abuse.

Sexual abuse is defined as nonconsensual sexual contact of any kind with an elderly person. Sexual contact with any person incapable of giving consent is also considered sexual abuse. It includes but is not limited to unwanted touching, all types of sexual assault or battery, such as rape, sodomy; coerced nudity, and sexually explicit photographing.

Emotional or psychological abuse is defined as the infliction of anguish, pain, or distress through verbal or nonverbal acts. Emotional/psychological abuse includes but is not limited to verbal assaults, insults, threats, intimidation, humiliation, and harassment. In addition, treating an older person like an infant; isolating an elderly person from his/her family, friends, or regular activities; giving an older person the "silent treatment"; and enforced social isolation are examples of emotional/psychological abuse.

Neglect is defined as the refusal or failure to fulfill any part of a person's obligations or duties to an elder. Neglect may also include failure of a person who has a fiduciary responsibility to provide care for an elder (e.g., pay for necessary home-care services) or the failure on the part of an in-home service provider to provide necessary care. Neglect typically means the refusal or failure to provide an elderly person with such life necessities as food, water, clothing, shelter, personal hygiene, medicine, comfort, personal safety, and other essentials included in an implied or agreed-upon responsibility to an elder.

Abandonment is defined as the desertion of an elderly person by an individual who has assumed responsibility for providing care for an elder, or by a person with physical custody of an elder.

Financial or material exploitation is defined as the illegal or improper use of an elder's funds, property, or assets. Examples include cashing an elderly person's checks without authorization/permission; forging an older person's signature; misusing or stealing an older person's money or possessions; coercing or deceiving an older person into signing any document (e.g., contracts or will); and the improper use of conservatorship, guardianship, or power of attorney.

Self-neglect is characterized as the behavior of an elderly person that threatens his/her own health or safety. Self-neglect generally manifests itself in an older person as a refusal or failure to provide himself/herself with adequate food, water, clothing, shelter, personal hygiene, medications (when indicated), and safety precautions. The definition of self-neglect excludes a situation in which a mentally competent older person who understands the consequences of his/her decision makes a conscious and voluntary decision to engage in acts that threaten his/her health or safety as a matter of personal choice.

Since many of the states that do have elder abuse laws have modeled them after the child abuse laws, there are often mandatory reporting requirements that in general include all health-care workers, with the same protections for reporting that exist under child abuse laws. In many ways, however, detecting elder abuse is even more difficult than detecting child abuse. Unlike children, who, after the age of five, must attend school and are inherently more social, many elderly live alone and might rarely venture into settings where abuse might be detected. Elders might even protect their abusers for fear that any alternative would be worse than their current status. In some states, if victims say they do not want corrective action, the state will abide by that decision as long as they are competent. However, in those states with mandatory reporting requirements that honor the elder's request, health-care providers are not relieved of their responsibility to file a report.[38]

At first glance, the threshold for reporting seems lower for adults than for children. That would certainly be true if the adult were competent and physically able to summon help. Yet many adult victims are as helpless as a child in protecting themselves, especially when they have low incomes, are physically fragile, have cognitive impairments, and experience depression—if only from knowing they are being mistreated by children or a spouse whom they helped and supported when they themselves were healthy.[35] Moreover, retaliatory battering is a genuine danger because adult protective services are so underfunded that they often are not able to provide the resources necessary to rescue elders without institutionalization. In fact, 30 percent of batterers inflict further assaults during prosecution.[39]

To conclude, in this chapter we began to explore caring for patients with an eye toward their wider good rather than toward only a narrowly defined medical good. Knowing when to take that wider good into account, and when it is inappropriate to do so, is an important dimension of professionalism, as the discussions of suffering and various forms of abuse made clear. In the next chapter we amplify this approach as it pertains to multicultural awareness. We also move into broader social issues about family, race, gender, and other aspects of personal identity and cultural diversity.

Discussion Questions

1. According to the World Health Organization (WHO), "Health is a state of complete physical, mental and social well-being and not merely the absence of disease or infirmity."[40] In effect, this definition equates patients' medical good (health, in the ordinary sense) with their total good. Do you find this definition inviting, given its "holistic" approach to health, or do you agree with critics that the WHO definition distorts our understanding of health and threatens to give health professionals too much authority in areas of life in which their training gives them no expertise?[41]

2. In the managed-care environment, productivity is measured in billable hours or other such methods that relate the time spent by the physical therapist to earned salary. This in turn limits the time we have with patients. Given these time pressures, (a) what are methods you have seen in the clinic by which physical therapists maximize their time with patients and continue to provide the kind of care discussed in this chapter, and (b) what other models of reimbursement can you envision that maximize the outcomes physical therapists achieve while being fiscally responsible? (Revisit this question in Chapter 9.)

3. Discuss the cases of Trevor and Tammy. What was the best way for the physical therapists involved to have dealt with their suspicions of abuse?

4. In your clinical affiliations, has anyone ever mentioned to you how you should respond in that environment to suspected abuse, including child abuse, elder abuse, or battered woman syndrome? If so, what was said? What do the laws in your state require (check with your local APTA chapter or review the state's practice act)?

5. Identify what you see as the primary dangers leading to burnout among health-care professionals. Are they due primarily to routine caring for patients, to inappropriate ways of caring, to control issues, to organizational management of providers, or to other factors? What countermeasures can professionals take to avoid burnout and to deal with it when it occurs? You might consult the interesting literature on burnout among professionals.[42–45]

6. Susan is a home health physical therapist who has been assigned a new patient, Mrs. Nicholas, who is a 72-year-old married woman recovering from two fractures of the bilateral upper extremities. Her husband of 41 years is in the home and, to Susan, seems cognitively to be in the very early stages of Alzheimer's disease. Because of Mrs. Nicholas's frail condition, Susan asks her about her nutrition. Mr. Nicholas answers for his wife and says that the problem is that she refuses to eat. Mrs. Nicholas purses her lips but refuses to answer the question when it is redirected by Susan. In taking the history, Susan asks Mrs. Nicholas how she sustained two broken arms. Mr. Nicholas replies that she tripped over the cat and fell in the bathroom. Susan asked Mr. Nicholas to leave the room so that she could work with Mrs. Nicholas, but he refuses, saying there is nothing that should be kept secret from him about his wife. Mrs. Nicholas does not respond. Susan believes that Mrs. Nicholas is being abused by her husband, but she is uncertain of how to respond. How would you advise Susan if you were her supervisor?

References

1. Cassell EJ. *The Healer's Art*. Cambridge, MA: MIT Press; 1986[1976]:47-83.
2. Gert B, Culver CM, Clouser KD. *Bioethics: A Return to Fundamentals*. New York, NY: Oxford University Press; 1997.
3. Cassell EJ. *The Nature of Suffering and the Goals of Medicine*. New York, NY: Oxford University Press; 1991:33.
4. Kleinman A. *The Illness Narratives: Suffering, Healing and the Human Condition*. New York, NY: Basic Books; 1988.
5. Frank AW. *The Wounded Storyteller: Body, Illness, and Ethics*. Chicago, IL: University of Chicago Press; 1995.
6. Nelson HL, ed. *Stories and Their Limits: Narrative Approaches to Bioethics*. New York, NY: Routledge; 1997.
7. Morris DB. *Illness and Culture in the Postmodern Age*. Berkeley, CA: University of California Press; 1998.
8. Sacks O. *A Leg to Stand On*. New York, NY: Harper & Row; 1984:105.
9. Spiro HM. What is empathy and can it be taught? In: Spiro HM, Curnen MGM, Peschel E, St. James D, eds. *Empathy and the Practice of Medicine*. New Haven, CT: Yale University Press; 1993:8.
10. Martin MW. *Meaningful Work: Rethinking Professional Ethics*. New York, NY: Oxford University Press; 2000:73. Cf. Koehn D. *The Ground of Professional Ethics*. New York, NY: Routledge; 1994.
11. Callahan D. The WHO definition of "health." *The Hastings Center Stud.* 1973;1(3).
12. Macurdy AH. Mastery of life. In: Young-Mason J., ed. *The Patient's Voice: Experiences of Illness*. Philadelphia, PA: F.A. Davis Company; 1997:11.

13. Veatch RM. *The Basics of Bioethics*. Upper Saddle River, NJ: Prentice Hall; 2000:41.
14. Martin MW. Professional distance. In: Martin MW. *Meaningful Work: Rethinking Professional Ethics*. New York, NY: Oxford University Press; 2000:82-100.
15. Purtilo R, Haddad A. *Health Professional and Patient Interaction*. 5th ed. Philadelphia, PA: W. B. Saunders Company; 1996:230-249.
16. The case is inspired by Purtilo R, Haddad A. *Health Professional and Patient Interaction*. 5th ed. Philadelphia, PA: W. B. Saunders Company; 1996:209.
17. Curzer HJ. Is care a virtue for health care professionals? *J Med Phil*. 1993;18:62. Some of the following discussion of Curzer is taken from Martin MW. *Meaningful Work: Rethinking Professional Ethics*. New York, NY: Oxford University Press; 2000:89-90. (Copyright held by Mike W. Martin.)
18. Anderson P. *Nurse*. New York, NY: Berkley Publishing; 1979:39.
19. Clark TJ, McKenna LS, Jewell MJ. Physical therapists' recognition of battered women in clinical settings. *Phys Ther*. 1996;76(1):12-18.
20. Dutton DG. *The Domestic Assault of Women: Psychological and Criminal Justice Perspectives*. 2d ed. Vancouver, Canada: UBC Press; 1995.
21. Hampton RL, Gullotta TP, Adams GR, Potter EH, Weissberg RP, eds. *Family Violence: Prevention and Treatment*. Newbury Park, CA: SAGE Publications; 1993.
22. Okun L. *Woman Abuse: Facts Replacing Myths*. Albany, NY: State University of New York Press; 1986:198.
23. Kalichman SC. *Mandated Reporting of Suspected Child Abuse: Ethics, Law and Policy*. Washington, DC: American Psychological Association; 1993:62.
24. U.S. Department of Health and Human Services. Health and Human Services Reports: New Child Abuse and Neglect Statistics. Available at: http://www.hhs.gov/news/press/2000pres/20000410.html. Accessed October 17, 2000.
25. Public Law 104-235, Section 111 U.S.C., 5105g.
26. National Clearinghouse on Child Abuse and Neglect Information. Reporting Procedures. Available at: http://www.calif.com/nccanch. Accessed October 2, 2000.
27. National Clearinghouse on Child Abuse and Neglect Information. Definitions of Child Abuse and Neglect. Available at: http://www.calif.com/nccanch. Accessed October 2, 2000.
28. Sagatun IJ, Edwards LP. *Child Abuse and the Legal System*. Chicago, IL: Nelson-Hall; 1995.
29. U.S. Department of Health and Human Services; National Clearinghouse on Child Abuse and Neglect Information. Child Abuse and Neglect: State Statutes and Elements. Available at: http://www.calif.com/nccanch. Accessed October 12, 2000.
30. Cal. Penal Code: 11166(a)–(c), (e)–(I) (West Supp. 1998).
31. U.S. Department of Health and Human Services; National Clearinghouse on Child Abuse and Neglect Information. What is Child Maltreatment? Available at: http://www.calif.com/nccanch. Accessed November 21, 2000.
32. Administration on Aging of the Department of Health and Human Services. National Elder Abuse Incidence Study. Available at: http://www.aoa.gov/abuse/report/html. Accessed on October 10, 2000.
33. Hickey T, Douglass R. In: Kapp M, ed. *Geriatrics and the Law*. New York, NY: Springer; 1992.
34. Pillemer K, Moore DW. Abuse of patients in nursing homes: findings from a survey of staff. *Gerontologist*. 1989;29(3):314-320.
35. Lachs MS, Pillemer K. Abuse and neglect of elderly persons. *N Engl J Med*. 1995;332(7):437-443.
36. National Center on Elder Abuse. Elder Abuse Laws. Available at: http://www.elderabusecenter.org/. Accessed October 20, 2000.
37. National Center on Elder Abuse. The Basics. Available at: http://www.elderabusecenter.org/. Accessed October 20, 2000.
38. Swisher LL, Krueger-Brophy C. *Legal and Ethical Issues in Physical Therapy*. Boston, MA: Butterworth-Heinemann; 1998:125.

39. Hyman A, Schillinger D, Lo B. Laws mandating reporting of domestic violence. *JAMA.* 1995;273(22):1781-1787.
40. World Health Organization, Preamble to the Constitution of the World Health Organization, *Official Record of the World Health Organization* 2, 100, 1946.
41. Callahan D. The WHO definition of "health." *The Hastings Center Stud.* 1973;1(3).
42. Pines AM, Aronson E, Kafry D. *Burnout.* New York, NY: Free Press; 1981.
43. Glogow E. Research note: burnout and locus of control. *Public Pers Manage.* 1986;15(1):79.
44. Maslach C. *Burnout: The Cost of Caring.* Englewood Cliffs, NJ: Prentice-Hall; 1982.
45. Schaufel WB, Maslach C, Marek T. *Professional Burnout: Recent Developments in Theory and Research.* Washington, DC: Taylor and Francis; 1993.

Respect for Persons and Diversity

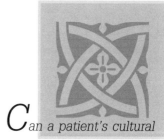

*C*an a patient's cultural beliefs supersede a therapist's duties of full disclosure and confidentiality?

Keywords

Cultural competence
Prejudice
Ethnocentrism
Racism
Sexism

Moral sensitivity
Affirmative action
Weak preferential treatment
Strong preferential treatment

Multicultural sensitivity and respect for diversity are expected of all professionals. In particular, health professionals should develop an awareness of cultural differences so they can assist all patients in improving their health and coping with chronic illnesses. In physical therapy this is partially implemented through *A Normative Model of Physical Therapist Professional Education* (version 97), which is the primary curricular content reference document for all physical therapy educational programs accredited by the Commission on Accreditation in Physical Therapy Education. Under "Professional Practice Expectations," the document specifies in detail the educational outcomes necessary for therapists to "be sensitive to individual and cultural differences when engaged in physical therapy practice, research, and education."

"Culture" is used here in a wide sense to refer to the characteristic beliefs, values, language, history, and shared challenges of groups of people. Culture is found in the groups with which individuals identify, including affiliations by ethnicity, nationality, religion, and sexual orientation. The American Physical Therapy Association, through its *House of Delegate Standards, Policies, Positions, and Guidelines*, unequivocally stated its position in HOD 06-98-14-06 (Program 04): "The American Physical Therapy Association (APTA) prohibits preferential or adverse discrimination on the basis of race, creed, color, sex, gender, age, national or ethnic origin, sexual orientation, disability or health status in all areas." In this chapter we discuss a cluster of themes concerning culture: respect for cultural differences, the nature of prejudice, sexism and feminism, the controversy over affirmative action, and respect for persons with disabilities. These topics pertain to respect for colleagues as well as to caring for patients, and so in this chapter we will integrate both of these dimensions of appreciating diversity.

 ## Multicultural Awareness

Patients' experience of illness, as well as their response to health-care professionals, depends in part on their cultural background. This is an increasingly important factor today as we move toward a more pluralistic view of our society. In the past it was expected that patients, and others, would assimilate into the dominant culture, learning its language and adopting its customs. Increasingly, however, the need for assimilation is being balanced with a pluralistic approach, in which members of minority cultures also preserve the basic elements of their ethnic identities. Pluralism is now valued for the diversity and enrichment it brings to a population, both socially and economically. In addition to these desirable consequences, pluralism is valued as part of respect for autonomy, moral rights, and human uniqueness. Equally important is a presumption that different cultures possess worth. As Charles Taylor writes, "It is reasonable to suppose that cultures that have provided the horizon of meaning for large numbers of human beings, of diverse characters and temperaments, over a long period of time—that have, in other words, articulated their sense of the good, the holy, the admirable—are almost certain to have something that deserves our admiration and respect, even if it is accompanied by much that we have to abhor and reject."[1]

Appreciating diversity means more than tolerance in the minimal sense of not interfering with the liberty of others. It also involves developing a "**cultural competence**" and willingness to interact in desirable ways with members of other cultures. As defined by Thorpe and Baker:

> Cultural competence is the ability to think and behave in ways that enable a member of one culture to work effectively with members of another culture. The components of cultural competence are: (1) awareness of one's own cultural limitations; (2) openness, appreciation, and respect for cultural differences; (3) a view of intercultural interactions as learning opportunities; (4) the ability to use cultural resources in interventions; and (5) an acknowledgment of the integrity and value of all cultures.[2]

The following case examples of cultural competence in health care, adapted from Geri-Ann Galanti's *Caring for Patients from Different Cultures*,[3] may risk encouraging stereotypes (prejudicial images) about groups, but we present them as rough generalizations that have numerous exceptions. As Galanti suggests, a stereotype functions as an end point in fixing how members of groups are viewed, whereas a generalization is a beginning point that indicates general trends that can be open to revision or wholesale dismissal in approaching individuals.[3(pp2-3)] Generalizations can be misleading, but they can also help guide us through a complex multicultural world.

Language

Mary Washington

Mary Washington, an elderly African-American woman, tenses slightly but noticeably, and stops making eye contact with a young white male therapist who had called her Mary when they first met. In her view, the therapist's failure to address her as Mrs. Washington demonstrated a lack of respect.

Would she have been offended if the therapist had been a black man? Perhaps, but perhaps not, thereby reminding us that even the most ordinary uses of language can carry unintended meanings as context varies. Moreover, many elderly white women might have responded exactly as Mrs. Washington did. Since health professionals cannot be expected to divine how new patients will respond to use of their first names, it might be best to assume that Mr., Miss, Mrs., or Ms. is more appropriate until a context of informality is established. It is also a safe assumption that members of minority groups that have suffered discrimination might have reasonable doubt that they will be fully respected within non-minority-dominated hospitals and other medical facilities.

Pain

Mr. Valdez and Mr. Wu

Mr. Valdez, a patient from Nicaragua, and Mr. Wu, a Chinese patient, are middle-aged men recovering from similar injuries and in need of the same physical therapy interventions. Mr. Valdez, however, complains far more about the pain he is experiencing, and prefers low-level exercises and more medication from the nursing staff than does Mr. Wu. The therapist assumes Mr. Valdez is a whiner, and this assumption influences his treatment of the patient.

In fact, cultural differences largely explain the patients' differing responses to pain. Asians are often socialized not to express pain so dramatically, and that socialization can also affect how intensely pain is experienced.

Religion

Jan Muh

Jan Muh, a young Buddhist monk from Cambodia who speaks little English, is scheduled to receive physical therapy for injuries received in a car accident. A female therapist enters his hospital room, greets him, places her hand on his injured shoulder, and asks him to sit up. Jan suddenly jumps away from her in panic, and the alarmed therapist calls for assistance. Relatives explain that, as a monk, Jan is not allowed to be touched by a woman. If he is touched, he is required not to look at her or make even the slightest movement in response, for to do so would be viewed as showing physical desire and breaking his religious vows. The incident that occurred would require Jan to pay great penance.

Nationality

Tom Takahashi

Tom Takahashi, a 60-year-old Japanese man, is in a hospital rehabilitation unit recovering from a stroke that significantly weakened his left side. He is doing well during physical and occupational therapy sessions, but regresses when his wife visits. Hospital staff discover that when Tom's wife is present in his hospital room, especially for long hours, he fails to do his prescribed exercises. At those times, his wife takes over all small tasks, such as brushing his teeth, shaving and dressing him, and even holding the bedpan for him, although the therapists had indicated he should begin getting up to use the bathroom. Tom's dependency on his wife is complemented by his barking orders at her. These behaviors are in accord with customs both the man and his wife accept. While the therapists wish to respect the couple's traditions, they also speak with them to work out an agreement about limiting the wife's presence in the room. ▨

Folk Medicine

Alicia Tran Phan

Alicia Tran Phan, a physical therapist who practices in a children's services program housed within the elementary and junior high schools of a large school district, is asked by a school nurse to work with a Vietnamese girl entering first grade. The girl suffers shoulder pains of unknown origin. The therapist immediately discovers dark red welts and scratches on the girl's arms, shoulders, and chest. Suspecting child abuse, Alicia alerts the authorities. In fact, the welts are caused by coin rubbing, a traditional folk remedy in many Asian countries. The therapy consists of vigorously rubbing a coin in prescribed patterns, typically radiating from the spine to the interstices of the ribs. The coin rubbing was not the source of the child's pain—it was instead an attempt to alleviate it, and it did not itself injure the child.

Today, coin rubbing is generally tolerated by Western health professionals as an "alternative" or "complementary" therapy. Earlier that was not so, as the following cautionary tale reveals:

> In 1975, during the first wave of refugee resettlement from Southeast Asia, a Vietnamese father in California brought his desperately ill son to an emergency department for treatment of advanced influenza. In an effort to treat the child at home as the first line of defense, the family had used traditional Southeast Asian coin-rubbing on him to bring out the fever . . . . Uninformed about this harmless and well-intentioned therapy, emergency department personnel contacted the police, who charged the father with child abuse and took him to jail. The child subsequently died due to complications from the flu. The father hanged himself in jail.[4]

Fortunately, tragedies like this are rare, and most cultural misunderstandings and gaffes are easily corrected or prevented through improved communication and multicultural awareness. The following case study illustrates how awareness and communication can bridge these differences.[5]

Krista and Jimmy

Krista had recently graduated from a physical therapy program and accepted a job in an area that served a large population of Native Americans. One of her first referrals for therapy was a four-year-old male named Jimmy, who was diagnosed with cerebral palsy/hemiplegia. Following her evaluation, Krista requested a meeting with the mother (who was present) to discuss the treatment goals and methods, including a home treatment plan. The mother agreed with her recommendations, and at the appointed time Jimmy came to the clinic with his mother, father, the child's uncle, and several unrelated friends. Krista was surprised by such a large group and worried about maintaining confidentiality. Uncertain as to how freely she could discuss the diagnosis, she asked to speak alone with the mother. The mother assured her that all of these people were involved in her son's care, and the actual agreement for care would come from the child's uncle. This comment raised a new concern for Krista: Consent for treatment had to come from the legal guardian—from the mother rather than the uncle. Still uncertain about how to proceed, she decided that if the mother wanted the others present, there probably was no confidentiality issue.

Krista made her presentation, explaining her findings and proposing a three-pronged approach. First, she would provide one-on-one therapy. Second, she would enroll Jimmy in a group she conducted each week. The group, she explained, was to engage Jimmy in a play setting with tasks that would complement her treatment in the individual sessions. The play would consist of games that allowed each child to compete individually with the other children in ways that motivated desirable responses. She planned to reward the children with stickers and small gifts they could select from the treasure chest when they won. The third approach was a home treatment program that the mother could administer to further enhance the treatment sessions. Krista alerted the family and friends that without intervention the child would continue to lose range of motion and would have great difficulty walking or being independent in self-help skills.

The family and friends listened quietly, and when Krista finished, there was a long silence. At first Krista wondered if they had understood her, but after a while the uncle politely explained that before treatment could begin, they would seek the help of the tribal healer. When he had performed the appropriate ceremony, they would return. The uncle stated that he was happy that Krista would work with his nephew, but he objected to the type of activities she had described for the play group. The responsibility for the home program would be shared by everyone in the room, not only the mother.

Krista, confused by the responses, consulted a senior therapist, Mary, who had practiced in the area for several years. Mary explained that family, in traditional Native-American culture, is broadly defined by a concerned community rather than by biological parents alone. Grandparents often attend to the spiritual concerns of the child, and an uncle will often assume responsibility for health-care decisions. Mary stated that activities for a child that stressed individualism and competition were not acceptable to many Native Americans, who believed that those activities separated the child from others. Group activities that were cooperative and facilitated relationships would be approved, but competition and notoriety through rewards would not be accepted. Mary also explained that often the families would seek the tribal healer because they believed in multiple causes of illness, not because they disbelieved the diagnosis or thought Western medicine was ineffective. As for the warning Krista had given, in the future she should speak only about the positive outcomes. The traditional belief was that negative thoughts and fears would impede the healing process. They should not be mentioned unless in the abstract third person, so that they were not personalized by the patient.

Although Mary's information provided Krista with more understanding, it did not by itself solve her dilemmas. Krista could yield on the confidentiality issue, but she felt conflicted about the consent for treatment coming from the uncle. She was convinced that a competitive play format would accomplish far more for the child. But perhaps most important, Krista felt that a frank discussion of possible negative consequences, just as much as positive outcomes, was essential to acquiring informed consent.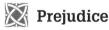

Sometimes the cross-cultural conflicts between provider and patient are deeply rooted. This is because cultural differences are not just beliefs but are entirely different "systems of meaning."[6] The first step in avoiding conflict is for the provider and patient to decide jointly on the goals of treatment without attending to the means by which those goals will be met. Once the goals are established, the means must be negotiated so that cultural differences are respected.

Krista solved the conflict over confidentiality by reasoning that if the mother wanted to share the medical knowledge, there was little difference between the mother telling others and their hearing it directly. In fact, there was less chance for misinterpretation if they all heard it from the same person at the same time. Similarly, Krista could reason that autonomy can be delegated to others by a competent person if the responsibility for the consequences remains with the person, not the surrogate decision maker. If the mother trusts the uncle enough to maintain this traditional decision-making pattern about health issues, then it would seem that it was her autonomous choice.

Krista might feel pressured by her perception of a legal system that requires the legal guardian's consent to treat. She might choose to explain to the mother her legal entanglement and ask the mother to confirm that the uncle had her permission to make health-care decisions for her child. She would then ask the mother to sign the required intake forms with the understanding that Krista would treat the uncle's concerns as though they were the mother's, noting that at any time the mother could resume that responsibility if she so wanted. Regarding the issue of competitive play, Krista could change the format to a group activity in which the goal would be to help others and to succeed as a group rather than as individuals. As for relaying negative outcomes as well as positive ones, she might reason that autonomous persons have the right to restrict the information they receive or to hear it addressed in a general rather than a personal context.

Prejudice

Prejudice, or bigotry, is the strongest obstacle to multicultural appreciation. Arguably, most bigotry is now covert (disguised, hidden). Yet bigotry that is overt (open, obvious) is still alarmingly frequent. Furthermore, as much bigotry manifests itself institutionally, embedded within social practices and organizational structures, as at the individual level. The institutionalization of prejudice often makes it difficult for individuals to recognize the degree to which they comply with the social values they have internalized. People with the best of intentions and a firm commitment to help others often mistakenly believe that the desire not to be biased automatically exempts them from prejudiced behaviors.

Ethnocentrism is the core of much prejudice. At some level, pride in one's own group is healthy, for it adds to one's sense of well-being and belonging. But far too frequently the group elevates itself by diminishing others. One symptom of ethnocentrism gone awry is that contributions by outsiders are ignored or unrecognized. For example, only in the past few years have the contributions by African-Americans to American culture been included in standard history texts in public schools. Contributions of gays and lesbians are still not generally acknowledged.

Persons born into ethnic or cultural groups that are in power inherit the values and even the language that helps maintain that power. More importantly, persons in the group holding power have privileges they did not individually earn, acquiring them simply because of the status of their group. They therefore might be unaware that not everyone shares in a certain ease of living, or they might reason that if others do not share their privileges it is because they lack initiative.

Being professionals and being in the cultural majority give most physical therapists a socially and economically privileged life, allowing them to live in areas that are considered to be safe and providing the necessary resources for their health and well-being. They also work to insulate them from understanding how others experience the world. Thus, when we say that we have no prejudice because we treat all others as we would want to be treated, we might fail to recognize differences relevant to the patient. Thereby, we might fail to take steps that contribute to their empowerment.

Before offering some general observations about the nature and sources of covert prejudice, whether of therapists toward patients or supervisors toward employees, let us mention a case of overt prejudice reported in 1999 by the *Los Angeles Times*:

Orange County Physician

An Orange County (California) physician and the health maintenance organization for which he works were being sued for causing emotional distress to a patient. The focus of the lawsuit was a routine physical exam, during which the physician asked the patient about her means of birth control. The patient replied that she did not use birth control because she was a lesbian. Following the exam, the physician suggested that she schedule her next exam with one of the other doctors in the office. When asked why, the physician said "he didn't approve of her gay 'lifestyle.' "[7] ◈

Evidently, the physician felt he had a right to refuse to provide treatment for gays, perhaps as an exercise of his religious faith or his personal conscience, or perhaps as part of the medical tradition of allowing physicians to refuse to accept individuals as patients (except in emergencies). At the very least, he was grossly insensitive in how he exercised his beliefs, given the emotional vulnerability of the patient whose body was being intimately examined by someone she thought she could trust.

We believe this case illustrates how highly intelligent and well-educated professionals can sometimes be overtly prejudiced. If others disagree, the case at least reminds us that as a society we have yet to reach a shared understanding of what prejudice is or of the many ways we can exhibit prejudice, either with or without awareness. Numerous studies, we might add, suggest that this case study is representative of a recurring bias on the part of some health-care providers.[8] A study conducted in 1992 found that nearly a quarter of physical therapists in Los Angeles County who provided home health services would prefer not to treat homosexual adults who were HIV negative.[9]

The Latin origin of "prejudice"—praejudicium—means to make a judgment based on prior experience. Although prejudice can involve prejudging someone favorably, such as assuming that a handsome man or beautiful woman must be talented, the greater threat to justice occurs when we prejudge negatively. Studies in cognitive psychology reveal that prejudice serves many functions, including predicting behavior and forewarning of dangers in addition to maintaining patterns of subordination.[10]

For example, in our increasingly complex world, we use on a daily basis mental shortcuts to guide our actions to avoid time-consuming investigations of our environment. These mental shortcuts, of which stereotypes are only one type, hasten our responses and contribute to our survival when rapid response is critical. When the shortcuts are constructed from insufficient data to predict a particular response, we typically obtain enough feedback from the situation to improve the shortcuts. As an example, say that in preparing for an outdoor sporting event we notice heavy cloud cover and decide to carry an umbrella. After carrying an umbrella to an event where there are clouds but no rain, we improve our working generalization to predict rain only when the clouds are gray. Had we more time, we could look at a barometer, take measures of humidity, temperature, and wind velocity, and calculate the probability of rain, but by then the event might be over.

In most cases these shortcuts serve us well enough. What happens, however, when we take these same mental shortcuts to estimate the behaviors of humans? Stereotypes—formed using limited variables to predict the behaviors of very complex beings—are often the result. They provide a certain "cognitive economy" that guides our choices.[11] For example, we might feel that short haircuts on women signify that they are masculine in their behavior, possibly rude, and certainly not socially refined. Because we have decided that this person is not someone we want to know, we are unavailable to them and do not participate with them in shared activities. As a consequence, the stereotype is never corrected because no new data are gathered to refute it.

Thus, in simplifying choices for a course of action, stereotypes typically minimize variance within a group and maximize differences between groups. Once these stereotypes or schemas are formed, we filter information to accept what fits the category, and we either do not recognize or do not accept information that does not fit. If we should be forced to interact with a woman with short hair and find her to be socially poised, feminine, and cordial, we decide that she is the exception to the stereotype and do not necessarily change the stereotype in our mind.

As ludicrous as it is to assume knowledge of a complex human being by knowing one variable, such as length of hair, we do it all the time. Multiple studies demonstrate that bias is unconsciously present even in those who do not want to be biased.[12] Without recognizing these unconscious biases, we cannot be genuinely fair, and we often end up implicitly supporting social practices of oppression that damage the victim's self-esteem and create a social stigma that further disadvantages the victim.

When power or institutionalization is added, prejudice is then labeled an "ism"—racism, sexism, ageism, and so on.[13] The inevitable consequence is to deny someone an opportunity, a service, a product, or any other desired good to which they have a right. In today's society, these "isms" are expressed more covertly than overtly, but that does not signal an end of oppression. It just makes prejudice more difficult to recognize and correct. Philosopher Marilyn Frye used the metaphor of a birdcage to express the effects of cultural biases on women, but the metaphor applies to all bigotries:

> Consider a birdcage. If you look very closely at just one wire in the cage, you cannot see the other wires. If your conception of what is before you is determined by this myopic focus, you could look at that one wire, up and down the length of it, and be unable to see why a bird would not just fly around the wire any time it wanted to go somewhere. . . . There is no physical property of any one wire, *nothing* that the closest scrutiny could discover, that will reveal how a bird could be inhibited or harmed by it except in the most accidental way.[14]

The contours of the cage—and that is what a social prejudice is—emerge only when we step back and see each wire as part of a wider gestalt.

Having emphasized cognitive sources of prejudice, we should note that prejudice often serves additional desires and needs. One such need is our desire to maintain self-esteem by affirming the superiority of groups with which we identify. P. Wachtel stated that, "A number of classic studies have documented that [racial] prejudice is far more likely among those whose status is low or declining than among those with high or rising status, who presumably have less need to find someone to place below them."[15] Another need is simply to be accepted as part of a group, embracing the group's tradition of prejudice as one aspect of membership. Still another need is to provide an outlet for inner conflicts, such as insecurities about sexual identity (for example, in the case of homophobia), or guilt and shame about one's failures (for example, the scapegoating of Jews by anti-Semites).

One need not be a psychoanalyst to have experienced firsthand the ease with which we project our own unacceptable desires onto other groups as a way to provide an outlet for our fears, frustrations, and aggression. Some would argue that attempts to understand the many forms of prejudice on a simple uniform model are bound to fail, for the inner dynamics of bigotry take many different forms depending upon personal needs and social structures.[16]

⊠ Racism

Up to this point we have made little specific mention of race. Many are now convinced that the idea of biologically different races—dividing up the one human race—is itself a product of racism. Indeed, the American Anthropological Association has recently called for the elimination of the term "race" in its discussions, finding that the category of "ethnicity" suffices to capture the relevant groupings. There is virtually no evidence supporting the idea of multiple biological human races, and the notion of discrete genetic packages that are unique to each race is a dangerous myth. In practice, "race," as most commonly used, is defined by skin color, hair texture, and other appearance variables. The genetic differences between the "races" are no greater than the differences between any two persons of the same race.[17-19] In particular, the only thing skin color predicts is location of one's ancestry relative to the equator. Prior health-care research which had described racial differences in disease and treatment had actually most often reported differences resulting from socioeconomic or environmental variables. In those few cases in which illnesses (i.e., sickle cell anemia) affect a disproportionate number of people from one ethnic group, it is most often because of a geographical region of origin, other than something "racially" inherent.

Of course, there is a "social construction" of race, in which individuals identify themselves and others as members of what they perceive as racial groups. Most people in the United States think of race as one of the four groups defined by census records as either (1) black, (2) white, (3) Hispanic, or (4) Asian. (The most recent census greatly expanded these categories, and allowed individuals to identity themselves by multiple categories.) There is, however, a more extensive listing under ethnic identity which speaks to such cultural variables as diet, smoking, and beliefs about wellness.

There is also a "policy construction" of race that uses racial categories to validate or refute discrimination based on social constructions of race. The policy construction of race is evident in policies as divergent as, on the one hand, Article 1, Section 2 of the U.S. Constitution, which mandated that African-Americans could be counted only as three-fifths of a person for purposes of taxation and representation, and the Civil Rights Act of 1964 on the other hand, as well as the more recent updates forbidding discrimination based on "race."

In fact, the perception of race by health-care practitioners has a profound influence on health-care decisions. Even after adjusting for socioeconomic factors and for the number of physician visits and health conditions, African-American and Hispanic children are less likely to receive prescription medication than are white children.[20] Also, even after statistical corrections for other variables, African-American children receive fewer surgical procedures than white children.[21]

Childhood living conditions, of which medical care is a component, have a profound effect on well-being and can produce a lifelong vulnerability.[22] In health care, minority-identified adults fare no better than their children. Perception of race has been a primary factor in disproportionate utilization of resources in situations involving a combination of causal factors, such as access, delivery, and usage. Here is a partial list of findings:

- Even when hospitalized, minorities receive fewer services than whites.[20]
- The more discretionary the procedure, the less likely African-Americans will receive it.[23]
- Whites are more likely to receive angiography and nearly twice as likely to receive bypass surgery or angioplasty than African-Americans, even when income and severity of disease are statistically controlled for.[24]
- African-Americans are more often assigned inexperienced therapists for psychotherapy and seen for shorter durations.[25]

- In hospital settings, African-Americans are two to four times more likely than white patients to have surgery performed by a resident rather than a fully trained surgeon.[21]

- Even after controlling for insurance and clinical status, whites are more likely than African-Americans to receive kidney transplants and be treated in the ICU for pneumonia.[22]

- African-Americans are far more likely to report that physicians do not provide them with necessary information about test results, medications, and prenatal care.[26]

- Perceived race was correlated with less timely follow-up by doctors after abnormal mammograms.[27]

- African-Americans receive lower quality care and are discharged in less stable condition than other patients.[28]

- African-Americans receive less intensive-care treatment for cardiac disease.[29,30]

In health-care research there has been a decreasing trend to include nonwhite subjects in research studies and in clinical field trial studies.[31] One interpretation of this disparate treatment and care is that the perception of race by health-care practitioners has a profound influence in health-care decisions because of the often unconscious biases associated with race. If this is true, then all practitioners need to be mindful of their biases and vigilant and corrective for the effect these may have in their personal and professional decisions.

 Sexism

The bias against women might be the most systemic bias in society because it is prevalent in every aspect of life, including the allocation of home responsibilities and the defining elements of personal relationships. Until the recent past, women "were expected to be continually dependent upon men—on fathers in childhood, on husbands as adults, and on sons in old age," writes D. Dunn.[32] This dependency was legally enforced by laws that forbade women from owning property, testifying in court, or having separate credit ratings from their husbands. Even the basic right to vote was denied women until August 18, 1920, when the 19th amendment to the constitution was passed. Even now, there is still no Equal Rights Amendment to the Constitution.

When a child is born, the first question usually asked by the husband, family, and friends is not about the child's health, but instead about the child's gender. That one variable significantly predicts a host of outcomes over a lifetime. For example, treatment of boys and girls within the education system differs greatly. Historically, starting in the early elementary grades, girls receive significantly less attention from their teachers than do boys, who flourish with the extra instruction.[33] Gender gaps in performance and interest start early and continue to widen, especially in the sciences. Although many of the gaps have decreased, new ones have opened. Thus, while the gender gap in math narrowed between 1992 and 1998, computer science became the new "boys club," with an enormous gender gap.[34] Graduate education did not see an equal number of women until 1984, and it was not until 1995 that the number of women in graduate school full-time matched that of their male counterparts.

Sexual harassment (discussed more fully in Chapter 8) is an obstacle throughout the educational process, and not only at the college level. In 1993, a poll found that four out of five girls in the eighth through eleventh grades had experienced sexual harassment, defined as "unwanted and unwelcome sexual behavior which interferes with your life."[34] Given the frequency of documented sexual harassment in the workplace, at present it appears to be a lifetime obstacle.

Education significantly impacts the earning potential of job candidates, including women, but the sexes are often far from equal when their earnings are compared. Women enter the market as enthusiastically as men: In 1994, 90.3 percent of females and 89.9 percent of males stated that being successful in work was "very important" to them.[35] Nevertheless, incomes differ between the sexes in all industrialized countries. The wage gap differs more in the United States than in a number of advanced countries, especially Canada, which has the most extensive pay equity policies in the world.

The table shown here provides an example of this (full-time) wage gap in 1998, after adjusting for levels of education.[35]

Gender	Bachelor's Degree	Master's Degree	Professional Degree	Doctorate
Male	$51,405	$62,244	$94,737	$75,078
Female	$36,559	$45,283	$57,565	$57,796

Even in academia, the differences are surprising. In the 1998–99 academic year, nearly 60 percent of full-time faculty on 9- or 10-month contracts were tenured; 67 percent of men were tenured and only 48 percent of women were tenured. Male professors made $9,000 more than female professors per year, male associate professors made $3,500 more than females in the same category, male assistant professors made $2,800 more, and male instructors made $1,600 more per year.[36]

Blended into salary differences, however, are considerations above and beyond personal bias. First, the kind of work that women do is often reimbursed at lower levels than work traditionally performed by men. This is not to say that the work is less important or less difficult to perform. Rather, the sex of the majority of workers in a particular field appears to influence the reimbursement rate in that field. Of course, there are other variables that influence wages, but something is awry when highly trained intensive-care nurses earn a fraction of the salary commanded by divorce attorneys, or when elementary school teachers barely earn enough to live above the defined poverty level.

Second, work behavior varies between the sexes. Men and women might have similar hourly wages, but on average, men work three or more hours longer per week than women, creating a difference in annual wages.[37] A. Bowlus also points out that women have a greater tendency to leave jobs and remain unemployed for extended periods because of pregnancy and other family matters—a phenomenon often referred to as "sequencing."[38] In turn, this tendency affects women's seniority and work experience, which are factors in reimbursement.

Yet even as these examples attempt to explain workplace bias, they only help to further define the social-family bias that women face. When a child is sick, it is the mother who is usually expected to stay home. When either the wife's or the husband's parents are ill or in need of continuing care, it is usually the wife who leaves her job to deliver the unpaid services. Even on a day-to-day basis, one reason women often do not work the extra two or three hours of overtime is that they spend multiples of that time taking care of their homes, children, family finances, food preparation, and cleaning. Given these dual jobs, it is not surprising that the Glass Ceiling Commission established by President George W. Bush found that between 95 percent and 97 percent of all senior managers in the top 1,000 industrial firms and the *Fortune* 500 were men.[39]

Women, like minorities, receive disparate health care. The nonreproductive health of women has largely been ignored, even when hormonal differences are especially relevant, as in medication dosages.[40,41] Women who are hospitalized for coronary heart disease are prescribed fewer diagnostic and therapeutic procedures and are 35 percent less likely to undergo coronary angiography or revascularization with adjusted odds.[42] In a study of 2,231 patients with myocardial infarctions, men were twice as likely—when clinical variables were controlled—as women to undergo invasive cardiac procedures.[43] Similar inequities arise in medical research. For example, an NIH study of 22,000 physicians to test the effect of an aspirin taken every other day to prevent coronary artery disease did not have a single woman in the study.[44]

The many documentations of gender bias in medicine are important in establishing a pattern of bias. For example, historically, studies have shown that men have received more extensive workups than women by male physicians for five common complaints.[45] And in a 1981 study using vignettes, unexpressive women were seven times more likely than unexpressive men to receive a psychological diagnosis.[46]

These biases in the health-care world pervade our everyday lives as well. We are bombarded with advertising that defines how women should look and behave, far more often than is done with men. The media objectify women, segmenting them into body parts and often portraying violence against women as sexy or entertaining.[47] Against this background, it is little wonder that the feminist movement began by lashing out at men as the principal cause of such injustice. After moving through its early stages, however, the feminist movement began to take on the productive task of identifying strategies needed to create a more just environment for women.

Bell Hook believes that the social, labor, and political injustices are in the end symptomatic of a fundamental assumption in need of correction. "Feminist effort to end patriarchal domination should be of primary concern precisely because it insists on the eradication of exploitation and oppression in the family context and in all other intimate relationships."[48] Yet feminists do not all speak with one voice. Indeed, an accurate short definition of feminism is now exceedingly difficult to provide because feminism takes so many different forms.[49] For example, feminism that highlights equal rights for women is now called "liberal feminism," referring to liberalism in the broad Enlightenment sense rather than its political meaning. (Many members of the Republican Party are feminists in this sense.) Feminists who link oppression to capitalism include Marxist and socialist feminists. There are postmodernist feminists, psychoanalytic feminists, multicultural feminists, and so on. Attempting an inclusive characterization, Susan Wolf suggests that "feminist work takes gender and sex as centrally important analytic categories, seeks to understand their operation in the world, and strives to change the distribution and use of power to stop the oppression of women."[50]

To illustrate just one area of strong disagreement among feminists, recall (from Chapter 1) Carol Gilligan's celebration of an ethics of care, which she linked to women's moral outlooks, and the ethics of justice (and rules), which she loosely tied to male ways of thinking. Some feminists see in Gilligan's work the promise of an illuminating new ethics focused on caring relationships, which are traditionally valued more by women than by men.[51] Other feminists, however, are highly critical of her care ethic, seeing it as reinforcing old stereotypes of women as the "gentle sex." Their view holds that, until care is a shared endeavor, it tends to perpetuate the existing power structure, which subordinates women. At the same time, many feminist ethicists agree with Gilligan that the approach to ethics that depends on universal principles ignores the social reality of women and only yields truly relevant and just outcomes to men; until women are not oppressed, they cannot fully participate as equals with men. In fact, these ethicists believe that a new ethic is needed that gives concern and support to the oppressed, not just to those whose well-being is improved. Until oppression is reduced, our continued focus on autonomy might strengthen those who are already privileged and powerful.[52]

S. Mullett contends that a feminist ethic should bring about a complex change in consciousness through three perspectives: "moral sensitivity," "ontological shock," and "praxis."[53] **Moral sensitivity** allows us to notice and acknowledge the enormous amount of violence and pain forced upon women, events so commonplace as to be perceived as "normal." **Ontological shock** is a double perspective that sees and understands the current social context but also imagines radical change and transformation. **Praxis** is the shift from "me" to "we" in the search for collective actions that can change the existing reality.

Mullett, like many other contemporary feminists, aims to foster awareness of the plight of women while offering an alternative to despair, rage, and self-pity. At the micro level—at the patient's bedside—this is translated into seeking assurances that women are indeed autonomous enough to know their own best good. A simple answer from a woman is not sufficient without knowing how much the answer is influenced by her duty to others, by her view of herself as negatively shaped by an unjust social perception, or by her assimilation of hospital staff's opinion about her worth.[52]

Affirmative Action

Nowhere are uses of social and policy constructions of race, as well as attempts to overthrow sexism, more controversial than in **affirmative action** programs, such as those used to determine both eligibility for admittance to programs in physical therapy as well as the hiring and promotion of professors of APTA-approved physical therapy programs. Advocates of affirmative action view it as a potent way to counter the continuing legacy of racism as well as sexism. Critics regard it as a contradictory attempt to seek justice by imposing injustice.

In its original meaning, affirmative action referred to taking positive steps to ensure equal opportunity for minorities and, subsequently, women. Quickly, however, affirmative action came to mean giving preference to members of these groups independently of equality in skill or background, whether in hiring, promotion, education, or training programs. **Weak preferential treatment** means providing the advantage to members of these groups when they compete against white males having comparable credentials. **Strong preferential treatment** means giving women and minorities an advantage even when they are less qualified than white males with whom they are competing. Both forms, especially the strong form, are controversial.

Historically, in the 1950s, affirmative action had its origins in a request by President Dwight Eisenhower to then–Vice President Richard Nixon, asking him to investigate charges of widespread discrimination based on race in the defense industry. Nixon generated a report that described the manner in which racial discrimination was perpetuated, but neither he nor Eisenhower acted on the information. When President John F. Kennedy took office in 1960, he issued Executive Order 10925, which stated in part that "the contractor will take affirmative action to ensure that applicants are employed, and that employees are treated during employment without regard to their race, creed, color, or national origin."[11(p163),54]

The first stage under this order was to correct the institutionalized racism that affected hiring. Despite Supreme Court rulings such as *Brown v. Board of Education of Topeka*, which invalidated the concept of separate but equal rights in education, priority in jobs and educational opportunities customarily went to whites, even when minority candidates possessed greater qualifications.[55] When it became clear that this step alone would not solve the problem, the Equal Employment Opportunity Commission (EEOC), the Economic Development Administration (EDA), and the Department of Housing and Urban Development (HUD), among other government agencies, set specific goals and time frames for achieving objectives.

Initially, quotas were developed for the specific percentages of jobs or college admissions that should be offered to minority candidates. The spirit behind the movement was to end the disadvantages that minorities and women had suffered for generations and to do so in a timely manner, recognizing the subtle and often covert methods of discrimination that continue even today. However, rigid quotas were struck down as unconstitutional in the 1978 Supreme Court case *Regents of the University of California v. Bakke*. The court ruled that an employer or university could use race as a factor in the selection process to achieve greater racial parity, but it could not use race as the only factor. Nor could it set rigid percentages for placements. Thus, affirmative action—which is now composed of a host of agency regulations, court decisions, and legislation— has been shaped at the intersection of the Constitution, the Civil Rights Act of 1964, and the Voting Rights Act of 1965.

Currently, the Office of Federal Contract Compliance regulations state that "regulations expressly forbid quotas or giving less qualified workers preference based on their race or sex."[11(p164)] However, under current federal guidelines, any federal contractor, which includes most major corporations, hospitals, and educational facilities, must keep records of the number of women and minorities at each strata of the organization and then do comparisons with the hiring pool in that area or employment catch basin. If there is a great discrepancy between the two, then the employer may initiate preferential hiring and promotion.[56] A court can impose these practices on a private employer and on state and local governments. At present, affirmative action plans contain one or any mixture of the following:[57]

1. Outreach programs that identify and recruit qualified minorities for opportunities.

2. Aid through financial incentives or technical assistance.

3. Mentoring that guides or coaches qualified candidates.

4. Treating race as an advantage factor in the selection process.

Some are now predicting that affirmative action will be abolished by the Supreme Court.[55(p191)] Nevertheless, affirmative action continues to be vigorously debated in the United States, with some in ardent support and others in bitter opposition.

Supporters of affirmative action contend that it is a powerful way to respect the rights to equal opportunity of women and minorities. The long history of discrimination is clear, and even the Supreme Court once endorsed slavery (in the Dred Scott decision) and segregation (in *Plessy v. Ferguson*). In addition, as we noted in the previous section, women were denied even the most basic rights, such as the right to vote, well into the 20th century. Institutionalized racism and sexism have not entirely disappeared, and race and gender biases continue to operate, consciously or unconsciously, in social and resource allocation. The only way to overcome the privileges of the white majority, which historically were significantly financed by the exploitation of minorities, is to compensate through race-conscious decisions in education, employment, and political apportionment. To be sure, once whites and minorities are on an equal footing, the laws should be abolished, but that achievement is still in the future. As summed up by President Lyndon B. Johnson with respect to race, "You do not take a person who, for years, has been hobbled by chains and liberate him, bring him up to the starting line of a race and then say, 'You are free to compete with all the others,' and still justly believe that you have been completely fair. Thus it is not enough just to open the gates of opportunity."[57(p17)]

Opponents of affirmative action admit that the history of racial bias in the United States is a tragedy, but they contend that we cannot correct the past by using the same methods that created the disparity. In their view, violating the rights of white males merely compounds injustice, since two wrongs do not make a right. To be sure, specific individuals who have been wronged have a right to compensation, but not by giving advantages to entire groups. The victims of the past are rarely the beneficiaries of corrective actions today, and those punished through lost opportunities were rarely the perpetuators. Moreover, opponents believe, preferential treatment programs are an insult to minorities because these programs create the social stigma that minorities and women cannot successfully compete without an advantage. The hostility these actions cause in whites, combined with the feelings of inferiority internalized by minorities by these methods, only deepen race-conscious feelings. In the long run, opponents declare, affirmative action promotes rather than hinders racism by generating a backlash of resentment and hostility.

Whether the supporters or opponents have the stronger case will be further examined in the Discussion Question section at the end of this chapter, but we add a few further comments here about the social controversy. At present, the social, political, and business responses to affirmative action vary widely. In 1997, the state of California, in its Proposition 209, amended the state constitution to forbid affirmative action preferences in hiring, contracting, or education. The state of Washington has taken a similar action. The Eastman Kodak Co. and Toys "R" Us, among others, have voluntarily initiated affirmative action programs because they feel it is imperative to match their consumer base in order to be market-savvy.[56(p22)] Procter and Gamble has an aggressive voluntary affirmative action program that not only recruits and hires minorities but also creates career pathways to move minorities up the management ladder.[57(p22)] Most universities remain convinced that racial diversity on campus has an important place in the educational process. *Academe*, which is the bulletin of the American

Association of University Professors, reports that nearly two-thirds of faculty believe that students benefit from racial and ethnic diversity on campus and that their universities value that diversity. More than 90 percent indicated that diversity in the classroom did not hinder the quality of students or the substance of class discussion.[58]

The Supreme Court has offered several comments to the effect that diversity on a college campus may be a legitimate goal. For example, Justice Lewis Powell asserted that diversity is vital to the "robust exchange of ideas," and that the selection of diverse students who are expected to contribute to the academic community was a permissible constitutional goal.[59] Justice Sandra Day O'Connor stated in *Wygant v. Jackson Board of Education* that "a state interest in the promotion of racial diversity has been found sufficiently 'compelling' at least in the context of higher education, to support the use of racial considerations in furthering that interest."[59] As this book goes to press, the Supreme Court is revisiting the issue of affirmative action in two cases involving the University of Michigan law school. Some have argued that academic programs for healthcare professionals have a special and perhaps compelling need for affirmative action. K. Deville proposes that there are three related reasons why diversity in medical education may be considered a "compelling state interest":

- It will increase the number of physicians who serve traditionally underserved patients and specialty areas;
- It promotes the robust exchange of ideas in medical education; and
- It will result in better medical care for minorities.[59]

At least five recent major research studies conducted since the 1978 Bakke case consistently show that minority physicians tend, in far larger percentages than their white colleagues, to practice in minority communities where there are insufficient primary care physicians and where they are more likely to serve Medicaid and uninsured patients.[60-64] Since the health of citizens is a concern for government, the methods aimed at addressing unmet needs should be supported when congruent with the law.

The profession of physical therapy might have especially compelling reasons for pursuing an affirmative action plan with regard to race. Although the United States is becoming more ethnically diverse, the field of physical therapy does not have proportional diversity among its practitioners. According to 1993 figures from the U.S. Bureau of Labor Statistics, 8.7 percent of physical therapists were from minority groups. And unlike nursing training programs (which are 15.4 percent minority), physician assistant programs (17.5 percent minority), and chiropractic programs (12.6 percent minority), which have similar prerequisites, similar curricula, and offer entry-level health-care degrees, there were proportionally far fewer minority students enrolled in physical therapy programs (3.7 percent).[65] By 1999, minority membership in the APTA was 8.9 percent, and minority student enrollment in physical therapy training programs in 1999–2000 was 12.9 percent.[66] Although there were undoubtedly multiple factors at play in effecting these changes, at least part of the success must be attributed to affirmative action strategies compiled and offered to all physical therapy educational institutions by APTA. These strategies included various outreach programs, such as informational sessions targeted to minorities, and minority recruitment efforts. Still, these data suggest that minorities remain underrepresented in physical therapy.

People with Disabilities

Given the nature of physical therapists' work, it is not surprising that practitioners have often been leaders in helping to change society's response to persons with disabilities. Therapists know firsthand the inaccuracy of stereotypes that stigmatize persons with disabilities with images of inferiority and devaluation. At the same time, therapists are human, and they occasionally lapse into subtle forms of prejudice themselves.

Consider, for example, the language sometimes used to refer to patients. One would hope that no therapist would denigrate patients by calling them "cripples" or "retards." Nevertheless, the climate of health-care work still leads some therapists, as well as physicians, to speak of their patients as "the quad" or "the knee," thereby reducing a person to a disability. As Susan E. Roush writes,

> The problem with this language is that it is not accurate; the *person* is not the *characteristic*. In addition, this language reinforces the limiting perspectives that a stigmatizing "mark" taints all other characteristics of a person. Another example of inappropriate language is the use of value-laden terms that again emphasize loss and negativity and ignore ability, such as "He is confined to a wheelchair" rather than "He uses a wheelchair for mobility."[67]

Editors of journals in physical therapy now take special care to ensure that authors avoid such reductions. Jules M. Rothstein, for example, notes that "Our journal [*Physical Therapy*] has long advocated the use of people-first language . . . . People have disease, impairments, and disabilities—they are not the sum product of their medical conditions. People have paraplegia—they are not 'paraplegics'!"[68]

Our language and our behavior regarding people with disabilities is a singular form of prejudice. We are all vulnerable to becoming disabled in a variety of ways, and at some level we all know this.[69] Rather than acknowledge that vulnerability, we lapse into insensitive language and behavior as a protective device against our unacknowledged fears. Among those less informed, the responses to the person with a disability range from avoidance to physical attacks. Even those from whom we would expect compassion sometimes falter when it comes to disabilities. For example, a private not-for-profit center for children with disabilities eventually had to advise the parents of the children they served to avoid shopping at the supermarket adjacent to the center. Apparently the market attracted a large number of worshipers from a nearby church, and with great frequency members from the church would approach these parents in the market and inquire as to what had been the nature of the sin committed by the parent to cause this disability.

The public's tolerance for disability is surprisingly low and even extends to disfigurements that have no functional significance. Consider John:

John

John was a professor who had years of experience both as a student and as a teacher. He had developed the social skills for each of those settings so that he easily made friends and rarely was treated with anything but a cordial social response. During a recent visit to his dermatologist, John was advised to apply a mild topical chemotherapy lotion on his face to remove cells that appeared likely to become cancerous. The physician had never witnessed an adverse response to the medication and so failed to check John or provide guidance in case he had a reaction. John's response was atypical and violent, leaving him temporarily discolored, bleeding, and swollen. John had already enrolled in a class at the local university, so he attended class just as he had done in the past. This time, however, he noticed a dramatic change in the way people responded to him. The professor and some of the students avoided eye contact with him, and only one student responded in a cordial way to his efforts to socialize. Within four weeks the discoloration and swelling had disappeared. The professor then began to address him in class and the other students socialized with him as they had done in other settings for years. ◈

If social response can be so dramatically affected by appearance, imagine the response to a functional disability, and then to a functional disability in which esthetics are compromised. Historically, persons with disabilities have been forced into poverty, even when they were capable of working, because they were unable to find an employer who would hire them. Largely through the efforts of the community of persons with disabilities, legislation has been enacted to promote fairness in employment.

By far the single most important legislation in this area is the 1994 Americans with Disabilities Act (ADA). This act is a powerful attempt to ensure respect for the rights of Americans with disabilities, estimated at some 50 million, including individuals working within the health-care professions. It covers access to public accommodations and employment rights. The act has generated some controversy, although nothing akin to that for affirmative action. In fact, it has enjoyed broad support, and although extensive litigation over its application is ongoing, the courts have largely supported it as compatible to rights of equal opportunity for individuals who have been subjected to severe discrimination. Accordingly, our aim is to outline some of the complexities of the act rather than to focus on controversy.

We will focus on Title I of the act, which deals with employment issues. Since its inception on July 26, 1994, Title I has covered all private employers with at least 15 employees who work at least 20 weeks in a calendar year, all city and state agencies, labor organizations, and employment agencies.[70] Although state employees can still sue their employers under state discrimination statutes, they may not do so under the ADA; this was determined by the U.S. Supreme Court's ruling in the case of *Board of Trustees of the University of Alabama et al. v. Garrett et al.* on February 21, 2001.[71]

The coverage of the ADA is broad in that it includes everything in employment, from job application procedures to disciplinary action and termination. The law applies only to qualified applicants and does not advocate preferential treatment or affirmative action, nor does it excuse poor performance. Its aim is to protect the right of qualified workers who have disabilities to compete for jobs and then to be successful in applying their skills.[72]

Disability is defined broadly in three distinct ways.[73] First, persons are disabled if they have a physical or mental problem that substantially limits a major life activity. Examples of such life activities, provided by the ADA, include walking, speaking, seeing, hearing, learning, sitting, lifting, and reading. Also included are any mental or psychological disorders. The fact that any of these conditions are controlled or cured by medications does not remove the ADA protection for that person because it protects from the lingering or even false perception of disease or disability.

Second, all individuals who have been substantially limited in the past are covered. This includes people who have had heart disease, cancer, or mental illness, even if cured.

Third, ADA extends to situations in which a problem is created by the attitudes of others. For example, managers violate the ADA when they refuse to promote a person with facial scarring to a position in which the individual will have contact with the general public. They would also be in violation if they fired an employee because they believed he or she was HIV-positive, regardless of whether the employee actually was HIV-positive or negative. The ADA makes it illegal to refuse a job to someone because the person's spouse or dependent has a disability, or if a roommate or friend suffers from a disease such as AIDS, or if the person does volunteer work with an organization focused on a particular illness such as muscular dystrophy or AIDS.

Just as the ADA uses a broad definition in its coverage for citizens, it is also broad in the coverage offered in the pre-employment and employment fields. The regulations focus on issues of equality with the provision of "reasonable accommodation." Reasonable accommodation is defined by the ADA as those accommodations that enable individuals to perform tasks at a satisfactory level, such as ramps, modified work schedules, and purchased devices to aid persons with disabilities.[70(p11)] The employer should consult with the employee about which items would help in the accommodation process, because the ADA specifies that accommodation must be based on an "individualized analysis."[74] M. Warnick states that, "In addition, courts have held that where the employee does not offer possible reasonable accommodation(s) during this interactive process, the employee cannot later claim that the employer failed to reasonably accommodate his situation."[75]

Employers are not required to make accommodations that cause a hardship, either financially or by severely disrupting the operations of the business. For example, if someone with vision problems can work as a waitress only on the condition that the restaurant lighting is bright, but the restaurant needs dim lighting as part of its ambiance, then the accommodation would be justifiably too expensive to the business.[73(p9/17)] As another example, a physical therapist unable to lift 25 pounds could probably be reasonably accommodated in a hospital setting where aides and assistants are available (especially since hospitals are specifically listed as "a place of public accommodation" under Title III of the ADA),[75(p37)] but therapists might not be reasonably accommodated if they do home health care and the employer would have to hire or appoint an aide to accompany them on a daily basis.

In the pre-employment area, job offerings must be posted so as to be available to persons with disabilities, and employers' human resource departments must be physically accessible to them. The process of applying must also be accessible. For example, if an applicant is blind, the company must provide someone to fill out the application at the instruction of the applicant. During the interview process, the employer may not ask any questions about a person's disability either directly or indirectly through general questions about one's health. The employer is free to ask all applicants if they can perform all key tasks listed in the job description. Key tasks are core items in the job description, not those that could be easily done by someone else. For example, if the receptionist job description includes the task of "carries letters to the mail room," when in reality the letters could easily be taken by the aide who goes to the mail room daily to pick up deliveries, a person with paraplegia should not be eliminated from consideration for that job.

If employers require a medical examination prior to employment, they cannot order that exam until after a conditional job offer has been made.[70(p10)] This is done to prevent employer bias and unnecessary elimination of a candidate. If the medical exam uncovers a disability that makes performance of the job impossible or jeopardizes the health and safety of others, then the offer can be retracted. However, this retraction is allowed only on three separate conditions: First, medical exams must be required of all employees in that category, not just applicants the employers suspect of having a disability. Second, the job is such that even reasonable accommodation will not make the employee's job performance possible. Third, the health and safety requirements cannot be subjective standards but rather ones on which experts would agree, and they must be based on science where it exists.[76]

As another example, a restaurant cannot refuse to hire someone who is HIV-positive simply because the supervisor believes the health and safety of the staff or the public are at risk. Such beliefs have been countered by the Centers for Disease Control and supported in *Abbott v. Bragdon* in 1998.[77] Similarly, physicians and any other health-care professionals cannot refuse to treat a patient who is HIV-positive because of fear of contagion.

If someone with a disability is hired, then regulations are focused on fairness in all areas of the employment. Employees with disabilities must be given the same opportunities for job performance and promotion as all others, again with reasonable accommodation. Their privacy must also be protected. Their disabilities can be divulged only on a need-to-know basis with their supervisors, safety personnel, and officials with the ADA.[70(p34)] If employees complain that accommodations are unfair to them, the only response managers can offer is that they are acting in compliance with federal law or acting for legitimate business reasons, without revealing the disability.[73(p9/25)] The employer cannot segregate employees on the basis of disability, which means that lunchrooms, restrooms, and social activities must be accessible. Employee benefits must be the same as those offered to all others. Insurance companies' "preexisting condition" clauses remain intact and apply to persons with disabilities, just as they would apply to any other employee. In fact, after reasonable accommodation, people with disabilities are to be treated as other employees.

If an employee with a disability behaves in violation of a policy that is logically applicable to that job, then employers can discipline that person, just as they would any other employee, even if the behavior is a manifestation of the disorder. Discipline or dismissal is not legal, however, when a dress code or conduct code is violated as a manifestation of the disability and when the violation does not affect work, other employees, or the public.[73(p9/26)]

Items that are not covered by the ADA vary greatly according to the reason they are not considered. Sexual orientation is not protected by the act because it is not a disability. Inability to read is not covered unless it is caused by dyslexia, and obesity is not considered unless it is the result of a glandular condition. Disabilities caused by illegal drug use are not covered if the person is still using illegal drugs. They are covered if the person is not using drugs and has participated in any type of rehabilitation attempt, even if self-administered, or if the individual is currently undergoing drug rehabilitation.[75(pp36-41)] Behavioral disorders, such as compulsive gambling or pyromania, and psychological characteristics, such as aggressive or threatening behavior, are not protected. Religious organizations that hire only members of their faith do not have to hire persons with disabilities who are not members of their faith.

To conclude, cultural competency requires far more than simple tolerance. It requires an understanding that can be achieved only by recognizing institutional, cultural, and personal biases. These biases negatively affect some individuals and unfairly advantage others. Whether overt or covert, prejudice can affect our health-care decisions unfairly. Such errors perpetuate the cycle of oppression that has prompted such remedies as affirmative action and the Americans with Disabilities Act.

Discussion Questions

1. How is cultural diversity treated on your campus, and how have you experienced it in hospital and rehabilitation settings up to this point in your education? Specifically, (a) Was diversity avoided, tolerated, or celebrated? (b) Were different elements of diversity treated differentially? For example, have you seen disparate treatment at your university and in hospital or rehabilitation settings for women, African-Americans, Latinos, Asians, gays and lesbians? Describe.

2. Discuss the Orange County physician who declined to provide future health care to his patient. (a) Is a health professional who feels uncomfortable touching a gay person prejudiced and homophobic, in the sense of having an irrational fear or hatred of gays? Is your answer the same about a health professional who is uncomfortable about touching Jewish people? Why or why not? (b) Can it reasonably be argued that the physician has a right to exercise his beliefs about homosexuality, particularly if his attitudes are linked to religious beliefs that homosexuality is "unnatural"? Why or why not? (c) Exactly what does "unnatural" mean in this context, and is calling homosexuality "unnatural" itself a sign of bigotry, whether at the level of individuals or organizations (such as religions)?[78]

3. Discuss the kinds of questions a feminist might raise with respect to the following case: "A 72-year-old woman with leukemia is considering whether she should refuse a second course of chemotherapy and wait for death with only home care and no further medical intervention."[79] The medical staff serving the woman is mostly male. The woman has spent a lifetime of service to others, and feels reluctant to be a burden on her daughter.

4. Present and defend your view about whether affirmative action in any form is morally justified or unjustified, both in general and in regard to physical therapy. Develop your arguments within the framework of one of the major ethical theories, such as rights ethics, duty ethics, and rule utilitarianism. Do you find the ethical theory helps resolve the issue, or does it merely provide a framework for addressing it? Discuss how rights ethicists might seek to balance the rights of white males (to equal opportunity) and the rights of

minorities and women (for example, to equal opportunity and to compensation for past wrongs) in a society where racism and sexism are still present. Whatever your position, take into account alternative proposals for remedying the lingering effects of racism and sexism in our society.

5. In the following case, written by Katharine Parry, discuss how therapy might become complicated because of the patient's religious beliefs. How might those complications be dealt with in a manner that respects the patient's beliefs while providing quality care?

> An elderly Cuban woman is diagnosed with rheumatoid arthritis. A priestess in the Santeria sect, she believes that the cause of her disease was a spell—cast by another person—that she had "stepped into" by mistake. She believes that by her accidental intervention, she prevented the death of the individual for whom the spell was intended. She believes her personal power reduced the power of the spell to something less dangerous.[80]

6. Critics argue that our society has gone too far in demanding "political correctness" by sanctioning an officially proper way of talking. They contend, for example, that there is nothing wrong with speaking of a person as "a victim of" or "suffering from" multiple sclerosis (instead of saying the person "has multiple sclerosis"). They acknowledge that this manner of speaking accents the disability and the problems it causes, but that in fact those problems are genuine and that politically correct language only leads to an elaborate game of pretense that disguises genuine problems and tragedies. Also, critics suggest it is perfectly acceptable, as a convenient abbreviation, to speak of "the stroke" in the next room or in intensive care, as long as such language is not used in front of these people or other patients. What would you say in reply to these critics?

7. Some critics argue that the productivity and competitive edge of American business are being seriously damaged by excessive government regulation, including the ADA. What moral arguments can be marshaled for and against their position, and what is your view?

8. In small groups, make a list of the unearned privileges enjoyed by white males in this society. How much consensus do you find in your group on this issue?

References

1. Taylor C. The politics of recognition. In: Gutmann A, ed., *Multiculturalism: Examining the Politics of Recognition.* Princeton, NJ: Princeton University Press; 1994:72-73.
2. Thorpe DE, Baker CP. Perspective addressing "cultural competence" in health care education. *Pediatr Phys Ther.* 1995;7(3):143.
3. Galanti G. *Caring for Patients from Different Cultures: Case Studies from American Hospitals.* 2d ed. Philadelphia, PA: University of Pennsylvania Press; 1997:19, 32, 40, 65, 122-123.
4. Julia MC. *Multicultural Awareness in the Health Care Professions.* Boston, MA: Allyn and Bacon; 1996:179. Cf. Nong TA. Pseudo-battered child syndrome. *JAMA.* 1976;623:2288.
5. The case is inspired by a chapter in Lynch EW, Hanson MJ, eds. *Developing Cross-Cultural Competence: A Guide for Working with Young Children and Their Families.* Baltimore, MD: Paul Brookes Publishing Compmany; 1992:89-115.
6. Jecker NS, Carrese JA, Pearman RA. Caring for patients in cross-cultural settings. *Hastings Cent Rep.* 1995;25(1):6-14.

7. *Los Angeles Times*, June 21:S1, S8.

8. Wilkerson A. Homophobia and the moral authority of medicine. *J Homosex.* 1994;27(3-4):329-347.

9. Murphy MB, Gammie K, Gabard DL, Browne P. *Willingness of Home Health Physical Therapists to Provide Care for People with AIDS.* [Master's thesis]. Orange, CA: Chapman University; 1993.

10. Katz D. The functional approach to the study of attitudes. *Public Opin Quart.* 1960;24:163-204.

11. Dworkin AG, Dworkin RJ. *The Minority Report.* 3d ed. San Diego, CA: Harcourt Brace College Publishers; 1999:8.

12. Cole KC. Brain's use of shortcuts can be route to bias. *Los Angeles Times.* May 1, 1995:A1, A8.

13. Ponterotto JG, Pedersen PB. *Preventing Prejudice.* London, England: Sage Publications; 1983.

14. Frye M. Oppression. In: Rothenberg PS, ed. *Race, Class, and Gender in the United States.* 4th ed. New York, NY: St. Martin's Press; 1998:148.

15. Wachtel PL. *Race in the Mind of America.* New York, NY: Routledge; 1999: 108-109.

16. Young-Bruehl E. *The Anatomy of Prejudices.* Cambridge, MA: Harvard University Press; 1996.

17. Gabard DL, Cooper TL. Race: constructions and dilemmas. *Admin Soc.* 1998;30(4):339-356. For a more thorough discussion, see Montague A, *Man's Most Dangerous Myth.* 6th ed. London: Sage Publications; 1997.

18. Venter JC, Adams MD, Myers EW, et al. The sequence of the human genome. *Science.* February 16, 2001;291:1304-1349.

19. Miestel R. Tiny disparities in human genes go a long way, studies find. *Los Angeles Times.* February 12, 2001:A1, A20.

20. Hahn BA. Children's health: racial and ethnic differences in the use of prescription medications. *Pediatrics.* 1995;95:727-732.

21. Yergan J, Flood AB, LoFerfo JP, Diehr P. Relationship between patient race and the intensity of hospital services. *Med Care.* 1987;25:592-603.

22. Williams DR, Lavizzo-Mourey R, Warren RC. The concept of race and health status in America. *Public Health Rep.* 1994;109:26-41.

23. Gittelsohn AM, Halpern J, Sanchez RL. Income, race, and surgery in Maryland. *Am J Public Health.* 1991;81:1435-1441.

24. Wenneker MB, Epstein AM. Racial inequalities in the use of procedures for patients with ischemic heart disease in Massachusetts. *JAMA.* 1989;261:253-257.

25. Levy DR. White doctors and black patients: influence of race on the doctor-patient relationship. *Pediatrics.* 1985;75:639-643.

26. Blendon RJ, Aiken LH, Freeman HE, Corey CR. Access to medical care for black and while Americans: a matter of continuing concern. *JAMA.* 1989;261:278-281.

27. Chang SW, Kerlikowske K, Napoles-Springer A, Posner SF, Sicles EA, Perez-Stable EJ. Racial differences in timeliness of follow-up after abnormal screening mammography. *Cancer.* 1996;78:1395-1405.

28. Kahn KL, Pearson ML, Harrison ER, et al. Health care for black and poor hospitalized medicare patients. *JAMA.* 1994;271:1169-1174.

29. Carlisle DM, Leake BD, Shapiro MF. Racial and ethnic disparities in the use of cardio-vascular procedures: associations with type of health insurance. *Am J Public Health.* 1997;87:263-267.

30. Peterson ED, Shaw LK, DeLong ER, et al. Racial variation in the use of coronary revascularization procedures: Are the differences real? Do they matter? *N Engl J Med.* 1997;336:480-486.

31. Jones CP, LaVeist TA, Lillie-Blanton M. "Race" in the epidemiologic literature: an examination of the *American Journal of Epidemiology,* 1921–1990. *Am J Epidemiol.* November 15, 1991:1079-1084.

32. Dunn D. Women: the 51 percent minority. In: Dworkin AG, Dworkin RJ, eds. *The Minority Report: An Introduction to Racial, Ethnic, and Gender Relations.* 3d ed. New York, NY: Harcourt Brace College Publishers; 1999:415-435.

33. Shields CJ. How schools shortchange girls. *Curriculum Rev.* 1992;3-5.

34. American Association of University Women, Educational Foundation; American Institutes for Research. *Gender Gaps: Where Schools Still Fail Our Children.* Washington, DC: Marlowe & Co.; 1999.

35. Outcomes of education. *Digest of Educational Statistics, 1999.* Chapter 5. Available at: http://nces.ed.gov/pubs2000/Digest99/chapter5.html. Accessed March 9, 2001.

36. Education Statistics Quarterly: Postsecondary Education. Available at: http://nces.ed.gov/pubs2001/quarterly/winter/postsecondary/p_section1.html. Accessed March 9, 2001.

37. Wannell T, Caron N. *The Gender Earnings Gap Among Recent Postsecondary Graduates, 1984–92.* Ottawa, Canada: Business and Labour Market Analysis Group, Statistics Canada; 1994.

38. Bowlus AJ. A search interpretation of male-female wage differentials. *J Labor Econ.* 1997;15:625-657.

39. Rosenblatt RA. "Glass ceiling" still too hard to crack, U.S. panel finds. *Los Angeles Times.* March 16, 1995:A1.

40. Krieger N, Fee E. Manmade medicine and women's health: the biopolitics of sex/gender and race/ethnicity. *Int J of Health Serv.* 1994;24:265-283.

41. Nadelson C. Ethics, empathy, and gender in health care. *Am J Psychiatry.* 1993;150:1309-1314.

42. Ayanian JZ, Epstein AM. Differences in the use of procedures between women and men hospitalized for coronary heart disease. *N Engl J Med.* 1991;325:221-225.

43. Steingart RM, Packer M, Hamm P, et al. Sex differences in the management of coronary artery disease. *N Engl J Med.* 1991;325:226-230.

44. Palca J. Women left out at NIH. *Science.* 1990;248:1610-1602.

45. Armitage KJ, Schneidermann LJ, Bass RA. Response of physicians to medical complaints in men and women. *JAMA.* May 1979;241:2186-2187.

46. Berstein B, Kane R. Physicians' attitudes toward female patients. *Med Care.* June 1981;19:600-608.

47. *Killing Us Softly 3: Advertising's Image of Women, with Jean Kilbourne.* Northampton, MA: 2000 Media Education Foundation; 2000.

48. Hooks B. Feminism: A transformational politic. In: Rothenberg PS, ed. *Race, Class, and Gender in the United States: An Integrated Study.* 4th ed. New York, NY: St. Martin's Press; 1998:581.

49. Tong RP. *Feminist Thought.* 2d ed. Boulder, CO: Westview Press; 1998.

50. Wolf SM, ed. *Feminism and Bioethics: Beyond Reproduction.* Introduction. New York, NY: Oxford University Press; 1996:8.

51. Holmes HB, Purdy LM, eds. *Feminist Perspectives in Medical Ethics.* Bloomington, IN: Indiana University Press; 1992.

52. Munson R. *Intervention and Reflection: Basic Issues in Medical Ethics.* 6th ed. Belmont, CA: Wadsworth/Thomson Learning; 2000.

53. Mullett S. Shifting perspective: a new approach to ethics. In: Boss JA, ed. *Perspectives on Ethics.* Mountain View, CA: Mayfield Publishing Company; 1998:17-22.

54. U.S. Government, Executive Order No. 10925, 3 C.F.R. 448, 449-450.

55. Spann FA. *The Law of Affirmative Action: Twenty-Five Years of Supreme Court Decisions on Race and Remedies.* New York, NY: New York University Press; 2000.

56. Rothenberg PS, ed. *Race, Class, and Gender in the United States.* 4th ed. New York, NY: St. Martin's Press; 1998:240.

57. Caplan L. *Up Against the Law: Affirmative Action and the Supreme Court.* New York, NY: Twentieth Century Fund Press; 1997:18.

58. American Association of University Professors. Does diversity make a difference? A research report. *Academe: Bulletin of the American Association of University Professors.* 2000;86(5):54-57.

59. Deville K. Defending diversity: affirmative action and medical education. *Am J Public Health.* 1999;89(8):1258.

60. Keith SN, Bell RM, Swanson AG, Williams AP. Effects of affirmative action in medical schools: a study of the class of 1975. *N Engl J Med.* 1985;313:1519-1525.

61. Komaromy M, Grumbach K, Drake M, et al. The role of black and Hispanic physicians in providing health care for underserved populations. *N Engl J Med.* 1996;334:1305-1310.

62. Nickens HW. The rationale for minority-target programs in medicine in the 1990s. *JAMA.* 1992;267:2390-2391.

63. Steinbrook R. Diversity in medicine. *N Engl J Med.* 1996;334:1327-1328.

64. Xu G, Fields SK, Lane C, Veloski JJ, Barzansky B, Martine CJ. The relationship between the race/ethnicity of generalist physicians and their care for underserved populations. *Am J Public Health.* 1997;87:817-822.

65. Gabard DL, Baumeister M, Takahashi R, Wells A, Canfield J. Barriers to potential non-white students in physical therapy. *J Phys Ther Edu.* 1997;11(2):38-45.

66. American Physical Therapy Association, Education Division, 2000.

67. Roush SE. Shifting the paradigm of disability. *PT Magazine.* June 1993:50.

68. Rothstein JM. Editor's note. *Phys Ther.* 1997;77(7):712.

69. MacIntyre A. *Dependent Rational Animals: Why We Human Beings Need the Virtues.* Chicago: Open Court; 1999.

70. Frierson JG. *Employer's Guide to the Americans With Disabilities Act.* 2d ed. Washington, DC: Bureau of National Affairs; 1995:6.

71. Board of Trustees of the University of Alabama, Garrett V, et al. No. 99-1240. Available at: http://www.supremecourtus.gov/. Accessed on March 7, 2001.

72. Silvers A, Wasserman D, Mahowald MB, eds. *Disability, Difference, Discrimination: Perspectives on Justice in Bioethics and Public Policy.* Lanham, MD: Rowman & Littlefield; 1998.

73. Steingold FS. *The Employer's Legal Handbook.* 3d ed. Berkeley, CA: Nolo; 1999.

74. Milrone JA. Reasonable accommodation in disability law. *PT Magazine.* March 1995:68-69.

75. Warnick MP. The ADA and the health care workplace. *J Med Pract Manag.* 1999;15(1):36-41.

76. Scott M. Letter to the editor. *JAMA.* 1999;282(12):1131.

77. White CC. Health care professionals and the treatment of HIV-positive patients: is there an affirmative duty to treat under common law, the Rehabilitation Act, or the Americans with Disability Act? *J. Legal Med.* 1999;20(1):1-44.

78. See Sullivan A. *Virtually Normal: An Argument About Homosexuality.* New York, NY: Vintage; 1996.

79. Munson R. Moral principles, ethical theories, and medical decisions: an introduction. In: Munson R, ed. *Intervention and Reflection: Basic Issues in Medical Ethics.* 6th ed. Belmont, CA: Wadsworth; 2000:54.

80. Parry K. Culture and personal meanings. *PT Magazine.* October 1994:44.

Meaningful Life and Death

*S*hould a physical therapist use charm and/or medical expertise to coerce a patient into forestalling a death that the patient has accepted?

Keywords

Meaningful life
Refusing therapy
Suicide
Rule of Double Effect
Natural Law Doctrine
Involuntary euthanasia

Nonvoluntary euthanasia
Voluntary passive euthanasia
Voluntary active euthanasia
Assisted suicide
Duty to die

Jim Yonemoto

Jim Yonemoto is a physical therapist employed at a hospital. He has been assigned a patient recovering from surgery for a total hip arthroplasty. The patient will need three weeks of therapy that will include active range of motion, strengthening, and gait training. Everything looks typical until the therapist learns that the patient has a life-threatening cancer. The nursing staff, in administering routine care, had noticed three darkly pigmented moles on the patient's back. A dermatologist was called in to do a biopsy, which led to a diagnosis of multiple-site stage-four melanoma. Further tests revealed that the cancer had invaded the lymph nodes. The information about the cancer has no direct implication for the services provided by the therapist, but does it have any wider relevance to how Jim should interact with the patient?

Some physical therapists rarely work with patients who have life-threatening illnesses, and other therapists, such as those in hospice care or in skilled nursing facilities, work with many. Either way, the topic of death is not incidental to therapists. Life-threatening diseases multiply anxieties in patients and their families, and sometimes they affect the therapeutic regimen. Moreover, therapists need to understand their own responses to death in order to communicate effectively with patients and to provide emotional support.

We begin by establishing a broad context for the meaning, or rather meanings, of death that bear on our shared humanity. Invariably, those meanings are linked to **meaningful life**—not in the sense of all human beings having moral significance, but in the sense of individuals experiencing their own lives as worthwhile rather than as worthless, pointless, or futile.[1] Why do we fear death? Which fears are reasonable? How should we respond to those fears in ourselves and others?

Next, we turn to practical questions about understanding and communicating with patients who have life-threatening diseases. We also discuss the dynamics of interacting with family members, especially when the patient is a child.

We conclude by discussing suicide, assisted suicide, and euthanasia. At first glance these topics seem removed from the work of physical therapists, yet these issues are becoming increasingly relevant to all health professionals. For example, what should a physical therapist do upon learning that a patient is planning an assisted suicide, or when a patient with whom the therapist has a long-term relationship "sounds out" views on assisted suicide? Which items should a therapist question before beginning treatment of a patient whose chart contains a "Do Not Resuscitate" (DNR) order?

Fear and Acceptance of Death

Within the context of humanity in general, most of us calmly acknowledge the need for death. An immortal species would quickly overpopulate the biosphere, destroying ecosystems that make possible ongoing cycles of new life. But on an individual level, particularly concerning ourselves and those we love, accepting death is more difficult. Understanding ourselves as part of a wider biological and social unit can be an important part of achieving acceptance, but it does not remove our fears of death. Most of the time those fears remain muted, as they did for Ivan Ilych, the protagonist in Leo Tolstoy's *Death of Ivan Ilych*. Ilych lived a comfortable, busy life in which his death was either inconceivable or at most an abstract possibility. Then, suddenly, he was struck with a life-threatening illness:

> In the depth of his heart he knew he was dying, but not only was he unaccustomed to such an idea, he simply could not grasp it, could not grasp it at all.
> The syllogism he had learned from Kiesewetter's logic—"Caius is a man, men are mortal, therefore Caius is mortal"—had always seemed to him correct as applied to Caius, but by no means to himself. That man Caius represented man in the abstract, and so the reasoning was perfectly sound; but he was not Caius, not an abstract man; he had always been a creature quite, quite distinct from all the others.[2]

Ilych gradually comes to comprehend and accept that he is dying. In doing so, he undergoes a moral transformation that yields a deepened appreciation of the importance of love and caring relationships. Initially, the appreciation is accompanied by regret about having failed to live a better life, but gradually it brings a reassuring sense that it is never too late to change how we relate to others. At the same time, he becomes tormented by the pretense of his family, friends, and even his physician, who have implied that he is simply ill, not dying, and would eventually return to normal life. Instead of providing hope and optimism, the pretense hinders the honest communication that Ilych desires, beginning with the simple acknowledgment that he is dying. It also leads others to stay away from him, especially at times when his suffering threatens to overwhelm him and when he is most in need of compassion and simple comfort.

Only Gerasim, a young household assistant, is able to provide support. Unobtrusive, yet willing to listen whenever Ilych wants to talk, Gerasim reassures him that he wants to help in any way he can. Sometimes what helps most are simple things, such as elevating Ilych's legs, or touching him gently but with a reassuring firmness. Other times Ilych's mood improves when he looks forward to the regular return of Gerasim, with his confident and reassuring presence. Gerasim's caring has a further influence in leading Ilych to reflect on the values that give life meaning.

Why Do We Fear Death?

This "why" is ambiguous: it might be a request for causes (influences, motives, explanations) or for reasons (justifications). Undoubtedly, the *causes* include genetic factors: fear of death manifests our biological will to survive and develop. The causes might also include social influences. Daniel Callahan, a prominent medical ethicist, outlines the evolution of our social responses to death.[3] Before modern medicine, illnesses leading to death were typically of short duration, in contrast to the chronic conditions experienced frequently today. The approach of death was something that was acknowledged, with death taking place at home among a gathering of friends and relatives and evoking support of the wider community. By the 20th century, nearly a complete reversal had occurred. Today, when death appears imminent, the dying are removed from their familiar surroundings to the sterile isolation of a hospital room, where they may be attended by one or two family members, depending on the visiting rules of the organization, until they die. Their bodies are immediately removed and taken to a funeral home, which applies a veneer of cosmetics to hide the appearance of death.

Another major social influence that has profoundly affected the way we view death is contained in the military metaphors used to define the purpose of medicine as well as how patients think about disease.[4] We wage wars on illnesses, and these wars gradually evolve into the ultimate war on death. Witness recent news articles describing the possibility of defeating death through genetic research. We are currently in a war against breast cancer, a war on Alzheimer's disease, and a battle against leukemia. These military metaphors imply that if we win enough battles, we might eventually win the war against death. But of course, death is inevitable.

The consequences of a war not won, an inevitable loss, are both institutional and private. Medicine often sees death as a defeat, an embarrassment to be ignored, disposed of quickly and quietly. As individuals, we view the dead as warriors who lost the battle. It would be simplistic to blame the medical profession for this transformation of death from a manageable event into life's greatest horror. All of us are co-conspirators when we demand all services that might extend our existence even for just an hour, regardless of the fact that the cost will be assumed by others. With the current cost of medical care, it is now possible for each generation not only to exhaust its own resources, but also to steal from its successor.

The causes that explain why we fear death are of great interest, but we are even more concerned with the "why" of *reasons*: What reasons are there that justify fearing death, and are they good reasons, all things considered? The Stoic philosophers of classical Greece and the Roman Empire exerted considerable ingenuity in portraying all fears of death as irrational. Epictetus was typical: "Men are disturbed not by the things which happen, but by the opinions about the things: for example, death is nothing terrible . . . [but instead] the opinion about death, that it is terrible, is the terrible thing."[5]

The Stoic ideal was to attain self-sufficiency and serenity by focusing life entirely on what is in one's power, especially beliefs and attitudes, and by not becoming emotionally upset by anything beyond that power. According to Epictetus, "If you would have your children and your wife and your friends to live for ever, you are silly; for you would have the things which are not in your power to be in your power."[5(p176)] True enough, how we perceive death shapes our fears about it. Our beliefs and values are under our control to a degree greater than we usually assume. Few of us, however, would purchase complete serenity at the cost of not caring deeply.

There are many different types of fears of death, some rational and some not, whose importance differs considerably among individuals. We might sort them into three general categories: fears of dying prematurely, fears of the process of dying, and fears about being dead. Cutting across these groupings is a distinction between fears about one's own well-being (based on self-interested reasons) and fears about the well-being of others (based on altruistic reasons).

The first category, fears about dying prematurely, comprises fears about dying before we or people we love have an opportunity for full and satisfying lives. Needless to say, these fears are eminently healthy and rational. It is tragic when young children die before they have a chance to develop fully, and tragic when young adults are killed before they have a full opportunity to develop their talents. It is also tragic when adults in their prime die before experiencing fulfilling love, meaningful work, or raising their children, and in general before living out a reasonable life plan. However, people fortunate enough to find inexhaustible joy in life might also regard death at any time as "premature." Upon reflection, however, most people accept the prospects of a "natural life span" that concludes with a "tolerable death," as Daniel Callahan suggests:

> My definition of a "tolerable death" is this: the individual event of death at
> that stage in a life span when (a) one's life possibilities have on the whole been
> accomplished; (b) one's moral obligations to those for whom one has had
> responsibility [especially one's children] have been discharged; and (c) one's
> death will not seem to others an offense to sense or sensibility [at least after a
> usual period of mourning], or tempt others to despair and rage at the finitude
> of human existence. . . . A "natural life span" may then be defined as one in
> which life's possibilities have on the whole been achieved and after which death
> may be understood as a sad, but nonetheless relatively acceptable, event.[3(p66)]

The second category of fears is focused on the process of dying, and includes fears of pain, disability, and suffering. It also includes fears about loss of control and self-determination—for example, anxieties about having to leave one's home to live in a medical facility. In most cases, pain can be controlled within tolerable limits with proper medical management, but loss of control overall renders us profoundly vulnerable and dependent, frequently inducing a sense of shame, or at least embarrassment. Like pain, death is intensely private, but in the context of a medical facility, privacy is lost. The constant unwanted intrusion of strangers threatens whatever dignity we might hope to keep until the very end.[6]

Some fears concerning the process of dying are linked to our relationships with people we care about: Will I become an emotional or financial burden on my family? Who will care for my children if I am hospitalized? Will my family be left with unaffordable debt? Will I become isolated and lose close contact with my family because they have jobs (and lives) to maintain? Some of these fears are exaggerated and can be alleviated by health-care providers by assuring patients they will receive support from caring professionals. While other fears about family and loss of control might be entirely justified, even then caring professionals can help simply by listening sympathetically when patients wish to talk (without intrusively forcing them to talk).

Perhaps the most complex of the fears about the process of dying is suffering, which encompasses more than physical pain. Callahan distinguishes between two levels of suffering:[7] at level one, he places the fear and dread of coping with the illness, which affects how that illness will impact the person's life and wholeness as a person; at level two, he places the more fundamental suffering that occurs as individuals try to find a purpose in their existence. Level one seems self-explanatory, but level two is more complex. Some individuals might have religious beliefs that help define their existence, but many others, even if they hold strong religious beliefs, still search for a sense of meaning and purpose in their individual lives.

The process of this search, or life review, can be something quite separate from a system of beliefs about an afterlife. J. Hardwig defines this process as "spiritual," although others might call it moral.[8,9] He contends that when the values and assumptions of a lifetime fail to coalesce into a meaningful unity, individuals undergo "spiritual suffering," which minimizes all other concerns about health care, including advance directives. There may also be a major depressive disorder involved that might resemble this type of spiritual suffering. Only a psychiatrist or someone similarly trained can distinguish the suffering characteristic of pathological "depression" from the suffering involved in examining life's meaning.

The third category of fears concerns those about being dead. For some people, these fears center on uncertainties about what happens to a person after death: Is there life after death, and what is it like? The uncertainties also include specific fears about the individual's own circumstances: What is my fate and the fate of people I love—perhaps heaven, or something else? Still another cluster of fears concerns anxieties about the possibility of one's sheer nonexistence.[10] These fears center on the permanent ending of one's present activities, relationships, and other interests that give life significance.

The Health Professional's Response

Patients are individuals with their own beliefs about these "existential fears." Many of these beliefs are formed in conjunction with the patient's religious principles, and every religion works out its own set of beliefs about what occurs at death. We do not delve into this area because religious discussions typically do not enter into physical therapists' care of patients, and often this type of discussion is inappropriate. Instead, care of patients requires being respectful of individuals' religious beliefs and practices that impact their coping with death and dying. Health professionals sometimes find it comfortable to avoid emotional engagement with death, even though (and partly because) they deal with it more often than most people. To some extent, as noted in Chapter 4, this emotional reserve functions as an aspect of professional distance that enables therapists to cope in difficult roles without burnout. Yet overdetachment is not the only or best alternative in caring for patients.

Much has been written about why physicians in particular too often abandon patients once death becomes certain. Dr. Sherwin B. Nuland's summary observations are insightful:

> [O]f all the professions, medicine is the one most likely to attract people with high personal anxieties about dying. We become doctors because our ability to cure gives us power over the death of which we are so afraid, and loss of that power poses such a significant threat that we must turn away from it, and therefore from the patient who personifies our weakness. Doctors are people who succeed—that is how they survived the fierce competition to achieve their medical degree, their training, and their position. Like other highly talented people, they require constant reassurance of their abilities. To be unsuccessful is to endure a blow to self-image that is poorly tolerated by members of this most egocentric of professions.[11]

Nuland adds that physicians have a powerful need to exercise control, and the threat of their patients' deaths comes as the ultimate threat to that sense of control. What is needed is a greater humility in the teeth of inexorable reality, as well as a form of medicine that keeps the patient's welfare paramount, not the ego of professionals.

Without being sentimental, many health professionals report that caring for dying patients can evoke and be guided by positive emotions of peace and acceptance of death as a natural process. Some even express a sense of privilege in being able to help people during their final hours.[12] They also report that the deepest frustrations, those that often cause burnout, come when medical care is used in situations in which there is no hope of benefit to the patient, or when an aloof physician who spends little time with patients is insensitive to their suffering.[12(p128)] Here, as is so often the case, healthy emotions are indicators of good medical care.

Helping Patients Who Have Cancer

"Cancer" is a frightening word. Because cancer is characterized by malignant tumors that potentially have unlimited growth and expansion, "cancer" connotes a life-threatening disease. Yet, cancer is not one thing. Like bacterial or viral diseases, there are over a hundred forms of cancer that vary greatly in form and severity. Many cancers are now curable or allow many years of healthy life. Others are more serious, as in the case of Marilyn French, the feminist activist and author of the bestseller *The Women's Room*.

Marilyn French

Marilyn French was diagnosed with metastasized esophageal cancer in 1992, when she was 61 years old. At the time, only one in five patients survived nonmetastasized esophageal cancer and no one survived metastasized esophageal cancer. Her oncologist told her that even with chemotherapy she had only one year to live. The oncologist was mistaken: French would prove to be one of those "miracle patients" who overthrow what medicine "knows" at a given time, possibly because she was given an experimental combination of concurrent chemotherapy and radiation. Yet, as suggested by the title of her memoir published six years later, *A Season in Hell*, she was to undergo a terrible ordeal. The chemotherapy and radiation treatments caused multiple side effects, including brain seizures that led to a 12-day coma, a heart attack, diabetes, and severe arthritis, not to mention spinal fractures when she went to a masseuse to relieve pain. It is likely she will need physical therapy for the rest of her life.

During her coma, an emergency room physician informed her family that she was dead, once again reminding us that medicine is something less than an exact science. Her living will specified no further medical interventions at that point, but her family ignored the document. Later, during an especially difficult time, she would express anger that the document had been ignored. Still later, after her condition improved, she would be grateful it had been ignored. ⬚

A central theme in French's memoir is the importance of maintaining hope when confronting serious illness. She found herself surprised by her own determination to survive: "In fierce blind insistence, I decided I had a chance to survive and would count on that."[13] She was also surprised by her capacity for hope well beyond what the evidence would seem to say was reasonable. Within hours of being informed that she had terminal cancer, she erased the word "terminal" from her consciousness and never used it in thinking about her disease or communicating with others about it. Although she prided herself on being a person who prizes truth, she engaged in what she later confessed was blatant self-deception about her chances of survival.

Another theme in French's memoir is the importance of health professionals' support of hopefulness, or at least their striving to not destroy a patient's hope.[13] To be sure, professionals must be honest in dealing with patients, whose fears are only magnified when they sense that essential information is being withheld. Nevertheless, French urges that the focus be on conveying an attitude of hope. She reports that her oncologist was exceptionally skilled but unnecessarily dour and pessimistic in dealing with patients, no doubt because most of his patients died. In sharp contrast to Ivan Ilych, she found herself in desperate need of health professionals who conveyed, through manner and style as well as words, a sense that things would improve.

French contrasts two physical therapists, selected from dozens who worked with her during years of chronic illness. One was the therapist who treated her while she was hospitalized for 20-minute sessions several times a week during recovery from her coma. Unable to support her head or sit up by herself, she was reduced to utter helplessness by muscles that had atrophied. She needed emotional support as much as physical support, but the therapist provided only the latter:

> She was young, efficient, and mechanical; she made no personal connection with her patients—not at least with me—and had no affect whatever. I am sure that to her I was just one more helpless elderly woman, but I have since met so many warm, devoted, caring physiotherapists that I wonder if she was in the wrong field. Still, she did her job. She urged me to walk holding on to a walker.[13(p149)]

Despite the fact that her weight increased enough for her to return home, she continued to need assistance, as her mobility was limited. She described herself as emotionally traumatized and as grieving for herself. A team of nurses and physical therapists would be central to her recuperation. Michael, the first therapist sent by the hospital, "was militantly cheerful and personally seductive; he employed charm to help his patients, especially elderly women. But I did not dislike him: his style was more agreeable than the mechanical style of the therapist in the hospital."[13(p157)] He also liked to give orders to the nurses about the requisite exercises; some of these orders French chose not to heed. Yet French came to trust him, to trust both his expertise and his commitment to her well-being. She would continue to seek his help and trust his judgment for many years.

At one point, French suddenly developed severe arthritis, which neither drugs nor electrical acupuncture helped. Michael said he could help her regain the use of her arm and hands, but the process would involve great pain. Without hesitation, French said, "Do it." The therapy consisted of sessions of an hour of exercises followed by a brief "torture time," in which Michael bent the joint until she heard the adhesions cracking. After four months she regained normal flexibility.

Professional manner and personal style in part reflect a therapist's unique personality, but in large measure they are the product of the development of communication and caring skills to respond to the special needs and personalities of patients. That growth takes time, of course, but it can be hastened by insights such as those Debbra Flomenhoft offers. Flomenhoft, who is a physical therapist and a survivor of cancer, points out that therapists' fears of saying the wrong thing, or of revealing too much, can lead to the far worse effect of avoidance that make patients feel not only isolated but rejected. "The content of the response, the specific words, is usually not important. The gesture of reaching out to the patient can speak far louder than words."[14]

Some of Flomenhoft's recommendations about caring responses in helping patients who have cancer include:

- "Viewing cancer as a chronic illness that most people live with for a long time can help to keep the disease in proper perspective," Flomenhoft says, by focusing on "living with cancer" rather than the more-usual "dying of cancer."[14]

- Cultivate a confident bedside manner, one that communicates that one can and will help. This bedside manner includes body language in the form of eye contact and a confident grip in touching a patient.

- Learn to be aware of your own feelings, to keep any disruptive feelings from interfering with helping. It is normal in caring for some patients to feel moments of anger, irritation, and frustration, as well as fear and self-doubt.

- Listen actively. When patients ask the hard questions, such as "Why me?" they do not expect health professionals to have the answers; instead they are expressing their grief, frustration, and anger. The appropriate response is supportive listening.

- Ask what a patient is feeling, rather than assuming you know. Kubler-Ross provided valuable studies about five stages of adjustment to death: denial, anger, bargaining ("If God will let me live, I will . . ."), depression, and acceptance.[15] Yet these stages are not sequential or universal. A patient might experience states of anger, depression, denial, and any number of other emotions over the course of a month or even a day.

- Rather than feeling pressure to initiate a conversation about cancer, pick up on patients' cues that they want to talk. When appropriate, adopt the patients' way of talking; for example, if they use the word "tumor" rather than "cancer," follow their lead.

- Touch matters. Like others, therapists vary in how demonstrative they are. Even at difficult moments, hugging might be neither necessary nor appropriate. Flomenhoft recalls how much it meant to her that when her physician had to convey the news that her tumor was malignant, he touched and stroked her ankle as he looked into her eyes.

- Echoing Marilyn French's observations, Flomenhoft advises finding a way to be both honest and hopeful, realistic and positive, at the same time. Hope is both curative (the placebo effect!) and adds meaning to the time remaining. Don't force a patient to "be realistic" when they choose even false hope as their way of coping.

- "Be careful not to isolate a patient, especially as death approaches," Flomenhoft emphasizes. "People are alive until the very moment of death, and time is particularly precious when it is limited."[14(p1234)] Even after treatment stops, try to maintain some contact, especially if you have worked for a long period with a patient, to prevent the patient from feeling abandoned.

Refusing Therapy

As discussed in Chapter 3, the general right to autonomy gives competent patients, or their designated surrogates, the specific right to refuse unwanted therapy. Unwanted therapy includes life-essential treatment as well as routine physical therapy during a terminal illness.

Henry and Sonia

Henry is a 76-year-old man in a private facility that combines skilled nursing and assisted living and takes both Medicare and private paying patients. He is there to receive care and physical therapy following a total hip replacement. Henry's wife of 58 years died two years earlier, and he has one surviving son who lives in another state. The son is married and has no children, and there has been no communication between them since the death of Henry's wife. Their relationship has always been distant, preserved at even this level largely to please his wife. Before his retirement, Henry owned a small but reasonably successful printing shop. He worked long hours, including most weekends. During this time he developed no meaningful hobbies or social networks.

His therapist, Sonia, saw immediately that he was withdrawn but capable of sustained conversations that demonstrated an uncommon level of self-awareness. During their early sessions Henry revealed many aspects of his life with surprising candor. He told Sonia that he did not follow any particular religion, but he considered himself to be spiritual and was trying to decide what was best for him at this time of life. The therapy progressed at a reasonable pace, but then Henry became progressively less interested in ambulation and more interested in talking socially with Sonia. After a month, Henry told Sonia that he did not want to do therapy any longer, but he would appreciate her stopping by occasionally for conversation.

Sonia explained that without therapy he was unlikely to become independent again. He would also run an increased risk of respiratory infection by remaining sedentary. Patients who do nothing, she added bluntly, fail to survive very long. She felt confident he would reconsider. Instead, he confided that he did not wish to live much longer. For him, life lost its meaning when his wife died, and now he could foresee only an increasingly dependent life. Although he has private insurance and a retirement portfolio more than adequate to meet his needs, he said he preferred to leave his money to his son, partly as repayment for his absence during his son's youth.

Sonia has admitted to herself that over the years she has seen a number of men and women who just seemed to give up after the death of a partner, and no amount of therapy seemed to make a difference. She senses that Henry is approaching death, but she is unsure of her professional role in helping him. Should she use their relationship as leverage to persuade him to continue therapy? ◩

We leave further discussion of this case to the Discussion Question section of this chapter, turning now to the broader context for understanding the moral and legal rights of Henry, and of all of us, to refuse life-extending treatments. Legal recognition of this moral right has been established gradually, through several decades of court rulings. Here are a few highlights.[16]

1976: The New Jersey Supreme Court ruled that the parents of Karen Ann Quinlan had a "right to privacy" that permitted them to have her removed from a respirator. A year earlier Karen had stopped breathing and slipped into an irreversible coma. The cause was never determined with certainty, and it is not clear whether a combination of drugs and alcohol played a role. Her parents requested that the respirator be removed, but because Karen was over the age of 21, they had to go to court to be appointed her legal guardians and to seek authority to remove her from the respirator. Although the request was denied by a lower court, the state's Supreme Court overruled the denial. (Such reversals at different levels of the court system, as well as close votes, have been typical of rulings concerning the ending of life.) The respirator was removed, setting a legal precedent that allows patients to refuse even the most essential life-saving technology. (Contrary to expectation, Karen did not die. She lingered for ten years in a vegetative state, but not "brain dead," sustained by intravenous nutrition and hydration.)

1977: California passed the Natural Death Act authorizing competent adults to sign "living wills" expressing their desires regarding "artificial" life support if terminal and "death is imminent." Other states quickly followed suit in establishing these "advance directives."

1981: *The Report of the President's Commission for the Study of Ethical Problems in Medicine* recommended a "whole-brain" concept of death, and the recommendation quickly shaped new state laws. Prior to this, the traditional legal definition of death used a heart-lung concept: that persons are dead when cardiopulmonary activity stops permanently. The new concept defined death as the cessation of all electrical activity in the brain. At that time, a person is considered legally dead, such that removal of life support is permissible. The new concept and laws have other legal implications, including the handling of permission to transplant organs (if so authorized by the individual or family), burial, cessation of health-care insurance, distribution of inheritance according to a will, and payment of life insurance to a beneficiary.

1990: The U.S. Supreme Court ruled in the Nancy Cruzan case, a landmark "end-of-life" decision, that the Fourteenth Amendment's "liberty interest" provides a constitutional basis for advance directives (such as living wills), in which an individual specifies which general types of medical procedures may be used, and for durable power of attorney documents, which designate a surrogate decision maker if a person becomes incompetent to make decisions about medical procedures. For the first time, the Court included intravenous nutrition and hydration as "medical procedures."

1991: A federal statute, the Patient Self-Determination Act, was enacted requiring health-care facilities that receive federal funds to inform newly-admitted patients about relevant state laws concerning refusal or discontinuation of medical treatment.

As these rulings suggest, the law has slowly moved toward recognizing greater legal rights of individuals to control treatment at the end of their lives. It should be noted that a living will by itself is not legally binding; it merely relays the patient's wishes. The durable power of attorney, however, has legal authority, and typically it is stipulated in that document that the designated surrogate decision maker is to follow the living will.

Nevertheless, recent studies suggest that, in practice, individuals often lack the control they believe they have. Only a small percentage of advance directives are being respected, for a variety of reasons: D. Grady states that "People lose or forge them; living wills are too vague to interpret; relatives disagree about what the patient wanted; hospital staff members mistakenly fear prosecution for terminating life support; or doctors overrule the family and refuse to stop treatment."[17]

One such case attracted national press coverage and generated two videos, *Please Let Me Die* and *Dax's Case*. These documented the refusal of medical personnel to stop treatment at the request of a competent patient, Dax Cowart.

Dax Cowart ◈

Dax Cowart was a pilot who was severely burned over two-thirds of his body in a propane gas explosion. He lost his sight, as well as the use of his hands, as a result of the accident. Painful treatments continued for over a year, and throughout this time he demanded that treatment cease and that he be allowed to die. He was examined by a psychiatrist who confirmed that he was competent, yet his demands were ignored. Although he later became a successful attorney, he still maintains that it was wrong to ignore his request to discontinue treatment.[18]

Cowart's case is not unusual. In a study involving 9,105 patients who were seriously ill, with approximately one-half receiving care before the enactment of the 1991 Patient Self-Determination Act and one-half after its enactment, it was "found that ADs [i.e., advance directives] did not result in a clinically relevant impact on resuscitation decision-making, even among those cases where intervention dramatically increased their documentation."[19]

Hamid

Hamid, a 71-year-old man with a history of lung and colon cancer, was admitted to the hospital with ataxia and headaches. An MRI was performed, and a brain tumor and hydrocephalus were discovered. With the help of a staff social worker, the patient completed a living will and informed his grandson that he did not believe that he would live and did not want surgery.

The patient began to exhibit new symptoms consistent with hydrocephalus, and emergency surgery was performed. He experienced respiratory failure and developed an extensive infection with a gram-negative organism in his spinal fluid. It was recorded in his chart, as was the existence of his living will, that the hospital's SUPPORT prognostic model predicted only a 10 percent chance of his surviving the next six months. Despite both documents, he spent 14 of his next 23 days of life in the ICU. "His wife noted that he would not 'want this,' but also that she 'could not bear to lose him.'"[19(p506)] At no point in time did the medical records reveal any discussion about his advance directive.

As this case suggests, and as noted in Chapter 3, the most difficult issues surrounding informed consent involve surrogate decision making in the cases of noncompetent adults and children. Yet there are also difficulties in the case of competent adults—for example, in interpreting DNR orders, a matter directly relevant to physical therapists.

If the DNR order has been decided by the medical treatment team because efforts to revive the patient would be futile—that is, they would not prolong life for any substantive time—then patient consent is not necessary. But, if the DNR order is issued without the consent of the patient or their legal surrogate when the resuscitation effort would likely be successful, it would be considered by most to be indefensible. When a physical therapist sees a DNR in the chart, deciding to honor it should be contingent on the answers to the following questions:

1. Was the order given because of medical futility?
2. If the DNR was ordered for reasons other than medical futility, did the patient consent?
3. Is the DNR signed and dated, and does it have the patient's name on the same page?[20]

Clearly, the first two items must first be confirmed with the originator of the DNR, not the patient. If there is any reason to doubt the authenticity of the response to the second item, the doubts can be resolved by talking with the patient. Item 3 is important because the therapist would wish to determine that the DNR was correctly intended for this patient, and that it was entered in the chart by someone with authority to issue the order. In addition, one should ask whether the order is dated, since relevant facts might have changed, rendering the order inappropriate. Unfortunately, some convalescent and skilled nursing homes inappropriately insert DNR orders into charts without the consent of the patient or their legal surrogate.

Suicide

What should a therapist do upon learning, or coming to suspect, that a patient is planning suicide? The specific context must be considered, as the following case suggests.

Mark and Dan

Mark was a 28-year-old Latino professional employed at the managerial level at the largest live theatre complex in Los Angeles. He worked long hours, and at first he attributed his fatigue to the pressure of a new theater season, a last-minute cancellation by a leading celebrity, and disappointing subscription sales for the new season. When he discovered a dark discoloration on his forearm, however, he decided to see his dermatologist. The dermatologist took a biopsy and questioned Mark about his HIV status. Mark said that he had not been tested because he had been sexually inactive for two or three years. He admitted that after his partner of five years left him with no explanation and no communication, he fell into a depression that work helped to alleviate. Recently he had considered dating again, but he lacked the energy for a social life. The dermatologist asked if he could draw a blood sample to be tested for HIV, and Mark agreed. At his next appointment the doctor informed him that he had Kaposi's sarcoma, a relatively rare skin cancer that was most often seen in persons with advanced HIV, which the blood test confirmed he had.

Mark had always been truthful; in fact, most of his friends chided him for being a little too honest. Consistent with his character, he informed his employer, physician, and dentist of his illness. He told his employer, hoping it would be understood why he needed time off from work to attend medical appointments and why he would need to reduce his hours from 60 to 40 hours per week. Understandably, his physician referred him to another physician who was more experienced in managing HIV. Less understandably, his dentist (whom he had been seeing since childhood) requested that Mark find someone else to attend to his dental needs. The dentist admitted to being afraid of the AIDS virus, despite knowing that standard precautions would protect him. Mark managed to find another dentist, but this was just the first of many encounters with professionals who treated him as a second-class citizen once they knew his sexual orientation and his HIV status.

Because he was in an advanced stage of AIDS, and because he could not tolerate the primary drug offered at the time because of adverse reactions, Mark's condition deteriorated quickly. The Kaposi's sarcoma appeared on his face and legs as well as on his back. Radiation and chemotherapy helped, but the lesions were still disfiguring. Fearing the effect on sales, his employer limited Mark's exposure to the public and essentially isolated him in his office. Mark decided that he simply did not have the energy to pursue legal redress, so he requested and received disability. The following week he called his parents, whom he had not seen—at their request—since he told them of his homosexuality. They stated that they were sorry but that he had brought this on himself and they would not be able to offer financial or other support. They also said that they would appreciate it if he would not say anything to their friends or his brothers and sisters.

Over the next two months the Kaposi's sarcoma re-emerged with renewed vigor and caused a blockage in the lymphatic system in his legs, resulting in swelling. His doctor recommended physical therapy for ADL and to assist with independent ambulation. Mark called on an old friend, Dan, who was a pediatric physical therapist, to help him find someone. Dan called several therapists working in home health care, but upon hearing Mark's diagnosis they stated that they did not think a patient could profit from their professional skills or that they were booked. Dan challenged two of the therapists, who had said that physical therapy would be ineffective for patients with AIDS, asking the therapists how a patient with AIDS differed from a patient with cancer, the elderly, or any other classification of patient in need of ADL and ambulating. The therapists said that they would not work with gay men even if they were HIV-negative.

Out of sheer frustration, Dan volunteered to help Mark after he finished work at the pediatric center, where he was chief physical therapist. Instructions on using a walker, wheelchair, toilet lift, and shower bench, along with gait training using crutches and a walker, all helped Mark achieve enough independence to manage. His friends provided some support, but they also had other commitments. As his T cell count dropped to below 50, Mark became terrified. He was disfigured, terrified of dying alone, and even more terrified of being dependent on others. He had neither the resources at this age nor the social support to anticipate much more than a protracted and painful death. The only person he really trusted was Dan, who had been reassuring and reliable, and with whom he had developed a deep friendship.

One day Mark informed Dan that he had requested and received 20 Seconal pills for back pain from two different physicians. He told Dan how much he had appreciated his help and his caring, but that he would like him to skip the next day. Dan knew what this meant, and he was unsure what to do. He could search for the Seconal and remove them, or he could call the doctor and inform him about what he thought Mark was going to do. Dan also considered staying with Mark until he died, so that he would not be alone. ▨

What should Dan do? Possible answers to this question will be explored in the Discussion Question section, and we will consider here the broader issue: What is suicide? The answer would seem clear enough: it is the intentional (not accidental) killing of oneself—voluntarily and with purpose. Yet in practice, what one counts as suicide depends in part on one's moral views about when killing oneself is justified. Suppose a physician's intention is to alleviate pain, at a patient's request, by requesting an increased morphine drip, and both the physician and patient know that it will kill the patient within a few days. This is considered an act of suicide by some, but others see it merely as an act of alleviating pain. For example, the Catholic tradition, which takes a strong stand against suicide, would justify the increased morphine dosage by appealing to a **"Rule of Double Effect,"** meaning, roughly, that an act that has a good and bad consequence is justified if the intent is solely to reach the good consequence (alleviating pain), not an unavoidable bad consequence (death). The Rule of Double Effect is a normative principle used to evaluate actions, but it also shapes how suicide is defined in this tradition.

Under the Rule of Double Effect, it is not the outcome that defines the rightness or wrongness of the action, but rather the intent. The rule attempts to distinguish between intended consequences and unintended consequences that are foreseen, and between direct and indirect consequences. Beauchamp and Childress outline four separate conditions necessary for the Rule of Double Effect to define an action as morally permissible:

1. *The nature of the act.* The act must be good, or at least morally neutral (independent of its consequences).

2. *The agent's intention.* The agent intends only the good effect. The bad effect can be foreseen, tolerated, and permitted, but it must not be intended.

3. *The distinction between means and effects.* The bad effect must not be a means to the good effect. If the good effect were the direct causal result of the bad effect, the agent would intend the bad effect in pursuit of the good effect.

4. *Proportionality between the good effect and the bad effect.* The good effect must outweigh the bad effect. The bad effect is permissible only if a proportionate reason is present that compensates for permitting the foreseen bad effect.[21]

By the Rule of Double Effect, if a pregnant woman develops a cancer in her uterus while pregnant, the surgeon may remove the cancer (in other words, the uterus) to save the woman's life, even though the abortion of the fetus is a foreseen consequence of removing the cancer. However, a surgeon may not induce an abortion to save a mother's life, as might be prognosticated if the mother's heart is failing as a result of the stress generated by the pregnancy.

Is suicide ever morally permissible? Ethical theories provide the language and general principles for discussing this question, but they do not by themselves provide the answer, which depends on the specific version of the ethical theory being applied. Consider rights ethics. Libertarians typically favor maximum freedom of choice for the patient, but other rights ethicists also emphasize the rights of family members, contributors to the social funding of medical care, democratically voted laws, and other issues. Similarly, act utilitarians usually favor allowing people to choose to lessen their suffering, including the suffering of being helpless and dependent, while rule utilitarians, who emphasize the possible abuses of a rule that justifies suicide, might object to some instances of suicide that act utilitarians accept.

Cutting across different types of ethical theories in this discussion is a striking contrast between two groups, liberals and conservatives (these terms are used here only in relation to suicide, not in their wider political senses).[22] Liberals emphasize freedom and being allowed to make one's own choices in matters that primarily concern oneself. Conservatives emphasize life as a gift that one has no right to misuse.

Liberals defend their view by emphasizing the principle of respect for autonomy. Clearly, there are many considerations facing a patient in determining how life should end. The quality of one's life might fall well below anything one finds tolerable. There can also be great suffering, including physical pain, which, in a minimum of cases, might be controllable only through heavy sedation. The cost of extended medical services might place a great financial burden on one's family, and even if the services are paid for by health insurance, some individuals might voluntarily prefer to see the services used to help others rather than themselves. Thus, the liberal viewpoint holds that, because there is no one mandatory way for all reasonable persons to balance such complexities, individuals should be allowed to make their own decisions.

Conservatives often ground their reasoning in appeals to religious faith. For example, Catholics appeal to the **Natural Law Doctrine** that says that humans have a "natural" (God-given) desire and goal of survival, which they view as violated by suicide and euthanasia. Liberals agree that we all have a natural desire for self-preservation, but they do not see that desire by itself as morally overriding the desire to end an unacceptable quality of life; they see the Natural Law as implicitly invoking religious doctrines that are not binding on everyone. In the arena of public discourse, conservatives have more influence when they argue that life is sacred and to be treasured no matter what one's religious beliefs. They reinforce this argument with the concern that the widespread practice of suicide, or even its toleration, will erode respect for human life. That appeal carries considerable force, even if liberals interpret respect for human life as encompassing death with dignity.

The differences between these liberal and conservative viewpoints are deep-seated, and it is unlikely that these opposing emphases will ever be reconciled. Perhaps some progress might be made by distinguishing between different types of situations in which individuals might consider suicide as an option. Thus, whereas Kant believed that suicide is never justified because it violates self-respect, Thomas E. Hill, Jr., a contemporary Kant-inspired ethicist, argues that suicide sometimes violates rational autonomy and other times manifests respect for it. He argues for this principle: "A morally ideal person will value life as a rational, autonomous agent for its own sake, at least provided that the life does not fall below a certain threshold of gross, irremediable, and uncompensated pain and suffering."[23]

Hill distinguishes seven types of suicide, the first four of which describe situations in which individuals fail to properly value themselves. They violate the ideal of respect for oneself as a rational person, whether or not they violate a duty:

1. *Impulsive suicide*: Persons commit suicide as a result of a brief but intense emotion, such as grief in losing a spouse or life partner, despair in losing one's job, or fear upon learning one has a serious illness.

2. *Apathetic suicide*: Persons commit suicide because of severe depression, whether temporary or chronic.

3. *Self-abasing suicide*: Persons are filled with self-loathing and commit suicide as a form of self-contempt or self-punishment.

4. *Hedonistic calculated suicide*: Persons commit suicide because they calculate that the future will probably bring more pain than pleasure.[24]

    Hill contrasts these situations with the following circumstances in which, he believes, suicide actually manifests, rather than violates, self-respect.

5. *Suicide to prevent subhuman life*: Persons commit suicide because they have good reason to believe that they will survive an illness physically alive but mentally destroyed, with life reduced to the level of a lower animal or vegetable.

6. *Suicide to end severe irremediable suffering*: Persons commit suicide when they are in intense pain that can no longer be controlled by medication, short of rendering them constantly unconscious.

7. *Morally principled suicide*: Persons act on justified commitments central to their moral integrity to help others and preserve that integrity.[25] An illustration of this situation is the case in which prisoners of war kill themselves rather than being forced to reveal military secrets to an enemy. Another example involves Captain Oates in Admiral Scott's expedition to

the South Pole, who, because of illness, walked out of his protected site to die in a blizzard rather than allow others on the expedition to risk their lives caring for him.

Assisted Suicide

Our views about suicide will, of course, largely shape our views about assisted suicide. If suicide should be opposed, then so should assisted suicide; if some suicide is morally permissible, then presumably some instances of assisted suicide would be, too. Yet assisted suicide raises new complexities, and one's belief that an instance of suicide is permissible by no means establishes that one is obligated to assist in it.

Sometimes assisted suicide is described as "euthanasia," but the meaning of that word is even more contested than the meaning of "suicide." Etymologically, "euthanasia" is derived from a Greek word for "good death," and most would define it as an altruistically motivated act of killing another person who has a terminal disease or injury and who is suffering greatly (understanding suffering here to include more than physical pain), or who otherwise has a very low quality of life. For most people, two categories of euthanasia lack any credible moral support: **involuntary euthanasia**, in which the patient has not been consulted or has refused the offer of euthanasia, and **nonvoluntary euthanasia**, in which the patient does not have the capacity to make an informed decision. In contrast, *voluntary* euthanasia occurs at the patient's request. It takes two forms: **voluntary passive euthanasia**, which is withholding or withdrawing treatment at the patient's request, and **voluntary active euthanasia**, whereby someone actively administers an agent that causes death.

Some people use "euthanasia" broadly to include assisted suicide, highlighting how it aids in a merciful death. Yet, others reject some of these ways of making distinctions between types of euthanasia. In particular, the American Medical Association defines euthanasia solely as voluntary active euthanasia, which it condemns. It considers voluntary passive euthanasia to be "letting die," which it sanctions when patients or their legal surrogates request it.

In any case, the line between killing and letting die (and also "helping die") is increasingly blurry. As an example, a physician is said to have "let" a patient die when, in response to informed consent, the physician removes the patient from a respirator. Yet turning off the respirator is surely an "act" in any ordinary sense, thus raising the issue of whether it is in fact active euthanasia.

The line between suicide (killing oneself) and euthanasia (assisted suicide) is also increasingly blurry. For example, is it suicide (with assistance) or active euthanasia when a physician intentionally prescribes a lethal dose of drugs, places them by a patient's bedside, and even helps lift the pills and a glass of water to a patient's mouth when the patient is too feeble to do so?

To some extent we will bypass these issues of definition by avoiding the term "euthanasia" as much as possible. In what follows, we will broadly use the term **assisted suicide** to include any action that helps persons intentionally bring about their own deaths. We also note that while the issue usually centers on "physician-assisted suicide," other health professionals are sometimes asked to participate, if only indirectly.[25-27] Consider the following case, which illustrates the fine line between simply knowing about a suicide and being drawn into participating in it in some way.

Randy and Paul

Randy is a 14-year-old patient with muscular dystrophy. His physical therapist, Paul, has worked with him intermittently for five years. During that time, Paul helped Randy and his family stall the inevitable reliance on a wheelchair, ordering adaptive equipment as necessary. Paul made it clear that an increasingly sedentary lifestyle using a chair would put Randy at greater risk for pulmonary complications, ultimately resulting in death.

Randy had developed a trusting relationship with Paul and often referred to him as the older brother he never had. Paul knew that eventually Randy would have to rely on an electric wheelchair to remain mobile. He was not prepared, however, for the confidence that Randy shared with him following therapy on a Thursday afternoon.

Randy explained that he was not just tired that day, but tired of constantly fighting to stay alive. He spoke of how difficult it was for him to see his family continue to sacrifice in order to provide him with things to make his life easier. He told Paul that he wanted a wheelchair, the cheapest they could find, and that he hoped that through an "accident" he could cause his own death. He explained to Paul that this was not a hasty decision; he had given it a great deal of thought, and if he waited much longer he would not be physically able to take his own life. He did not want years of gradually losing one skill after another, leaving him as dependent on his parents as when he was a newborn.

At the time, Paul said nothing to the parents. When he returned for the next appointment, he was disappointed to hear Randy repeat his desire with a calm resoluteness that led Paul to believe he had reached a firm decision.

Paul was torn for several reasons. First, he did not want to betray Randy's confidence. There were few people in Randy's life as important to him as Paul. It seemed to Paul that Randy had made an informed choice and that he should have governance over his life, including the ending of that life. But Randy was only 14 years old and not considered legally autonomous. Moreover, if he went along with Randy and told the parents that Randy was physically unable to do any more than he said he could do, Paul would be lying and undermining their legal surrogate decision-making responsibilities by withholding vital information from them. What course of action can Paul take to retain Randy's trust, respect his autonomy, and also respect the legal and moral obligation his family has to protect Randy's best interest? And what *is* Randy's best interest? ▨

We leave these queries for further exploration in the Discussion Questions section at the end of the chapter. We turn now to the case of legally competent adults, who are the primary focus of the debate over assisted suicide. Marilyn French contemplated suicide more than once during her ordeals, but each time she chose to continue living. However, she never wavered in her belief that people have a right to end their lives under extreme conditions if they so choose. She also believed people have a right to receive assistance in committing suicide, if they need the assistance and if someone is willing to help. Her views are not atypical. Only a few decades ago, opinion polls showed most people strongly opposed suicide and assisted suicide under almost all conditions. In contrast, today the opinion polls show a marked shift in attitudes, almost a complete reversal statistically, and few social issues evoke such wide interest and concern.

The courts have moved in a similar direction. The rulings listed on pages 127–128 concerning refusal of therapy are relevant when thinking about assisted suicide. For example, prior to the 1990 Nancy Cruzan ruling, many would have argued that to remove intravenous food and water constituted euthanasia, or perhaps suicide, if Nancy had written a living will requesting the removal. The court ruling essentially redefined the removal as constituting a special case of refusing therapy, which, since the Quinlan ruling in 1976, had been recognized as legal. The following are several additional rulings that are especially relevant to the present debate over assisted suicide:

1997: The U.S. Supreme Court ruled there is no constitutional "right to die." It left open the possibility, however, that the Court might in the future consider (carefully written) state laws allowing physician-assisted suicide as compatible with the Constitution.

1998: Oregon's law legalizing physician-assisted suicide went into effect. During 1998, 15 people with terminal illnesses used legally prescribed overdoses of drugs to kill themselves. The Oregon law (the "Death With Dignity Act") was passed in 1994 but had to survive lengthy legal challenges, many of which were renewed following the change in federal administrations after the general election of 2000. Stringent conditions of the act include the requirement that both a primary-care physician and a consulting physician agree that a patient has six months or less to live. It is also required that patients make two oral requests, followed 15 days later by a written request. The physician is then authorized only to prescribe a lethal dose of drugs and to indicate how they are to be taken, not to use more active means such as lethal injection.

1999: Dr. Jack Kevorkian was convicted of second-degree murder for giving a lethal injection to a man with amyotrophic lateral sclerosis (ALS). Dr. Kevorkian had successfully avoided prosecution for assisting in the suicides of about 120 people during the 1990s. The public was divided about his campaign to legalize assisted suicide. Some viewed him as heroic; others saw him as reckless, especially given his brief contact with the patients he assisted. He might have continued with his campaign for many years, but instead he decided to emphasize his cause by moving from assisted suicide to active euthanasia and then sending the tape of the proceedings to the television show *Sixty Minutes*, which broadcast excerpts from it.

Should Assisted Suicide Be Legal?

The same clash of conservative and liberal outlooks concerning suicide arise regarding legalizing assisted suicide, but additional factors need to be considered. Given the strong differences between conservative and liberal viewpoints on this issue, whatever social policies and laws emerge will be partially a matter of compromise among people having reasonable differences and partially a matter of politics within a democratic setting. Compromises, however, presuppose that opponents can discern evidence of cogent reasoning on the other side of the issue, even if one does not agree with the reasoning.

Within democracies, the centrality of individual autonomy would seem to favor the liberal position, which is to pass laws giving individuals maximum freedom to make their own decisions about suicide. At the same time, legalizing assisted suicide invites abuses and new dangers. Thus, it is not uncommon for some individuals who disapprove of assisted suicide to favor laws that allow it (as with abortion). Nor is it uncommon for individuals who approve of assisted suicide in some situations (for example, extreme and unremediable suffering) to oppose legalizing it. They are not upset that some physician-assisted suicide occurs behind closed doors, but they fear that a public law would tend to invite abuse and erode respect for life. Their critics insist that abuse is more likely behind closed doors. In *Washington v. Glucksberg* (1997), the U.S. Supreme Court appeared heavily swayed by the fear of abuse: "In legitimating the state's fear that legalizing assisted suicide would simply be the first step on a slippery slope leading to involuntary euthanasia, the Court cites statistics demonstrating the high proportion of cases in the Netherlands in which patients were killed without their explicit request or consent."[28]

In general, what are the possible abuses and dangers? It's possible that individuals might choose suicide based on mistaken diagnoses or prognoses, of the sort illustrated in the Marilyn French example. Greedy family members might pressure individuals into a suicide decision they otherwise would not make, or even bribe a dishonest physician to influence the patient to choose an early death. A climate of harsh and intimidating "managed care" might create subtle pressures to "choose" assisted suicide as a felt obligation.

Indeed, John Hardwig has argued that there can be a "**duty to die,**" or a duty to take one's own life—notions that critics of assisted suicide find alarming. He builds his case largely on the catastrophic consequences imposed on families when the terminally ill elect to pursue all possible medical interventions despite a minimal expectation of prolonging life and a marginal quality of life ahead. Those catastrophic consequences include physical exhaustion of the caretakers and financial indebtedness that robs the caretakers of their own retirement funds, their children's education, and loss of all their savings and homes. He argues that "families and loved ones are bound together by ties of care and affection, by legal relations and obligations, by inhabiting shared spaces and living units, by interlocking finances and economic prospects, by common projects and also commitments to support the different life projects of other family members, by shared histories, by ties of loyalty."[29,30] As a consequence of these ties, Hardwig says, the sick have responsibilities to their loved ones to not destroy their futures by making healthcare decisions as though only they alone would suffer the consequences of those decisions. Hardwig's proposal goes beyond a simple refusal of treatment to embrace planned suicide. He states: "Ending my life if my duty required might still be difficult. But for me, a far greater horror would be dying all alone or stealing the futures of my loved ones in order to buy a little more time for myself."[29(p42)]

Although Hardwig presents a forceful argument, most scholars feel that at best one could argue that avoiding catastrophic effects on caretakers is admirable, but not a duty. Some scholars see significant dangers in his proposal. If there is a duty to die, then others might argue that they have a right to have the patient commit suicide. Even the weakened idea that suicide is sometimes admirable, though not a duty, could easily pressure individuals into an unwanted action. Abuses for the sake of inheritance are not difficult to imagine. At a more general level, liberal laws might create a climate in which society is less willing to fund expensive terminal care as costs continue to escalate.

Even without abuses, some are alarmed by the prospect of physicians changing their traditional role of healer to the role of expediter of death. They fear an adverse effect on professional commitments and negative changes in patients' attitudes toward their physicians. Moreover, nearly everyone agrees that health professionals should never be required to assist in a suicide when doing so violates their moral convictions. But would legalization put pressure on health professionals to participate in acts they disagree with, especially where they have long-term relationships with patients?

All involved in the debate agree that the possibility of abuse and adverse side effects is genuine. However, those favoring legalization point out that all laws are imperfect, but when balancing the positive aspect of individual freedom with any negatives, individual autonomy tips the scale. Proponents of legalization believe that, with stringent regulation, the abuses can be minimized, and that any abuses can be balanced against the greater good through the legal system. They point to the likelihood that assisted suicide will be chosen by only a few individuals, as now occurs in Oregon and in the Netherlands, where knowing that it is an option brings comfort to many who are terminally ill even though they opt to continue to live. Opponents of legalization object that the risks are simply too great, that legalizing assisted suicide will merely speed the "slippery slope" toward increasing dehumanization and callousness about life. For many, suicide is simply inherently immoral.

Daniel Callahan, who, as we noted earlier, has argued for greater acceptance of death in our society, nevertheless has expressed great concern about efforts to legalize assisted suicide. He proposes that, as an alternative, all patients be informed that there are at least five stages in treatment that they can choose. In all these stages, relief of pain must be available: In stage one, the patient can refuse all health-care intervention, including preventive measures, and seek only relief of pain; in stage two, a patient can experience the diagnostic phase of treatment but refuse any curative efforts; in stage three, the patient can participate in the diagnostic phase of care and pursue medical treatment only if it promises a high probability of positive results with minimal unpleasant side effects; in stage four, diagnosis and any treatment that offers even a low probability of success can be pursued but with the understanding that if in the course of treatment there are any unexpected negative reactions, then treatment will stop; and in stage five, all medical treatments can be sought even if there is only an extremely remote chance they will be successful.[7(pp204,205)]

We have focused in this chapter on the issues surrounding meaningful life and death because of their inherent human interest and their occasional central importance, even though they do not arise in the everyday work of most physical therapists. We also focused on these issues because they highlight the interplay between the medical and total good of patients, a theme important in the previous two chapters as well. In the next chapter we will turn to more mundane but still crucial concerns about honesty at the workplace and conflicts of interest—concerns that also begin to widen our attention to societal issues about health-care management.

Discussion Questions

1. Referring to the case of Henry and Sonia on page 126, discuss what Sonia should or might permissibly do regarding her patient, Henry, who refuses treatment.

2. Referring to the case of Mark and Dan, discuss what Dan should or might permissibly do regarding his patient Mark, whom he knows is planning suicide. In doing so, present and defend your view concerning when, if ever, suicide is morally permissible. Take into account the different kinds of situations distinguished by Thomas E. Hill, Jr. Also, discuss John Hardwig's view that in some circumstances it is not only permissible but a duty to die.

3. Consider a hypothetical situation in which we imagine Marilyn French bringing up the topic of suicide with Michael, the physical therapist who had provided home care for her for several years. Assume that French is competent and not clinically depressed. Which of the following options are morally permissible for Michael to pursue, and why?

   a. Say nothing, perhaps with an accompanying raised eyebrow, alarmed glance, or sharp glare.
   b. Interpret her remarks as an expression of momentary frustration, and immediately help restore her hope by saying that things are all right and that she is improving.
   c. Alert her physician or a family member, urging them to immediately find a psychotherapist to help French or even to consider institutionalizing her (actions that some might consider a betrayal of French but that others might view as being in her best interests).
   d. Discuss the topic calmly with her, expressing himself in a manner that makes clear that her views are what matter in the situation.
   e. Offer to help, perhaps in finding a physician willing to assist her suicide, or become further involved himself—an option that might have very serious legal repercussions and involve risking his career.

4. A 12-year-old child who suffered burns over 70 percent of his body was not expected to live. The hospital's physical therapy staff performed the debridement (removal of dead or contaminated tissue/skin) while the boy was placed in a whirlpool on a stretcher. They then performed range of motion exercises to keep the joints mobile. The parents, who were in denial and believed their son would survive, gave consent for the procedures. They supported any treatment offering hope that the child might live and make a functional recovery. The child screamed and pleaded with the therapists to do nothing but the whirlpool—to leave the dead skin on and not hurt him. The nursing staff believed the physical therapists should be less diligent in removing the skin and as a consequence cause less pain. The physician, however, expected the same quality of care given to everyone else.

   When asked by the therapists to witness the suffering that the aggressive debridement was causing, the parents replied that they couldn't bear to watch their child in pain. The physical therapists followed the physician's directives, but later, after the boy died, they questioned whether they made the right decision and whether they should have done more to heed the child's requests. What more could the physical therapists have done? Should they have been less aggressive in their therapy, even though doing so would defy both the physician's orders and the parent's wishes?

5. Discuss how the Rule of Double Effect might be applied to the following example: Jody and Mary are conjoined twins who share one heart and one set of lungs. Mary was born with severe brain damage and survived only because of Jody's healthy heart and lungs. Doctors want to separate the twins because without the separation both twins will die within six months. If they are sepa-

rated, however, Mary will almost certainly die. The family, who are devout Catholics, cite their religious faith in opposing the surgery. They cannot condone the killing of Mary to advantage Jody.[31]

6. In the eyes of the law, people used to be considered dead when their hearts and breathing stopped (the "heart-lung" criterion for death), but now people are considered legally dead when they lack all brain activity (the "whole-brain" criterion). Critics insist that this is a moral issue rather than simply a medical delineation, and that the current legal definition is far too narrow to allow individuals to express their moral convictions on the issue.[16(p206)] For example, they argue that Karen Ann Quinlan was dead, as a human being, during the decade in which her body was sustained with intravenous nutrition and hydration, even though during those years she had some measurable electrical activity in her brain but existed in a vegetative state. Some of these critics argue that persons are dead when they permanently lose consciousness (the "higher brain" criterion), even if some electrical activity in the brain continues. Others argue that persons are dead when they lose all ability to interact in meaningful ways with the world, even if they retain consciousness (the "personhood" criterion). What is your view, and what arguments can be offered to resolve the issue?

7. Marilyn French urged health professionals to never squelch a patient's hopes. She did not distinguish among different objects of hope, such as: (a) hopes for survival, (b) hopes for a meaningful future (however brief), and (c) hopes for specific improvements. In this connection, consider the case of Reynolds Price, himself a distinguished writer and teacher of writing. Intense radiation treatment for a spinal cancer left him unable to walk, but he was convinced he would eventually walk again. After three days of working with him, Wilkie Thomas, one of his first physical therapists, told him firmly (and accurately) that he was paraplegic and that walking was an unrealistic goal.[32]

   Distinguish some hope-preserving and hope-destroying ways of conveying such news to a patient, marking the distinction between different kinds of hopes. (As a postscript: After a brief period of despair, Price went on—as no one could have foreseen—to have the most productive period of his writing career. He reports that the decisive positive influences were the support he received from health professionals and especially the contact he had with other severely injured patients in a rehabilitation program.)

8. For some time, active euthanasia has been practiced in the Netherlands. Research the recent literature about the extent of abuse and other undesirable side effects that have occurred. How would a utilitarian assess the extent of these abuses, in the Netherlands and potentially in the United States? (Take into account that virtually no social policy can escape some abuse, and abuses already occur secretly in the United States right now.) What might a rights ethicist or a duty ethicist say in response to the utilitarian assessment?

References

1. Klemke ED, ed. *The Meaning of Life*. 2d ed. New York, NY: Oxford University Press; 2000.
2. Tolstoy L. *The Death of Ivan Ilych*. Trans. Solotaroff L. New York, NY: Bantam; 1981:93.
3. Callahan D. *Setting Limits: Medical Goals in an Aging Society*. New York, NY: Simon & Schuster; 1987.

4. Sontag, S. *Illness as Metaphor and AIDS and Its Metaphors*. New York, NY: Doubleday; 1990.

5. Epictetus. *The Enchiridion*. In: Kirk R, ed. *Marcus Aurelius*: Meditations; *and Epictetus*: Enchiridion. Chicago, IL: Henry Regnery; 1956:172.

6. Freedman B. Respectful service and reverent obedience: a Jewish view on making decisions for incompetent patients. *Hastings Cent Rep*. 1996;26(4):31-37.

7. Callahan, D. *The Troubled Dream of Life: In Search of a Peaceful Death*. Washington, DC: Georgetown University Press; 2000:100.

8. Hardwig, J. Spiritual issues at the end of life: a call for discussion. *Hastings Cent Rep*. 2000;30(2):28-30.

9. Helminiak DA. *The Human Core of Spirituality: Mind as Psyche and Spirit*. Albany, NY: State University of New York Press; 1996.

10. Becker, E. *The Denial of Death*. New York, NY: Free Press; 1973.

11. Nuland SB. *How We Die: Reflections on Life's Final Chapter*. New York, NY: Vintage; 1995:258.

12. Zalumas J. *Caring in Crisis*. Philadelphia, PA: University of Pennsylvania Press; 1995:101.

13. French M. *A Season in Hell*. New York, NY: Ballantine Books; 2000:36.

14. Flomenhoft D. Understanding and helping people who have cancer: a special communication. *Phys Ther*. 1984;64(8):1232.

15. Kubler-Ross E. *On Death and Dying*. New York, NY: Macmillan Company; 1969.

16. Munson R., ed. *Intervention and Reflection: Basic Issues in Medical Ethics*. 6th ed. Belmont, CA: Wadsworth/Thomas Learning; 2000:190-211.

17. Grady D. At life's end, many patients are denied peaceful passing. *New York Times*. 2000(May 29):A1.

18. Cowart D, Burt R. Confronting death: who chooses, who controls? A dialogue between Dax Cowart and Robert Burt. *Hastings Cent Rep*. 1998;28(1):14-24.

19. Teno J, Lynn J, Wenger N, et al. Advance directives for seriously ill hospitalized patients: effectiveness with the Patient Self-Determination Act and the SUPPORT intervention. *J Am Geriatr Soc*. April 1997;45(4):507.

20. Sim J. *Ethical Decision Making in Therapy Practice*. Oxford, England: Butterworth-Heinemann; 1997:104.

21. Beauchamp TL, Childress JF. *Principles of Biomedical Ethics*. 5th ed. New York, NY: Oxford University Press; 2001:129.

22. Prado CG, Taylor SJ. *Assisted Suicide: Theory and Practice of Elective Death*. Amherst, NY: Humanity Books; 1999:14.

23. Hill TE. Self-regarding suicide: a modified Kantian view. In: Hill TE. *Autonomy and Self-Respect*. New York, NY: Cambridge University Press; 1991:95.

24. This summary of Hill's views follows Martin MW. *Everyday Morality*. 3d ed. Belmont, CA: Wadsworth; 2001:338.

25. Battin MP, Rhodes R, Silvers A., eds. *Physician-Assisted Suicide: Expanding the Debate*. London, England: Routledge; 1998.

26. Battin MP, Mayo D, Wolf SM. *Physician-Assisted Suicide: Pro and Con*. Lanham, MD: Rowman & Littlefield; 1999.

27. Beauchamp TL, ed. *Intending Death: The Ethics of Assisted Suicide and Euthanasia*. Upper Saddle River, NJ: Prentice-Hall; 1996.

28. Kaveny MC. Assisted suicide, the Supreme Court, and the constitutive function of the law. *Hastings Cent Rep*. 1997;27(5):33.

29. Hardwig J. Is there a duty to die? *Hastings Cent Rep*. 1997;27(2):36.

30. Hardwig J, Hentoff N, Callahan D, Churchill L, Cohn F, Lynn J. *Is There a Duty to Die?* New York, NY: Routledge; 2000.

31. Miller M. Agonizing over who lives, dies. *Los Angeles Times*, September 11, 2000:A1.

32. Price R. *A Whole New Life: An Illness and a Healing*. New York, NY: Plume; 1995:99.

Honesty and Conflicts of Interest

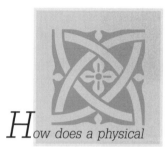

How does a physical
therapist uphold ethical standards when a
managed-care employment contract conflicts with
the best interests of patients?

Keywords

Conflicts of interest

Role responsibilities

Episodic conflicts of interest

Systemic conflicts of interest

Business standards vs. professional standards

Transdisciplinary team

Problematic physical referrals

Gifts

Simone Thomas

Simone Thomas is a physical therapist at Valley Memorial Hospital, where she is a respected clinician known for her skill in treating orthopedic injuries. She graduated in 1984 and remains current in her field by attending and giving continuing education courses in orthopedic management. Her son is a high school senior who has received a partial scholarship to Yale University. To finance the balance of his tuition costs, Simone has decided to start a private home health practice operating at night and on weekends and specializing in orthopedic management and treatment. She formed this business after noticing that the current managed-care contracts do not allow an optimal number of physical therapy treatments. She notifies many of her patients that they can continue treatment with her as private patients after their managed-care benefits lapse, and that she can see them in their homes. This arrangement is especially helpful to patients for whom there are functional limitations to daily activities. But Simone is caught off guard when one of her friends suggests that she discuss this plan with the supervisor, since she seems to be entering into one or more conflicts of interest. 🗷

Conflicts of interest are sometimes difficult to discern, especially because the self-interest involved often distorts judgment. We begin by providing a definition of conflicts of interest, not with the hope of removing all vagueness, but to highlight key areas where vagueness and ambiguity arise in practice. Next we distinguish some of the systemic conflicts of interest within a managed-care environment. Then we sample some of the recurring conflicts of interest in physical therapy: physician referral, equipment and supplies, gifts, and teaching and research.

Defining and Evaluating Conflicts of Interest

Conflicts of interest are situations in which individuals have interests that significantly threaten their role responsibilities, or that would do so for a typical person in their role.[1] This is a very broad definition, and three of its features deserve clarification: role responsibilities, interests, and typical persons.

Role responsibilities are well-delineated duties attached to formal assignments within organizations or social practices such as the health-care professions. In the present context, they refer both to the particular duties assigned to physical therapists at their jobs as well as to therapists' general professional duties.

Interests include all benefits to the professional, as well as altruistic concerns. Most conflicts of interest involve competing interests in business or professional life, such as a therapist's accepting personal inducements from a salesperson to use a particular product, engaging in moonlighting for a competitor's company, or making a heavy financial investment in a competitor's company (without an employer's permission). But our definition is broad enough to include involvements in private life that threaten professional responsibilities, such as alcohol and drug abuse.

Not all "conflicting interests," however, constitute conflicts of interest.[2] For example, a parent who is torn between wanting a divorce and wanting to remain with her spouse in order to provide support for her children is caught in an ethical dilemma involving conflicting interests, but she is not in a conflict of interest. However, a parent coaching her daughter's soccer team is often faced with a conflict of interest because of her desire to keep her child playing for as much time as possible while at the same time needing to keep her child on the bench for the well-being of the team. The difference is that in the second case an interest threatens her role responsibilities as coach.

Finally, our definition distinguishes between individuals and *typical persons*. Consider a judge of such exceptional integrity that we know she would be fair in adjudicating a dispute involving a family member. However, the judge is still considered to be in a conflict of interest in such a case because a typical judge in that situation would be at risk of failing to fulfill her role responsibilities. Thus, the judge is obligated to avoid even the *appearance* of a conflict of interest. Similarly, the APTA *House of Delegate Standards, Policies, Positions and Guidelines* (HOD 06-99-25-08, section B) declares that members of the board or the board-appointed body should not participate in discussions of a case if there is a relationship which would prevent them from acting impartially "or that reasonably would tend to cast doubt on the member's ability to act impartially." Conversely, some professionals are inclined to lose "professional distance" in particular areas, perhaps because of their religious beliefs, whereas a "typical" professional would not. Hence the definition refers to both the individual involved and to typical individuals.

We are primarily interested in routine and recurring types of conflicts of interest, ones that arise with frequency. Recurrence takes two forms, however. **Episodic conflicts of interest** are those conflicts that arise from choices made voluntarily—for example, the choice to coach the soccer team on which one's child plays, or, in the case of physical therapy, giving and accepting personal gifts on the job. In contrast, **systemic conflicts of interest** arise from the very structure of professions and other social practices. For example, there is an ongoing temptation in all professions with a fee-for-service reimbursement system to provide unnecessary services to clients in order to increase profits. Conversely, there is the ongoing temptation to limit services in a capitated reimbursement system, as we will discuss later.

Some systemic conflicts of interest are inescapable and morally tolerable— short of overthrowing or radically modifying social practices and economic systems (which can generate new systemic conflicts). To be sure, some ethicists do stipulate that the expression "conflict of interest" refers only to morally objectionable situations, which explains why the expression typically carries unsavory connotations. But notice that ordinary usage allows us to say that parents who coach their children's teams are in a conflict of interest. As another example, the Federal Aviation Administration (FAA) permits designated engineers working for airline companies to serve as FAA inspectors on the airplanes the engineers help build.[3] This is a clear conflict of interest, in that the engineers' loyalty to their companies could threaten their duties to be impartial inspectors. Yet the conflict of interest is acceptable because the complexity of airplanes and the limited resources of the FAA make this the most workable arrangement for inspection. Similarly, the Commission on Accreditation in Physical Therapy Education includes physical therapy faculty from already accredited programs on its on-site review teams when a school is being considered for accreditation. The reason for this is similar to that in the FAA case: it takes someone fully informed about educational theory and the discipline of physical therapy to judge accreditation worthiness. It is expected that the faculty on the review team will disregard the fact that every accredited program is a potential competitor for students.

In general, conflicts of interest are *tolerable* when the relevant systems (institutions, economic structures, etc.) are morally permissible, when effective procedures for overseeing abuses are in place (laws, self-regulation within professions, consumer-group publications), and when the relevant parties voluntarily accept the arrangement. For example, we largely take for granted the economic systems of Western democracies that combine, in varying degrees, capitalism (free enterprise), government regulation, and professional self-regulation.

Calling a conflict of interest tolerable, we should add, does not banish moral concern about threats to responsibilities. Parents who coach their children remain open to criticism for making biased judgments. Similarly, inescapable conflicts of interest call for conscientiousness by committed professionals and vigilance by disciplinary structures.

In general, however, there is a strong presumption against preventable conflicts of interest in the professions. Why is that? One reason is clear from the definition: conflicts of interest threaten responsibilities, potentially undermining professional integrity. Another reason is that even the appearance of conflicts of interest can endanger the trust of patients and the public. And yet another reason is that most conflicts of interest involve deception and other failures of truthfulness. All these values—integrity, trustworthiness, and truthfulness—are aspects of honesty, which we therefore adopt as the central guiding value in thinking about conflicts of interest.

Regarding episodic conflicts of interest, alternative moral responses include the following options: (1) escape from them, typically by relinquishing the conflicting interest that threatens the role responsibility, (2) avoid them in the first place, (3) disclose them to appropriate parties (such as employers, clients), or (4) take other steps, as appropriate, even if it is only exercising special caution to ensure role responsibilities are properly met.[4] We will discuss which options are appropriate in particular situations.

Health care exists because individuals are vulnerable and need help. Furthermore, harm caused by mistakes frequently cannot be undone, unlike mistakes made in financial or legal matters. As a result, disclosure of conflicts of interest is generally not enough. To undermine the trust on which care is built is to diminish the care itself, regardless of whether professionals profit financially or not. Unlike law or banking, in which it is desirable for all parties to be vigilant and in which full disclosure helps assure that vigilance, the primary concern and focus in health care is for the patient to achieve better health or function. This concern is often in response to a sudden illness that finds the patient uninformed about the best course of treatment and hence needing to trust the judgment of providers. Thus, to minimize threats to patient trust, there is a strong presumption that therapists and other health-care professionals should do everything possible to avoid conflicts of interest related to patient care.

Thus, defining a situation as a conflict of interest raises a red flag, but it does not indicate how the flag is to be waved. As an analogy, consider deception, discussed in Chapters 2 and 3. All deception raises moral questions, but the questions are sometimes easily answered and other times sharply contested. Deception is permissible in a game of poker; it is obligatory when it is the only way to prevent a criminal from taking an innocent life. However, its moral status is debatable when it is used to conceal personal sexual matters. Similarly, when and why conflicts of interest are morally objectionable are questions that need to be explored contextually, such as within the current system of managed care.

Systemic Conflicts within Managed Care

The most basic systemic conflicts of interest center on the primary good served by the profession. Described in general terms, this good is shared by all health fields: to promote health while respecting patient rights. Described more specifically, the good served by physical therapy treatment is to restore persons to more functional, pain-free, and independent lives, as well as to help prevent injuries and pain in the first place. Three interwoven questions arise immediately: (1) When is health-care intervention warranted and at what level? (2) Who defines acceptable outcomes—the patient, the provider, or the reimbursement organization? (3) What is the cost, and who pays?

Most of us—healthy and functional with respect to the expectations of others, our age, and our level of activity—could profit from physical therapy services in preventing (proper body mechanics) or even improving such areas as balance and gait. Who defines the threshold for such services? If left to patients, all will draw a different line in the sand. Even where there is obvious disability, some patients are quickly resigned to a life of needless dysfunction; others want athletic skills rather than mere average abilities. Needs for physical therapy can be highly specialized, even within the specialties recognized by the national organization and achieved through extensive training and monitored clinical experience. For example, within sports medicine, some physical therapists specialize in treating only professional dancers and the unique injuries and risks associated with that profession.

As with physicians, therapists' primary conflict of interest is centered in the entrepreneurial method of reimbursement and the acquisition of medical services. All health-care providers affirm an ethic of beneficence and equality (serving all patients to the best of one's ability) and an ethic of equity (service according to a patient's ability to pay or a plan's pre-negotiated equity format), but equality and equity can conflict in nuanced ways. In addition, each of the methods of reimbursement carries with it potential conflicts of interest between whatever service is provided (or denied) and the financial well-being of the provider.

Like most professions, physical therapy generates systemic conflicts of interest centered on the therapist's dual roles of adviser and provider.[5-10] Thus, most professionals advise clients about options, help decide the best course of action, and then provide the services. The implications of adviser-provider conflicts differ according to the payment systems within which health professionals function, and those systems are presently and continuously in the midst of turmoil. Many options are being considered, but the two main categories are fee-for-service and managed care.

In traditional fee-for-service systems, the provider has a systematic incentive to advise for unnecessary services, thereby raising costs dramatically. Fee-for-service tends to bring higher costs for patients, unnecessary tests, and unnecessary procedures. The provider's self-interest leads to setting goals and timetables which will harvest the maximum payment even as patients and insurance companies desire to restrict cost as much as possible. Under the fee-for-service system, it is not uncommon for therapists in private practice to earn yearly incomes that are multiples of the national average. The goals, objectives, frequency, and duration of treatment are largely at the discretion of the therapist, expressed to and endorsed by the referring physician. Yet, in the vast majority of cases, the therapist's discretion works in the interest of the patient.

Joan Gibson defines managed care as any delivery and reimbursement system which attempts to control the following: (1) the clients served, (2) the range of benefits and services offered, and (3) costs.[11] Managed care has evolved as a significant health-care system since the congressional passage of the Health Maintenance Organizations Act of 1973, but its earliest roots were in the 1900s.[12] In theory, it is organizationally configured as a composite of the most productive elements of business theories. In truth, managed-care systems' cost structure for providing services constitutes a systematic incentive to *not* advise patients of all needed services and thus minimize usage of services. Capitation is based on paying according to numbers of members in the health plan rather than on usage of services. In a managed-care environment, the conflict of interest is between the duration of treatment in the best interest of the client and what is permissible (reimbursable) under the managed-care plan. The move to managed care generates many conflicts for physical therapists in their role as advisers: Should the therapist counsel the client about the true potential and risk in the minimal care that is being reimbursed? Should the therapist inform patients of options that might produce beneficial results but at extra cost for the provider? Should the therapist proceed so as to limit client expectations and thus meet standardized pathways and time frames?

At its core, then, the primary conflict of interest in a managed-care situation is between **business standards and professional standards**.[13] The table on page 147 provides a brief look at some of the common values characteristic of a profession and those of business.

Characteristics of a Professional	Business Values
1. Makes decisions by means of general principles and theory.	1. Select clinical pathways to reduce variability and increase efficiency.
2. Has unique knowledge.	2. Shared knowledge is versatile, therefore more efficient.
3. Status is awarded by accomplishments.	3. Competition enhances profit and acquisition of power.
4. Decisions made on behalf of the client/patient.	4. Actions should yield reasonable or maximal profit.
5. Authority is accepted only from colleagues.	5. Managers should be trained in business theory.

Therapists might be employees of managed-care organizations or provide a contracted service for the organization. The contracted-service arrangement relieves the managed-care organization of having to provide fringe employee benefits as well as of having to meet requirements governing the employer-employee relationship. Within this contractual arrangement, the business model is coercive when it "deselects" health professionals, including physicians and physical therapists, because of their so-called "excessive" resource utilization.[14] Under this arrangement, services can be limited contractually, both directly through gag orders and indirectly by providing incentives to limit care, such as those inherent in capitated plans, or even by replacing trained professionals with less costly and less-trained employees.[11(p131-138), 14(p139-152)] Most contracted services are subject to discontinuance for any reason, by either side, and are not subject to the due process review or the same laws governing an employer-employee relationship. Hence, contentious or resource-demanding providers are likely to find themselves without a job and without a method to appeal.

Legally, providers are caught between judicial rulings and a managed-care corporation's right to end contracts at any time and for unspecified reasons. In *Wickline v. California,* 1986, the court made it clear that if the provider did not try to negotiate against an adverse limitation in coverage that would adversely affect the patient, the provider would be held accountable for an unfavorable outcome.[14(p144)] In effect, the court demanded that professionals make decisions by way of advocacy for the patient, even if business policy points in the opposite direction.

John

John is a therapist with a contract to provide services to the patients of Sheraton Managed Care. Sheraton is very clear in its contract that John is to follow the critical pathways. He can treat patients fewer times if warranted, but he cannot extend additional care without approval. He is not free to refer patients to outside therapists, nor is he in any way to "undermine" the credibility of the care offered by Sheraton Managed Care.

In the course of treating a 42-year-old man for injuries resulting from multiple gunshot wounds, John realizes that his patient should have the care of a physical therapist with expertise in treating the hand. He also realizes that he will not be able to help his patient reach his potential within the number of visits approved by Sheraton Managed Care.

Sheraton has never honored any of his previous requests for extensions. If John does not petition for an extension and the patient is harmed—for example, he cannot return to employment—then John may well be liable for the harm. But another petition from him might reduce the likelihood that his contract will be renewed and even put him at risk for dismissal. If he informs the patient that he needs a therapist with an expertise in hand therapy, and if the patient then demands from Sheraton the expertise John recommends, John will most certainly be dismissed. However, if John uses his social skills and convinces the patient that he is getting the very best care, it is unlikely there will be any negative repercussions for John. Integrity, trustworthiness, and truthfulness are all at risk in this environment. ⊠

While the contracted service model is coercive to the provider, it is also deceptive to the patient because it encourages withholding important information. These contracts often embed many items of information typically not available to the public—for example, economic incentives and disincentives to physical therapists and physicians, treatment options under the plan, and gag orders (forbidding providers to tell patients) on expensive procedures.

Working as an employee of the managed-care organization also carries its own threat to the delivery of optimal care. Managed-care structures typically have six features that create a mixture of benefits and potential problems:[15]

1. Managed-care corporations frequently use teams, often preferring *trans-disciplinary* teams. Although therapists have long worked in teams, the teams are most often multidisciplinary or interdisciplinary. In the multidisciplinary team, representatives from different disciplines share common general goals for the patient, even though each discipline supplies only its own specialized skills. In the interdisciplinary team, the disciplines share common goals but the activities are synergistic and overlapping. For example, the physical therapist might request that the occupational therapist and speech therapist position the child in a particular way to maximize stretch on the hamstrings. In turn, the speech therapists might request that all disciplines use words with three or fewer syllables when addressing the patient. Team meetings are occasions where requests are conveyed, goals are decided, and everyone is updated on the patient's status.

   In the **transdisciplinary team** model, more highly integrated care is provided, and activities and techniques are taught across disciplinary lines. If the patient is primarily cared for by an occupational therapist, that therapist might receive instruction from physical and speech therapists to implement their respective professional programs. This model has been encouraged in many institutions as a means of cost containment. Yet professional objections have been voiced concerning occasions when unexpected patient responses occur and the caregiver does not have the theory base to respond appropriately. Some therapists reject this model because they believe it sacrifices quality care and because it might violate the state-defined scope of practice for each participating licensed profession. In the APTA *House of Delegate Standards, Policies, Positions and Guidelines*, it is stated in HOD 06-99-12-05 that "The American Physical Therapy Association (APTA) opposes the concept of the cross-trained professional practitioner, defined as 'a health care practitioner who is cross-trained in area(s) of practice in which the individual is neither educated nor licensed.' " Therapists who have had success using this model caution that the standards of practice must be reviewed and discussed well in advance of implementing them to determine their appropriate scope.

2. Managed-care structures combine administrative and clinical duties. Although this combination creates variety in the workday of some, for many others it displaces the care they would prefer to give to patients.

3. Managed-care companies train people only in what they need to know and standardizes treatment for greatest efficiency, such as through critical pathways. This practice tends to limit the understanding of the clinician relative to the overall distribution of resources within the organization, thereby lessening fully informed advocacy for patients. The uniqueness of individual patients is not always best served by a singular approach that minimizes professional judgment.

4. A managed-care environment maximizes team efforts at problem solving. This is a positive feature when it is understood to be consultative problem solving, with professionals still in charge of the decisions relative to their expertise. If, however, the group decisions override individual professional decisions, the therapist must spend significant time building power and influence within the group to ensure effective advocacy for the patient.

5. A managed-care environment rewards team effort rather than individual skill development. Rewarding team productivity treats all contributions within the group equally, even though typically the value of contributions varies considerably—especially in a rehabilitation setting.

6. Managed care links all evaluations ultimately to customer (patient) satisfaction. Its retail approach to health care can displace the most important element in medicine—professional standards of practice. Patients may be pleased if they are attended to and treated with respect in attractive settings, as with retail sales, and the telephone calls made by the receptionist or nurse to inquire about how the patient feels after hospitalization might be influential in surveys of satisfaction, but such calls or décor do relatively little to ensure competent care. The patient typically does not know what care, procedures, and medications would provide maximal health benefits, so their expressed satisfaction is uninformed, particularly in the elements of care that are most critical to their health.

Regardless of the employment relationships within the managed-care environment, the primary responsibility of physical therapists is to their patients: to provide quality services and products at reasonable costs, within the constraints of respect for autonomy. In addition to issues of cost, quality, and control, there are related considerations about honesty and maintaining the public trust, which require avoiding even the appearance of objectionable conflicts of interest. There are also responsibilities to employers, to coworkers, and to the general public. Exactly when these responsibilities are threatened requires close attention to context, enlightened by a broad understanding of human propensities.

Overall, in our judgment, the current managed-care system encourages providers to offer a minimum level of care, not an optimal level. While economic realities cannot be ignored, concern for the patient must remain paramount. When patients would probably profit from additional treatment, they should be so informed. Defending the adequacy of a managed-care pathway that is not appropriate for a given patient is dishonest. Therapists should not sign contracts that restrict expression of professional opinions, or gag orders, any more than physicians should.

The APTA *Code of Ethics* and *Guide for Professional Conduct* offer guidance, although they leave specifics to the judgment of individual practitioners. The guide explicitly forbids certain types of conflicts of interest (without using the expression). For example, section 7.1 states that "A physical therapist shall never place her/his own financial interest above the welfare of individuals under his/her care."

✖ Physician Referral

Historically, physician referral has been one of the most discussed conflicts of interest in physical therapy. At one time physical therapists worked most often directly under physicians' supervision. As physical therapy became increasingly professionalized, and therapists' required skills were greatly augmented in both diagnosis and treatment, there was a strong move toward private-practice therapy. As a result, **problematic physician referral** arrangements were established that allowed physicians and physical therapists to profit, particularly when physicians were paid simply for making referrals.

The practice had serious potential for abuse, as was widely appreciated by the early 1980s. It often constituted kickbacks that significantly increased costs to patients, adversely affected judgments about quality of services, and threatened public trust. A consensus developed that referral was not a service from which physicians should be allowed to profit. In 1983, the APTA forbade physical therapists from entering into arrangements that allowed physicians or other referring practitioners to profit from simply making a referral.

Philip Paul Tygiel cited many instances in which patient rights were abused when physicians profited from referrals.[16] The instances included prescribing unnecessary services, on the part of both physicians and physical therapists; low-quality care as a result of physicians not considering the appropriateness of the specialization of the therapists they used; and denying patients the therapists they preferred. In one case study, an orthopedic surgeon employed a physical therapist who, although well trained in treating spinal conditions, did not have expertise in hand therapy—even though hand surgery was a primary component of the surgeon's practice. Hand therapy and the custom splinting frequently required is a highly specialized area of practice for both physical and occupational therapists. The surgeon nevertheless referred his patients to the therapist in his employment, even though patients frequently had to be referred later to one of four qualified hand therapists in the community because the surgeon's favored therapist lacked the special skills needed. The later resplinting by a qualified therapist was an additional cost to the patient.

The APTA *Code of Ethics* has since been clarified and strengthened to forbid physical therapists from entering into many problematic referral relationships. However, regardless of how carefully a code is constructed, it is not possible for a single document to anticipate all possible variations on a common theme. For example, consider a case in which the husband is a physician and the wife is a physical therapist. Although legally their practices are separate, and therefore withstand the APTA definition of conflict of interest, their joint income is enhanced by referrals from the physician husband to his therapist wife. The physician responds that he wants his patients to receive the best physical therapy care available, and he believes that is provided by his wife. Clearly, there is a possibility for abuse. Disclosure to patients by the physician or therapist should be supplemented prior to the first appointment with a listing of other therapists in the area with similar training. Section 7.3 in the APTA *Guide for Professional Conduct* appears to support the spirit of this recommendation: "A physical therapist shall disclose to the patient if the referring practitioner derives compensation from the provision of physical therapy."

Referral issues have become somewhat more convoluted in managed-care situations in which the senior physicians in a health maintenance organization (HMO) are also its owners. Profit is still the concern, but this time underuse rather than overuse of physical therapy poses the more serious offense. The dilemma is compounded by the dependent role of the physical therapist. In some states, such as California, the physical therapist can evaluate or treat a patient without a physician's referral, but in the vast majority of states, insurance carriers will not reimburse the patient or therapist without the referral. As a result, therapists are financially wedded to physicians even though they themselves are increasingly skilled and professional enough to be capable of making independent physical therapy diagnoses and treatments. This financial tether has the potential to bind the professional judgment of the therapists to a menu of physician-acceptable options.

Equipment and Supplies

Frequently, physical therapists make equipment for patients, such as splints and seating inserts. Therapists who work with patients know their specific needs and have the specialized knowledge to order equipment. In private practice it is not usual for the therapist to charge patients for materials and the time used to construct the equipment. These therapists often supply equipment at a lesser cost than do specialized vendors, but not always.

Therapists who fabricate equipment for patients often cite patient benefit as the primary motivation. Because equipment, especially splints, needs to be custom-made, therapists argue that it is more time efficient and ultimately contributes to a better product when therapists do the fabrications. They do not have to take the time to communicate in detail the patient's needs to a fabricator. They also point out that fabricating a piece of equipment enables them to respond to unanticipated variables, to change the specifications of the equipment, and to implement those changes immediately.

Many therapists charge only for the cost of the materials, plus their customary practice rate, to generate the equipment. There are companies dedicated to the creation of these appliances, however, and these companies are quick to point out that this practice robs them of needed income for tasks they are specifically trained to perform. But perhaps the greater problem is the appearance of a conflict of interest. Therapists can easily fill any downtime with equipment fabrication, thereby securing a steady income in private practice. Hence there is the temptation to create a market for equipment within the therapist's patient population, which could not possibly get the exact appliance without going to another therapist who also manufactures equipment. The appliances are so uniquely a blend of the patient's need and the therapist's goal of correction that without the therapist's input, an outside vendor would be unable to adequately meet the patient's needs.

Therapists also should not have a major financial interest in the company that supplies them with products they use in practice. Yet there is an interesting dilemma inherent in this advice. Since, in general, people are advised to invest in companies or markets with which they are familiar, it would seem to be good business practice for therapists intent on securing extra financial security to invest in companies whose products they know to be better than the competition's. So, even though therapists may own stock in those companies from which they make purchases, they are driven by the commitment to provide the best supplies. As a result, stock ownership is inherently objectionable only if it becomes excessive or if the company supplies inferior products or offers direct kickbacks—as defined by reasonable guidelines within organizations and the profession.

⊠ Gifts

The importance of conflict of interest, as well as of context, enters centrally into a discussion about gifts. Principle 4.4 of the APTA *Guide for Professional Conduct* states, "A physical therapist shall not accept or offer gifts or other considerations that affect or give an appearance of affecting his/her professional judgment."

Precisely what does this mean? The intent is not to forbid all gifts, even though such a prohibition might be necessary in some settings, such as the defense industry, in which gifts from contractors to government officials are essentially banned altogether. In physical therapy, like many other professions, hard and fast rules on gifts can cause unexpected negative consequences. For example, many gifts from suppliers, or vendors, are "reminder items" that have negligible monetary value. But as a tool to enhance a relationship, their value cannot accurately be measured in dollars. Instead, their value must be considered relative to the subtle influence on the relationship and related decisions. The American Medical Association (AMA) allows small gifts, and anyone who has attended a health profession conference in this nation has experienced how widespread this practice has become. At APTA and other health-related conferences, the trend has been to move away from promotional gifts which can be used with patients and instead toward gifts specifically for the therapists, often without any relationship to the products the vendors sell.

Other gifts raise different concerns, both in their acceptance and rejection. In most physical therapy settings, the therapist is engaged with the patient over significant periods of time, and the quality of that time is enhanced by collaborative goal setting and assessment—tasks that frequently build a social as well as professional relationship. Patients often see the therapist as their primary advocate and their primary hope for restoration of function. As a result, gifts from patients to therapists are common, especially in pediatric settings, and often insignificant in their cost—for example, drawings, homemade cards, or a box of chocolates. Whereas with vendors such small gifts might be objectionable because they may be intended to influence therapists in the products they purchase, gifts from patient to therapist can actually strengthen a component of care.

It is also true that in some cultures gifts are given to health-care providers out of custom and appreciation, without any intent to acquire more or better services. To refuse such a gift is considered an insult. Refusal symbolically says the gift and the giver are unappreciated, and thereby disrupts the patient-therapist relationship. Since the type of work that therapists perform requires maximum effort and cooperation from the patient, any action which diminishes the trust with the patient potentially diminishes the effectiveness of the intervention.

At the same time, no therapist is immune to attempts by patients to influence them to provide more services as appreciation for a gift. Patients sometimes try to influence therapists to continue treatment past the point at which, in the therapists' judgment, the patient has the capability of benefiting from treatment. Many patients believe that as long as the therapist continues treatment, hope for significant recovery or restoration of function exists. Certainly no one wants patients to abandon realistic hope, but patients and loved ones should not cling to false hope when doing so undermines efficient use of services or equipment. In these ways, gift giving and receiving are caught in a subtle interplay of hope and honesty in ways that call for good judgment rather than fixed rules.

The cost of a gift is one guide to its intent, albeit a fallible one. For example, gifts must be assessed in relation to the economic situation of patients rather than to its value to the therapist. What appears to be a large gift to a therapist may be an inexpensive expression of appreciation by a patient, while for another patient the same gift would be a considerable sacrifice. In all these cases one must assess the intent based on the history of the relationship and what is known of the patient.

Despite such moral subtleties of gift giving and receiving, in practice the difficulties are not insurmountable. Claudette Finley offers several criteria that cover most cases:[17] Gifts should be expressions of gratitude, not manipulation or coercion; they should have minimal monetary value; they should not significantly shape relationships with vendors; they are best when they benefit people in need; their cost should not be passed on to patients; and, most important, one should be willing to disclose the gift to interested parties.

 ## Teaching and Research

Physical therapists who are also professors have new roles and hence new potential conflicts. Professors of physical therapy experience enormous demands from research and consulting requirements that can threaten teaching responsibilities. Exactly how much time, effort, and skill professors are morally obligated to devote to the teaching role is contestable, thereby inviting a temptation to give more attention to prestige-promoting activities such as writing and research for publication, at a considerable cost to students. But there are threats to research as well, and in general the temptation to enhance personal income, job security, and prestige presents threats to role responsibilities in academia as they do to patient treatment.

There are also episodic conflicts of interest in the teaching arena. One area of concern, for example, is sexual affairs between teacher and student. Do such affairs threaten professors' ability to grade fairly—threatening it sufficiently to call for a university policy forbidding affairs with current students? In our view, the answer is decidedly yes, and that applies not only to the university environment but also to clinical instructors in the clinic setting who teach students as a part of the university program. But others disagree, and many schools do not have policies forbidding such affairs. Values of freedom, sexual and otherwise, are invoked to prevent anything stronger than legally mandated sexual harassment policies. At the very least, however, it is important for universities to give careful attention to this issue and to develop policies after full discussion.

Additional conflicts of interest arise in accepting, rejecting, and supervising student internships. Curricula in programs accredited by the Commission on Accreditation in Physical Therapy Education (CAPTE) are required in section 2.7.2 of the "Evaluative Criteria for Accreditation of Educational Programs for the Preparation of Physical Therapists" to provide "sufficient quality and quantity of clinical education experiences to prepare students for practice." An emerging problem, however, especially in a managed-care environment, is that many therapists are simply refusing to take students because of productivity standards that leave little or no time to supervise the student, thereby adding to universities' difficulties in finding appropriate internship experiences. To further complicate matters, government regulations are constantly in revision. When administrators of Medicare–Part B determined that covered services could not be rendered by students, including physical therapy and medical students, clinicians had to either find new patient experiences for interns or withdraw as student clinical supervisors. At the other end of the spectrum, students in some facilities were sometimes treated as revenue-generating personnel with little, if any, supervision. Since the latter is the only situation over which the educational facility has governance, many schools regularly interview students and conduct on-site clinic visits to ensure that students receive supervision and are not used solely to increase revenue at the expense of the safety of patients. However, as clinical sites continue to diminish, temptations increasingly arise for educational institutions to rationalize inadequate supervision as preferable to creating expensive new university-sponsored clinics to supply needed clinical experiences.

The selection of candidates for educational programs is currently of great concern as well. Periodically, the number of applicants to schools of physical therapy decreases, in particular when managed care institutes cost-saving measures that directly impact the employment opportunities for and salaries of therapists. Meanwhile, the number of accredited physical therapy programs in the United States has increased, rendering some schools unable to fill their class quotas. Like most businesses, university departments are staffed and funded on the basis of anticipated enrollment and accompanying tuition revenue. Compounding the dilemma, academic programs are encouraged by APTA, or even given suggested deadlines by APTA state chapters, to convert existing programs to doctoral programs. This is a transition with considerable cost in terms of labor and material resources.

Taken together, these pressures intensify schools' dual need to select competent students who, upon graduation, will be able to pass licensure examinations, while at the same time keeping enrollment levels adequate to assure the survival of the department. These educational institutions serve as the gatekeepers to the profession and have a duty to populate it with competent professionals, and while some schools have responded to these financial threats by increasing their recruitment programs, it is feared that as competition increases for a diminished pool of applicants, compromises in admission standards are inevitable.

Even the method of selecting candidates is controversial. Basic academic abilities and skills needed to complete the academic program are obviously needed, but what additional qualifications are required? Should the educational institutions focus only on recruiting future clinicians when there are other areas of the profession, such as research, that are seriously deficient? Given the extremely diverse areas of specialization within clinical applications—combined with the employment opportunities in teaching, supervision, and case management—the task of defining valid admission criteria is daunting. Restricting the student population too narrowly does a disservice to the profession, but to apply no standards invites inappropriate academic recruitment to fill revenue needs.

In all university teaching, research responsibilities are important in their own right, in addition to their general contribution to education. The profession of physical therapy is criticized for failing to provide documentation that treatment methods pass accepted standards of scientific inquiry for efficacy, and professors share a responsibility to help remedy that. Practitioners also have this duty, but the conflicts are significant. Especially in a managed-care environment, therapists' first obligation is to provide the best care to the patients who depend on them. Patient loads and allotted time typically eliminate any hope of conducting valid scientific enquiry in the true experimental model. Even quasi-experimental models require more time and planning than most therapists in clinical practice can be expected to accommodate.

In the university setting, faculty in physical therapy carry heavier teaching loads than most other faculty and have very limited resources to finance research studies, either at a public or a private level. The focus of research dollars remains on the most expensive elements of health care, namely pharmacy and surgical interventions.

Even when funds and opportunities are available, double-blind studies have been opposed on the grounds that it is unethical to deny treatment to persons participating in the study. These grounds are valid only when it is known that the treatment has an effect. Controlling for bias in research is essential, given the placebo effect of treatment and researcher bias in therapy. In the absence of that knowledge, we have to question the ethics of providing care that may be of no benefit to tens of thousands of patients, as well as the ethics of carrying opportunity costs to the patient, either by denying alternate care that might provide some benefit or by simply avoiding the costs incurred. There is also the suspicion that research is neglected because it might reveal that certain procedures are ineffective, resulting in possible elimination of some components of practice in physical therapy.

The study of conflicts of interest provides a prism for exploring both the core commitments of, and differences between, individual professions, and nowhere is that more true than in physical therapy. We have highlighted some of the enduring issues in this area, focusing on those related to the public good served by physical therapists (such as provider-adviser conflicts), and also those arising from historically contingent institutional structures and economic settings (such as managed health care). Although we have commented on possible solutions, often the primary challenge is to identify and keep salient key areas in which conflicts of interest recur and are especially likely to cause harm. In the next chapter we will comment further on understanding wrongdoing in conflicts of interest and elsewhere.

Discussion Questions

1. Referring to the chapter's opening case study, identify the conflicts of interest inherent in Simone Thomas's proposal. Are all the conflicts morally objectionable, or would they be tolerable under certain conditions? Discuss.

2. In an advertisement for a new profitable leg brace, a physical therapist endorses the equipment and discusses how it has helped hundreds of her patients. In truth, however, the therapist has had little direct involvement with the braces, apart from being allowed to purchase stock, at a substantially discounted rate, in the company producing the braces. After consulting the APTA *Guide for Professional Conduct*, discuss under what conditions this endorsement and ad would constitute an objectionable conflict of interest. Under what conditions would it be a tolerable conflict of interest?

3. Bill is a hospital administrator in a location that still has a substantial number of patients who pay independently (fee-for-service) for treatment, and he oversees a physical therapy clinic whose revenue has steadily eroded.[18] He calls the clinic director, Mark, and suggests that he expand the number of procedures used per patient visit and thus increase the reimbursement, or else be prepared for decreased staffing in the future. Reluctantly, but feeling strong loyalty to his staff, Mark encourages his staff to increase overall modality (procedure) utilization. Identify the conflict of interest involved in this case, and present and defend your view about whether Mark acted ethically or unethically. If you cannot determine an answer, what further information would you need to know?

4. Marsha has maintained a profitable and expansive private practice since the early eighties. Despite an excellent reputation, she has not been successful in negotiating a rate with the largest local managed-care company that would be an amount adequate to cover her costs and generate a reasonable profit. The last time she spoke with the company's representatives, they suggested that, to be awarded a contract with the managed-care company that would allow her to make a reasonable profit, she should decrease patients' length of stay and be more willing to rely on patient self-administered home treatment programs when their functional abilities improved. Marsha feels her therapists are at their ideal performance level now, but she knows that fiscally the company's recommendations make sense. What conflicts of interest, if any, do you see in the company's proposals?

5. Trevor is a physical therapist assistant at a private practice named Care Unlimited. He is also the owner of the practice and employs 12 physical therapists and 5 physical therapist assistants. Partly because of reduced revenues and partly because of personal beliefs, he instructs the physical therapists to work "smarter" by using the assistants as much as possible to free them up to evaluate and establish the treatment programs for more new patients. During an especially busy day, he is in the clinic when one of the assistants, Shannon, comes to him and says that she will have to dismiss a patient for the day because a change in the patient's status warrants a different course of treatment. However, the patient's physical therapist is busy with a new patient and will not be available to consult with them on the issue in a time frame that will work for the patient. Trevor reviews the patient's chart, he and Shannon agree on an alternate treatment program, and he instructs her to change the program and to treat the patient. What conflicts of interest are apparent in

this situation? What arguments and documents should the physical therapists offer? What arguments and documents should Shannon offer?

6. Considering the inherent conflicts of interest that arise in both fee-for-service and capitated reimbursement plans, what type of reimbursement plan would most diminish the conflicts related to method of reimbursement? Explain your answer.

7. If you were given the opportunity to speak with a congressional leader on matters related to health care, what policies and laws would you recommend to regulate managed care in the area of conflict of interest? Keep in mind that in the current political environment, managed-care corporations, just like any other business, must be allowed to satisfy shareholders by generating a profit.

8. Is direct access to physical therapy a realistic alternative to physician referral? Why are the insurance companies resistant to direct access to physical therapy? What needs to occur within the profession for current students and practitioners to engage in direct access?

9. Physical therapy programs throughout the United States have been hard hit by the combination of increased programs and a stable or even diminished pool of student applicants. What safeguards, if any, could be established to ensure that the quality of practitioners is not diminished by programs that lower their standards to fill their student openings? If changes are offered, should they occur at the state or federal level or should they come from the APTA?

References

1. Martin MW, Gabard DL. Conflict of interest and physical therapy. In: Davis M, Stark A, eds. *Conflict of Interest and the Professions*. New York, NY: Oxford University Press; 2001:314-332.
2. Margolis J. Conflict of interest and conflicting interests. In: Beauchamp TL, Bowie NE, eds. *Ethical Theory and Business*. Englewood Cliffs, NJ: Prentice-Hall; 1979:361-372.
3. Martin MW, Schinzinger R. *Ethics in Engineering*. New York, NY: McGraw-Hill; 1996:221.
4. Davis M. Conflict of interest. In: *Encyclopedia of Applied Ethics*, vol. 1. San Diego, CA: Academic Press; 1998.
5. Kipnis K. *Legal Ethics*. Englewood Cliffs, NJ; Prentice-Hall; 1986.
6. Green RM. Physicians, entrepreneurism and the problem of conflict of interest. *Theoretical Medicine*. 1990;11:287-300.
7. McDowell B. *Ethical Conduct and the Professional's Dilemma: Choosing Between Service and Success*. New York, NY: Quorum; 1991.
8. Rodwin MA. *Medicine, Money, and Morals*. New York, NY: Oxford University Press; 1993.
9. May L. Conflict of interest. In: May L. *The Socially Responsive Self*. Chicago, IL: University of Chicago Press; 1996:123-138.
10. Davis M. Conflict of interest revisited. *Business and Professional Ethics Journal*. 1993;12(4):21-41.
11. Gibson JM. The ethics of managed care. In: Bennahum DA, ed. *Managed Care: Financial, Legal and Ethical Issues*. Cleveland, OH: Pilgrim Press; 1999:131-152.
12. Spidle J. The historical roots of managed care. In: Bennahum DA, ed. *Managed Care: Financial, Legal and Ethical Issues*. Cleveland, OH: Pilgrim Press; 1999:11.
13. Swisher LL, Krueger-Brophy C. *Legal and Ethical Issues in Physical Therapy*. Boston, MA: Butterworth-Heinemann; 1998:204.
14. Rubin RH. Gatekeepers and gatekeeping. In: Bennahum DA, ed. *Managed Care: Financial, Legal and Ethical Issues*. Cleveland, OH: Pilgrim Press; 1999:142.

15. Bennahum DA, ed. *Managed Care: Financial, Legal, and Ethical Issues*. Cleveland, OH: Pilgrim Press; 1999.

16. Tygiel PP. Referral for profit. In: Mathews J, ed. *Practice Issues in Physical Therapy*. Thorofare, NJ: Slack, Inc.; 1989:35-43.

17. Finley C. Gift-giving or influence peddling: can you tell the difference? *Phys Ther*. 1994;74(2):143-147.

18. Purtilo R. Modality utilization: readers respond. *PT Magazine*. July 1996:72-78.
Case study written by Ron Hruska, M.P.H., P.T.

Integrity and Wrongdoing

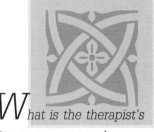

*W*hat is the therapist's and employer's obligation to root out and expose harassing or irresponsible behavior in the workplace?

This chapter explores compliance issues that arise in situations in which professionals make wrong decisions even though it is reasonably clear what is required of them. We begin with sexual harassment, including harassment of patients by therapists, harassment of therapists by other employees, and inappropriate sexual behavior by patients toward therapists. Then we move on to drug abuse by professionals and the problems of fraud in the health-care industry. Following these topics, which constitute only a few of many concerns, we turn to a discussion of how we can both understand and prevent wrongdoing. Throughout this chapter we comment on appropriate responses to wrongdoing by others, and in the concluding section we discuss whistle-blowing, which is by far the most controversial response to wrongdoing.

Sexual Harassment

Sexual harassment is an abuse of power involving sex. It is objectionable primarily because it violates individuals' autonomy—their right to pursue their interests without harmful interference by others.[1] Typically, it inflicts harm on people at a time when they are especially vulnerable in their roles as either patients or employees. In many instances, an element of coercion is present, often employed when, for example, employees feel their jobs are at risk, or when patients perceive that the quality of care is dependent on their compliance with inappropriate requests. Beyond coercion, harassment leads to a violation of patients' trust that professionals will provide them with optimal care.

When the media make the general public aware of abuses, an organization or an entire profession may be adversely affected. Thus, the APTA's *House of Delegate Standards, Policies, Positions and Guidelines* states clearly in HOD 06-99-17-06 (Program 17) that "Environments in which physical therapy services are provided, or in which the work of the American Physical Therapy Association and its components is carried out, should be completely free of sexual harassment."

Sexual harassment occurs in many contexts, three of which are: (1) sexual harassment of employees within organizations, whether engaged in by supervisors, coworkers, or workers outside the organization; (2) sexual harassment of patients by therapists; and (3) sexual harassment of therapists by patients. We begin with sexual harassment within organizations because it is defined and dealt with extensively in the law, court rulings, and federal regulations.

Harassment Within an Organization

Sandra

Advanced Care is a private physical therapy practice in operation since 1989 and owned by Paul Sanford. The practice has been highly successful by adapting to the multiple changes that have occurred since the practice started. There are 14 full-time therapists, 4 physical therapist assistants, and 3 physical therapy aides. The staff has always been predominantly male, and currently only one female therapist is employed there. Sandra started about three months earlier and is already considering leaving the practice, even though she likes the pay, the hours, and the patient load.

She tells a close friend that her office, which is actually a cubicle, provides no protection from the constant bantering of the other therapists. The men have never treated her unfairly nor disparaged her, but their conversations constantly reference their sexual adventures and fantasies. She has never considered herself a prude, but she finds their comments both distracting and offensive to women in general. When she told the owner about her concerns, he advised her to not listen to the discussions, that men will be men, and that there was nothing he could do. She can relocate to another job, but she wonders if she has any other options. Her friend suggests she might be dealing with sexual harassment.

Legal protection against sexual harassment is founded on the federal Civil Rights Act of 1964, although that act was not originally intended to cover gender discrimination.[2] The original bill was introduced in Congress to end discrimination in employment based on religion, race, color, and national origin. Gender was not included until it was attached at the last minute in an amendment by Southern conservative opponents who felt certain the addition would cause the failure of the entire bill. After being voted into law, the gender component of the act was ignored. The first head of the Equal Employment Opportunity Commission (EEOC), which was the agency charged to enforce the act, stated that the sex discrimination portion was a joke. In fact, the first regulations classifying sexual harassment as a form of sexual discrimination were published many years later, in 1980, under Eleanor Holmes Norton, the new director of the EEOC. It took six more years for the U.S. Supreme Court to confirm that sexual harassment was indeed a form of sex discrimination, in its ruling in *Meritor Sav. Bank v. Vinson* (1986). The issue garnered national attention in 1991 when, during the Senate confirmation hearing for Supreme Court nominee Clarence Thomas, attorney Anita Hill charged that Thomas had sexually harassed her when she worked for him at the Justice Department. After the hearing, about one-third of Americans believed Anita Hill's claim, but two-thirds of Americans believed Clarence Thomas, paving the way for his confirmation as a Supreme Court justice. Nevertheless, as a result, sexual harassment became a topic indelibly etched on the public's consciousness.

The EEOC defines sexual harassment in the workplace as follows:

> Unwelcome sexual advances, requests for sexual favors, and other verbal or physical conduct of a sexual nature constitute sexual harassment when submission to such conduct is made either explicitly or implicitly a term or condition of an individual's employment, submission to or rejection of such conduct by an individual is used as the basis for employment decisions affecting such individual, or such conduct has the purpose or effect of unreasonably interfering with an individual's work performance or creating an intimidating, hostile or offensive working environment.[3]

Subsequent court rulings have often combined the first two situations in the EEOC definition into a category called "quid pro quo" (this for that, or getting "something for something") cases, including threats of harm and offers of benefits at the workplace. The last situation in the definition is now often called a "hostile work environment." Thus, the two main categories are now distinguished as:[1(p441)]

Quid pro quo: Unwelcome sexual advances, requests, or other sexual conduct that are made a condition of employment, promotion, pay raise, or other job benefit.

Hostile work environment: Unwelcome sexual advances, requests, or other conduct that may unreasonably interfere with work performance or create an intimidating or offensive work environment.

The courts have interpreted both these categories very broadly. Thus, quid pro quo sexual harassment includes all unwelcome sexual offers even if they occur only once. Hostile environment harassment includes any feature of the workplace that could lead employees to feel their ability to work or to compete fairly is in jeopardy. For example, suppose a supervisor or coworker makes inappropriately explicit sexual comments. It is not necessary that anyone be the target of the comments. The EEOC has stated that "the victim does not have to be the person harassed but could be anyone affected by the offensive conduct."[2(p1,19)] This conduct includes language and jokes which make for a "sexually poisoned workplace," posting pornographic or sexually oriented pictures, solicitations for sexual favors, or name calling focused on a person's gender.[2(p2,3),4]

A familiar defense of employers in sexual harassment cases is that some workers are excessively sensitive, to the point where they react irrationally to even a mildly sexual innuendo by a coworker. What standard do the courts use to rule in such cases? The interpretation of exactly what counts as sexual harassment is made from the perspective of a "reasonable person," a "reasonable woman," or a "reasonable victim," depending on the court.[5,6]

Most recently, the standard has been expanded to cover any form of same-sex harassment as well. The Supreme Court, ruling in *Oncale v. Sundowner Offshore Services, Inc.* (1996), made it clear that sexual harassment can be between persons of the same sex regardless of motive. This ruling struck down the prior federal court position that same-sex harassment could only occur in the presence of sexual desire, thus defining it only when the aggressor was homosexual: "Harassing conduct need not be motivated by sexual desire in order to be actionable, and the standards in same-sex cases will be the same as in opposite-sex cases: whether the sex-based conduct is sufficiently severe and pervasive to create an objectively hostile or abuse work environment."[7] Based on the *Oncale v. Sundowner* ruling, gays and lesbians will likely have federal as well as state protection from sexual harassment in the workplace.

What if managers simply say they were unaware of the problem and hence should not be held responsible for the actions of their employees? In the eyes of the court, managers are still responsible because their job is to know what goes on in the workplace, and negligence does not absolve them of that responsibility. The standard that applies is that managers "knew or should have known." To avoid liability, employers must prove they used reasonable care to prevent and correct harassing behavior, and also show that the victim unreasonably failed to take advantage of preventive and corrective action.[8] If for any reason managers retaliate against an employee who has alleged sexual harassing behaviors, then they have committed a second offense under Title VII of the Civil Rights Act of 1964. However, under federal law, individual managers are not liable for damages, unless, of course, they are the perpetrators. Yet some states, including New York and Illinois, have imposed personal liability on the manager.

In all cases in which sexual harassment charges are pursued through the EEOC, the victim must exhaust administrative remedies before the EEOC will give its permission for a lawsuit. Of course, one can skip the EEOC altogether, depending on the state, and file for compensatory and punitive damages through civil court. In all states, the victim can sue through civil court for damages due to defamation or emotional distress. Thus, at the very least, every employer should:

1. Publish a written policy forbidding sexual harassment.

2. Implement a complaint procedure with clear prohibition on retaliation.

3. Set up programs to train all current and future employees about the policy and complaint procedures.[9]

Harassment of Patients

We turn now, more briefly, to sexual harassment of patients by therapists. Such categorically forbidden behavior flagrantly violates the autonomy of patients who have chosen to seek therapy—and who have decidedly not chosen to serve as objects of someone's sexual gratification. Patients trust that professionals will set aside their self-serving motivations in order to provide quality health care. The rare therapist who violates that trust is harming patients at a time of great emotional and physical vulnerability. The trust of colleagues, both within the organization and within the profession as a whole, is also violated, because when the abuse comes to light, negative publicity harms both the health-care organization and the entire profession.

What about situations in which sexual attraction is mutual and appreciated? In such instances it would seem there is no victim and hence no harm. One troublesome issue, however, concerns the genuineness of the relationship. Formal roles (therapist, patient) can eclipse important values that support lasting committed relationships often desired by one or both parties. Furthermore, even if we have no interest in protecting the genuineness and duration of relationships, the organization might be harmed. A health-care service environment is tightly focused on the services and equipment linked to the delivery of care; it has nothing to gain by allowing behaviors contrary to its mission, and problems arise all too often as relationships go awry. Thus, failed romantic relationships in the employment setting are a frequent cause of charges of sexual harassment, as one party keeps pursuing a relationship unwanted by the other. Failed relationships are also a source of violence in the workplace.[10]

Taken together, these considerations support a complete ban on any kind of sexual relationship between professional and client. Yet, would such a ban violate the autonomy and the sexual freedom of consenting adults? After struggling with this question, the American Physical Therapy Association *Guide for Professional Conduct* adopted an approach that forbids all sexual relationships with current patients while allowing consenting adults to pursue a relationship after formally ending the professional-client relationship. Section 2.1(c) of the APTA *Guide for Professional Conduct* states: "A physical therapist shall not engage in any sexual relationship or activity, whether consensual or nonconsensual, with any patient while a physical therapist/patient relationship exists." This leaves open an option previously mentioned in the guide but omitted from its latest revision: "In the event that a physical therapist and patient are about to begin a sexually intimate relationship, the therapist shall expeditiously disengage from care of the patient and coordinate the transfer of care of the patient, as appropriate, to another provider." This alternative attempted to take account of sexual freedom between consenting adults, which is assumed in the current guide. We would caution, however, that patients' vulnerabilities can extend beyond the time the therapist provides professional services.

Harassment by Patients

Now consider the far more common problem of sexual harassment and other inappropriate sexual behavior by patients toward physical therapists. Therapists, male and female alike, are especially at risk for these behaviors because of the close physical contact and prolonged private communication with patients. In addition, because of their physical disabilities and complex psychological states that may be triggered by medications, feelings of isolation, and damaged self-esteem, patients frequently experience a need for reassurance that they are desirable and lovable.

The statistics are dramatic. According to a study conducted in Canada, 92.9 percent of surveyed practicing physical therapists experienced some level of inappropriate patient sexual behavior in the work environment.[11] Of those, 32.8 percent of female physical therapists and 37.5 percent of male physical therapists experienced severe inappropriate sexual behavior by patients. Over 66 percent of students in physical therapy, by the end of their training, encountered inappropriate sexual behavior by patients. In the United States, a national study published in 1997 found that 86 percent of physical therapists experienced some form of inappropriate sexual behavior by patients and 63 percent reported at least one incident of sexual harassment by patients.[12]

Patient harassment of therapists occurs at several levels.[12] Mildly inappropriate sexual behavior by patients, characterized as suggestive stories or solicitations for dates, are frequently best handled by ignoring or being nonresponsive to the behavior, thus escaping from the conflict. Moderate (deliberate touching, direct propositions) and severe (forceful fondling and attempts to secure sexual intercourse) inappropriate sexual behavior present the therapist with much more difficulty—and sometimes temptation.

In these cases, disclosure to appropriate parties, and notations on the patient's chart, usually secures a just outcome. In difficult cases, patients can be reassigned to a new therapist. However, many therapists fear that administrative efforts will downplay the offense or even blame the therapist for contributing to the situation. This may be because administrators are often preoccupied with patient satisfaction to keep the market share necessary for survival and profit. Portrayal of the organization or individual therapists to the public as repressive, lacking a sense of humor, or just being plain hard-nosed does not increase subscription rates or ensure continuing contracts. To counter these perceptions, many therapists ignore patients' inappropriate behavior and fail to report it to supervisors, fearing that their own integrity might be brought into question. Indeed, therapists who complain about patient behavior to supervisors are frequently regarded as whistle-blowers who reveal an institutional secret. Some therapists are left without any realistic means of protecting themselves or achieving fairness.

The institutional response should focus on the long-term survival of the organization. That means recognizing that the health-care worker should be afforded the same legal protection from patients as from coworkers. Substantial numbers of therapists simply will not stay in an employment setting where their personal integrity is compromised. When therapists are harmed by patient behaviors, the quality of care is diminished, either through avoidance or through stringent risk-reduction efforts. To meet expectations of quality care and to maintain a stable workforce, health-care organizations must make clear to patients and staff that sexual harassment policies extend to patients as well as to staff.

If a patient sexually harasses a therapist, the supervisor is responsible for taking immediate action to prevent recurrence, even if the employee does not complain. Attorney and physical therapist Ron Scott suggests that responsible steps include the following:

- Investigating the victim's complaint.
- Counseling the offender to cease and desist from further sexual harassment of victim.
- Transferring the patient to another therapist's care.
- Consulting with other health professionals, the referring physician, human resources management, or an EEOC official, as appropriate, for advice.
- Removing the patient who continues to sexually harass staff from the clinic.[13]

Drug Abuse by Professionals

Stuart and Marcie

Stuart is a senior therapist at St. Joseph's Hospital and has recently finalized a traumatic divorce. He is always on time for work, but he is obviously "not with it" until nearly noon. This, and the fact that he forgets to attend to even the most basic matters, such as charting, are unlike his performance in the department during the prior six years. Marcie, another physical therapist, told some of her peers that an occupational therapist in the department had a patient who complained that Stuart smelled of alcohol when he treated her that morning. Other therapists had noticed a real change in the quality of Stuart's work, but they had not seen anything that put patients at risk. Together, they wondered what they should do, for the sake of both Stuart and future patients.

Substance abuse and substance dependency are concerns in all professions, but especially the health professions.[14] Psychoactive drugs, both legal and illegal, permeate our society. Given the nature of their work, health professionals often have knowledge of and easier access to drugs than most citizens. Moreover, the work of professionals often involves a high stress level, if only because of continual striving for excellence in performing complex tasks. And abuse of drugs by professionals is easy to ignore, cover up, or rationalize, given the image of "druggies" as entirely unlike highly educated and socially contributing individuals.

Do employees have a privacy right to use and even abuse drugs without penalty from one's employer or interference by colleagues as long as they do their jobs? If so, random drug testing—and the penalties it imposes—is presumably unjustified even though it is widely practiced today. Is substance abuse utterly irresponsible—something that should be reported to appropriate authorities?

Defenders of a strong right to privacy in drug use argue that adults should be allowed to pursue their freedom unless they harm others. They consider many current drug laws excessively punitive, and they object to the now common practice of allowing employers control over their employees' privacy by using mandatory drug tests. As noted in Chapter 2, this Harm Principle is defended by libertarian rights ethicists, but its most powerful defense was given in utilitarian terms by John Stuart Mill. In *On Liberty*, Mill argued for "one very simple principle":

> That principle is that the sole end for which mankind are warranted, individually or collectively, in interfering with the liberty of action of any of their number is self-protection. That the only purpose for which power can be rightfully exercised over any member of a civilized community, against his will, is to prevent harm to others. His own good, either physical or moral, is not a sufficient warrant.[15]

Mill argued that each of us is best able to make decisions about our own happiness and self-fulfillment. Often we make mistakes, but even those mistakes can strengthen our capacities for choice, insight, and emotional development. Accordingly, Mill strongly opposed nearly all forms of paternalism regarding competent adults, including government control of alcohol and other drugs, although he allowed government the right to tax and provide other disincentives to drug use. He favored protecting the freedom to use alcohol and drugs as rights—rights that within his utilitarian framework are areas of freedom deserving protection.

For their part, libertarian rights ethicists appeal more directly to basic human rights of liberty to defend a strong privacy right in matters of alcohol and drugs. Regarding the workplace, they argue that as long as individuals do their jobs according to expectations, employers have no right to interfere with their drug use by imposing mandatory drug tests.[16] In their view, health professionals and other employees are paid to perform at a certain level of excellence, and when they fall below that level they are open to disciplinary action for the behavioral failure, whatever its cause. However, if employees perform effectively while at work, libertarian rights ethicists believe employers do not have the right to use mandatory random drug testing to monitor employees' use of drugs away from the workplace.

Most critics of drug testing do allow some exceptions, however. Consistent with Mills's Harm Principle, they acknowledge that testing is justified when workers using drugs impose a clear and present danger to other persons. This exception would seem to apply to many health professionals who could do great damage to patients if their judgment becomes drug-impaired. Defenders of strict laws governing drug abuse and drug testing in the workplace go further in emphasizing these dangers to patients and to others. Serious addictions, whether to cocaine or to alcohol, are a time bomb waiting to explode, even when they do not impose a "clear and present danger" at a given moment. Certainly in the long run, worker productivity is threatened, but in the health-care environment much more than absenteeism and decreased energy are at stake. There are genuine dangers to patients.

Even if the extent of privacy rights regarding drugs were clear, the entire debate over drug use is complicated by many questions. One important question is whether we should view drug abuse and addictions as forms of sickness, to which medical approaches apply, or as acts of wrongdoing, to which moral attitudes apply. The **therapeutic trend** is the tendency to adopt health-oriented attitudes and approaches to problems earlier viewed in moral terms. This trend unfolded on many fronts throughout the twentieth century, but nowhere was the trend more dramatic than in the perception of addictions. The official view, first endorsed in the 1930s by Alcoholics Anonymous, is that alcoholics have a disease, and this same view has been adopted toward many other addictions, from drugs to pathological gambling. Psychiatrists now label substance dependency a "mental disorder"—a form of impairment or distress occurring when three or more of the following criteria are met during a 12-month period: (1) tolerance (the need for greater amounts of the drug to achieve the desired effect); (2) withdrawal effects; (3) taking more of the drug than intended; (4) unsuccessful efforts to cut down or control use of the drug; (5) spending much time obtaining, using, and recovering from the drug; (6) giving up important activities in using the drug; and (7) continuing use of the drug despite knowing the harm it is causing.[17]

Critics of the therapeutic trend argue that this specification of substance abuse is nothing more than a description of the loss of control involved when individuals fail to meet their responsibilities to maintain rational supervision of their lives. Harmful addictions, according to critics, are bad habits for which individuals remain morally accountable. They are habits that can take on a life of their own, becoming "central activities" that powerfully shape the lives of individuals, as well as leading to cognitive distortion and adverse physiological effects.[18,19] Nevertheless, even the law holds addicts accountable for the damage they cause, even though at the time they might not be fully in control of their actions. Thus, by the time intoxicated persons get into a car, they might be literally out of control but they are fully accountable before the law for drunk driving and any injuries caused. Even therapeutic perspectives necessarily regard individuals as responsible for seeking and cooperating with available help.

Probably a Janus-faced moral and therapeutic view of addictions is needed, but our society has yet to work out such a nuanced view.[20] As just one of many examples of our society's confusion about this question, consider two recent California laws. The "Three Strikes Law," implemented in 1994, made lengthy prison terms mandatory for commission of a third felony, and since drug abuse is a common felony, California prisons were immediately loaded beyond capacity with drug offenders. Then, in 2000, the public passed Proposition 36 by a two-thirds margin, sending nonviolent drug abusers into mandatory therapy instead of prison (beginning in July 2001). Insofar as substance abuse and dependency are viewed as sicknesses, Proposition 36 can be seen as a form of paternalism that forces sick people to get help. Alternatively, the proposition can be viewed as affirming that use of illegal substances is still a crime for which individuals are brought before the law even though those individuals are not morally blameworthy, but rather sick and in need of therapy.

The clash of moral and therapeutic views enters into one of the most difficult decisions professionals sometimes must make: what to do when a colleague is abusing drugs. Is the colleague a wrongdoer who should be reported to an employer or other authorities before causing serious damage to patients, or a victim of a sickness and as such in need of sympathetic help? Often the answer seems to be a combination: the professional is doing something wrong but also needs help, at least until a point is reached at which the professional refuses help and pursues a destructive course that requires forcible intervention.

Ruth B. Purtilo considers the following case:

> Suppose that during the past few months you have seen a drastic change in your colleague AB, who lately has a disheveled appearance and is unable to remember even simple things. Something clearly is wrong. Every time you approach AB about this, he says he is okay; however, several incidents in the last week have convinced you that he is putting patients at risk. One patient even took you aside and suggested that AB was "acting kind of strange," but the patient would not elaborate. You strongly suspect AB has a substance abuse problem.[21]

What should you do? Purtilo argues that usually a combination of compassion and firmness toward the colleague is needed. She recommends the following steps be taken: First, gather information discreetly, trying to balance the need to confirm and document your concerns with the protection of AB's privacy. Talk with and seek advice from trusted colleagues, again while trying to maintain confidentiality. Second, identify and weigh the conflicting duties that invariably create an ethical dilemma in such situations, including duties to protect patients, duties to AB and other colleagues, and duties to one's organization. In the situation, which is most important? Third, consider all reasonable options, including morally creative ways to resolve the dilemma. Fourth, proceed with courage and attempt to minimize harm to all involved.

Ron Scott believes that licensure regulations or state or federal law should mandate that peers must report providers who are impaired because of the potential risk to patients.[22] This position is supported by Principle 9.1 of the *Guide for Professional Conduct*, which states "A physical therapist shall report any conduct that appears to be unethical, incompetent, or illegal." However, at what point is the provider incompetent, and just how much impairment is cause for action? After recovering from the flu or a cold, probably no one is optimal, but does being less than optimal constitute a threat to patients?

In some situations, group interventions prove effective. R. Coombs states, "A caring group of family, friends, and other associates, all carefully rehearsed, surprise the addict in a meeting in which they tell him or her how the addictive behavior adversely affects them."[14(p168)] Other times, having a trusted friend, perhaps oneself or another colleague, speak with the drug-impaired professional is enough. In extreme situations, the best route might be to blow the whistle on the individual by filing a formal complaint with one's employer or other authority. All these choices carry risk, but there can also be serious risks in doing nothing.

Fraud

Troy

Troy has been with Buena Vista Rehabilitation for three years, and during that time his patient load grew to the point where he had few appointment times available for new patients. Administrators are pleased with his work and especially pleased with the profit ratio of Troy's department. Nevertheless, administration has maintained a freeze on hiring because of the marginal profit of the institution as a whole. Rather than have patients go without care, Troy initiated several group activities, one of which was a knee therapy group. The group consisted of eight patients who were at the same approximate stage in their rehabilitation. The patients did exercises together at Troy's instruction while providing encouragement to each other. At each session the patients reviewed their home programs, asked questions, and expressed any concerns.

The group was a success in several ways. Patients liked working together, not only for the effective therapy, but also for the additional social benefits and for the information they gathered from other patients. Troy was pleased because the patients did well, and the one class opened up seven appointment times for him. Even though he knew that Buena Vista was in marginal financial trouble, Troy did not want to lose the revenue from these patients that would have been gained had they been seen individually. He therefore billed Medicare for each patient under the CPT code for individual therapy. Since an appreciable amount of time was spent on the home program reviews, he also billed this activity under CPT 99071, which is a code for educational materials, since there is no reimbursement code for oral review of home programs.

Prior to its implementation, Troy had reviewed the group idea with the department chair, who instructed him in the Medicare codes and billing format. From Troy's perspective, the patients received necessary treatment and the department was rewarded at a rate that made financial survival more likely.

It was estimated that in 1999, in the Medicare program alone, improper payments of $13.5 billion accounted for about 8 percent of the total $169.5

billion of reimbursements.[23] The improper payments frequently occurred when care was billed but never delivered, when noncovered services were coded as covered services, or when charges were "upcoded" to represent a higher level of service than was actually performed. In general, such activity is labeled **fraud,** which is the intentional misrepresentation (by commission or through the omission of relevant information) of eligibility or the services or goods delivered. **Abuse** occurs when reimbursement is sought for treatments or goods which are medically unnecessary, excessive, or inappropriate.[24] Such abuse calls into question the moral integrity of the practitioner, and even of the profession when it occurs frequently. Since financial resources are limited, any effort to unfairly claim payment suggests that unless taxpayers bear the responsibility of payment, patients in need of services will have to be denied. In recognition of the social consequences of this form of theft, the APTA *Code of Ethics* strictly forbids fraud and abuse under Principles 2, 3, 4, 7, 8 and 9.

Professional codes of ethics are not the only standards violated. Fraud, depending on whether it is with private or public insurance, violates federal or state laws in addition to licensure regulations.[22(pp127-129)] For example, in the case, Troy is probably guilty of Medicare fraud, and, since he mailed the requests for reimbursement, he is also probably guilty of mail fraud. If he submitted the claims electronically, there is a separate federal law which covers the use of telephone lines for fraudulent purposes.[25] If he lies about his actions or makes false statements, he has committed a separate felony under the False Claims Act. Even though he was given bad advice by his superior, he remains personally culpable. Ignorance of regulation is no defense.

Troy's supervisor is probably guilty of conspiracy, both because he facilitated the fraud and because he failed to report Troy's illegal activity. Any peer who had knowledge of the fraud and failed to report it is also guilty of conspiracy. Even if his supervisor had not advised Troy and had not been told what had occurred, the supervisor would still have been charged with conspiracy under the "knew or should have known" standard.

Health-care reimbursement systems are becoming increasingly protected from abuses other than fraud. For example, kickbacks for goods, services, or referrals—either receiving them or giving them—is prohibited under the federal Health Insurance Portability and Accountability Act of 1996. Physical therapists have paid fines and some have served prison sentences as well as expulsion from the APTA and the loss of their licensure.

Although deliberate fraud might appear to be easily detected, there are institutional and covert forms that are not always apparent. For example, some facilities maintain patients regardless of their ability to profit from therapy until the third-party payments are exhausted.[26] Only when funding is exhausted do they discharge the patients. As another example, some providers exhaust the coverage under one diagnosis and then assign a new, untruthful, diagnosis to receive extended reimbursed treatment.

Not all misrepresentation clearly rewards the provider. In some publicly funded therapy, such as children's services, continued therapy is contingent on continued documented progress. When therapists exaggerate or even create improvements for the sake of continuing therapy, they might be acting upon what they perceive to be the best interest of the patient. In some cases, patients do plateau, only to later improve. Therapists sometimes express the fear that unless they continue seeing the child, they will not know if the child has just reached a plateau or reached maximum potential. Sadly, the cost of futile treatment, regardless of whether it is intermittent or continuous, is passed on to the children who are on the waiting lists. The longer they wait, many feel, the more narrow the window of opportunity for treatment to be maximally effective. The better approach would be to regularly audit the child who has ceased to make genuine progress and reintervene if lack of progress is indeed just a temporary phase of development. A new patient from the waiting list could at least be assigned a home treatment program.

Common to most types of fraud and abuse, however, is the effort to put the welfare of patients secondary to that of providers. One type of fraud is the delivery of services that are not medically necessary or appropriate. Some treatments in physical therapy have little if any empirical proof of efficacy, raising questions about the standard of "medically necessary and appropriate care." How close is the profession of physical therapy to institutional fraud when we offer and charge for treatments which have no proven efficacy, and are in fact in doubt, such as coma stimulation and cognitive retraining?[26(p3)] If the "ostrich with its head in the sand" is not a defense for fraud or conspiracy in fraud because of the "knew or should have known" principle, then the profession must aggressively seek to produce research studies that address effectiveness of treatment methods. Without that validation, the integrity of the entire profession is at risk.

The historical context for the absence of evidence-based treatment is complex. Physical therapy is a relatively young and emerging profession that has focused its attention on treatment. Educational programs have historically screened applicants to accept only those likely to develop excellent clinical skills. Clinicians, especially in the managed-care environment, rightfully claim that even though the educational process taught them how to do research, there is neither time nor financial support for this endeavor. Clinicians will also often state that they went into the profession to treat, not to do research. Treatment validation, they insist, should fall to the academic faculty, who can use the university resources to do the research. On the other hand, the faculty respond that they have heavy teaching loads, heavier than other disciplines, and as a consequence have less time to conduct the large randomized sample investigations that are needed. Besides, they will say, clinicians are ideally placed to understand the treatments that need to be investigated and how they should be investigated.

Both sides express part of the truth. Nevertheless, a duty to produce the needed research can only be realized when the duty is assigned. In all likelihood, that duty belongs to both the clinicians and academicians in partnership, each supplying their expertise and resources. As the profession matures, the educational units must realize that screenings for classroom positions should not screen out those who would prefer to teach or conduct research.

Explaining Wrongdoing

In the novel *Middlemarch*, George Eliot explores how easily, and yet how gradually and unthinkingly, professional commitments become compromised. Professionals are motivated to meet their responsibilities, but they are also motivated by compensation issues—personal benefits such as earning a living, acquiring great wealth, gaining power and authority, and maintaining prestige. In some individuals, compensation motives become entirely dominant and lead to wholesale corruption.[27] More often, however, they exert their influence in more subtle ways, gradually eroding commitments to the public good served by the profession.

In Eliot's book, Dr. Lydgate moves to the town of Middlemarch, confident of his own good character. It is not that he is complacent about ethics—on the contrary, he begins by setting a higher ethical standard in his medical practice. In the provincial town, other physicians routinely take a percentage back from pharmacists for their prescriptions. The physicians also dispense drugs, allowing them to make a double profit, once in prescribing and again in filling the prescription. Unlike his peers, Lydgate discerns the inherent conflict of interest in such practices. Nevertheless, he is overly assured about his own incorruptibility. He also happens to share his wife's expensive tastes in a house and furniture, and he implicitly expects his peers to appreciate his superior class background.

Gradually his debts mount to the point where he is forced to take out a large loan from the local banker, whom he has been warned will misuse his influence for personal advantage. As he continues to live beyond his means, Lydgate becomes ensnared in a complex web of events that creates a strong appearance of wrongdoing. Specifically, he prescribes a medicine that is misused by the banker to contribute to the death of the banker's former business partner, who is blackmailing the banker. Through it all, Lydgate is caught unprepared for his vulnerability to mundane corrosions of moral commitment: "He was amazed, disgusted that conditions so foreign to all his purposes, so hatefully disconnected with the objects he cared to occupy himself with, should have lain in ambush and clutched him when he was unaware."[28] Like most of us, he simply lived his life in different directions that are not comprehended together—with "numerous strands of experience lying side by side and never compar[ing] them with each other."[28]

Eliot helps us appreciate how character and circumstances intertwine, and hence how both enter into understanding wrongdoing. She appreciates how social explanations and character **explanations of wrongdoing**, as we might call them, are complementary in helping us explain wrongdoing in the professions.

Social explanations explain wrongdoing by defining the structural features and outside pressures that create temptations for professions not to meet their responsibilities. The features might be systemic, such as the inherent tensions we have discussed within managed-care practices. Or they might be episodic, specifying particular features of the jobs and situations in which individuals choose to work.

Character explanations explain wrongdoing by identifying personal faults. Sometimes these explanations are dismissed as simplistic "bad apple explanations," in which certain individuals are cast as villains. It is true that bad apple explanations are usually (though not always) inaccurate and naive ways of understanding wrongdoing. Yet, character explanations assume more subtle forms. We can draw a distinction between global and situational character explanations that parallels the distinction between systemic and episodic social explanations. *Global character explanations* are the bad apple explanations, which are only rarely plausible. In contrast, *situational character explanations* refer to specific faults that lead to specific kinds of failings in particular situations. As Eliot reminds us, character is not all good or bad; it is "spotted" with faults and strengths.[28(p149)] Moreover, these faults and strengths change over time: "Character is not cut in marble—it is not something solid and unalterable. It is something living and changing, and may become diseased as our bodies do."[28(pp734,735)]

Character explanations might be sorted into three several broad categories, each with several subheadings: (1) bad preferences, (2) lack of rational self-control, and (3) moral indifference.[29,30]

Bad preferences are morally harmful intentions and undesirable desires. One subcategory is **preferential immorality**, in which a professional, aware of what is morally required, simply prefers the personal benefits that come from wrongdoing over doing what is right. An example would be knowing that morality forbids fraudulent billing of medical costs and yet engaging in fraud for personal gain. Another subcategory is **perverse immorality**, in which the professional believes that what is in fact immoral is moral. An extreme example is bigotry, in which one believes that particular groups of people are less than fully equal human beings. Another example is the sexual harassment of vulnerable victims for sexual-aggressive gratifications.

Lack of rational self-control means a lack of sufficiently strong moral motivation to do what one knows is right because it is right. **Weakness of will** (or moral weakness) is the most familiar subcategory. For example, one knows that one should avoid taking an expensive gift from a salesperson, and one has some desire to maintain one's professional integrity, but the temptation overrides this desire. Signs of weakness of will include experiencing conflict passions at the time, or feeling guilt afterward. **Moral negligence** is another subcategory, in which one's judgment becomes blurred through thoughtlessness, carelessness, and lack of due care. This distortion of judgment might be reckless (knowing), but more often it is inadvertent. An example of inadvertent moral negligence is found in the conflicts of interest that Simone Thomas, in the example opening Chapter 7, was about to enter.

Both forms of lost self-control are often accompanied by *self-deception*, in which we refuse to acknowledge to ourselves truths that are important in our situation. This refusal can take several forms:

> Self-deceivers might (a) evade understanding by blurring their grasp of what they know, (b) evade attention through systematic distraction, (c) evade belief via willful ignorance or rationalization, (d) evade cogent argument by disregarding evidence, discounting relevant facts, or refusing to let oneself see clearly what follows from what, (e) evade appropriate emotional responses and attitude adjustments by using emotional detachment, (f) evade appropriate action using self-pretense.[31]

Eliot traces many of Dr. Lydgate's failures to his excessive vanity, which motivates him to deceive himself about the extent to which he is vulnerable to temptations: "Lydgate's conceit was of the arrogant sort ... massive in its claims."[28(p149)]

Finally, **moral indifference** is lack of concern for the well-being of others (or oneself). Obviously this lack of concern overlaps with the previous categories, but it is also a distinctive problem. One of its subcategories is **amorality**, a general refusal to apply moral principles to one's life. An extreme example is the sociopath who lacks any sense of moral right and wrong.

Another subcategory, more germane to the professions, is **moral detachment**: having general moral concern but failing to apply that concern in particular situations, usually because one is disillusioned, burned out, or overwhelmed with personal difficulties. This should not be confused with appropriate professional detachment, discussed in Chapter 4, that enables one to avoid excessive or improper emotional entanglements with patients. But certainly overdistancing can lead to moral detachment.

To explain wrongdoing is not to excuse or forgive it, contrary to the proverb that "to understand is to forgive." That proverb has a point in cautioning us against self-righteous and hypocritical condemnations of others, itself a form of (perverse) immorality. But understanding why professionals engage in wrongdoing is important in making moral assessments. It is also important in finding ways to prevent or minimize wrongdoing.

Whistle-blowing

In discussing sexual harassment, drug abuse, and fraudulent billing, we commented on some of the appropriate or even obligatory responses to wrongdoing by others. We now consider perhaps the most controversial response by professionals to others' wrongdoing: **whistle-blowing**. In recent decades, whistle-blowing has received considerable attention in professional ethics discussions, and for good reason. Almost invariably, some professionals are aware of, or have grounds to suspect, instances of malpractice, negligence, and other forms of wrongdoing within organizations. As professionals, they are charged with serving the good of their clients, and also the wider good of the public as it bears on their professional roles. At what point are professionals morally permitted, and even morally required, to "blow the whistle" by reporting the problems to appropriate officials? And even though there are responsibilities to blow the whistle, and yet also severe penalties for doing so, are there moral rights to whistle-blowing that deserve support and legal protection by government, professional societies, and others?

To begin with, what exactly is whistle-blowing? Its critics define it pejoratively, as disloyalty and as "ratting on" the company and colleagues. Its advocates sometimes define it honorifically, as the heroic act, based in humanitarian motives, of warning the public of dangers. We prefer to adopt the following neutral definition, which does not assume that whistle-blowing is either justified or unjustified, or done with good or bad motives, thereby leaving these matters for moral inquiry:

> [Whistle-blowing is] the actions of employees (or former employees) who identify what they believe to be a significant moral problem concerning their company (or other corporations they deal with), who convey information about the problem outside approved organizational channels or against strong pressure from supervisors or colleagues not to do so, with the intention of notifying persons in a position to take action to remedy the problem (regardless of whatever further motives they may have beyond this intention).[29(p139)]

As defined, whistle-blowing might be *internal*: information is conveyed to higher authorities within the organization. Alternatively, it might be *external*: information is conveyed outside the organization, perhaps to a journalist or a government official. Also, whistle-blowing can be *open*, in which one identifies oneself as the source of the information, or *anonymous*, whereby one withholds one's identity. A mixed case occurs when one reveals one's identity to a journalist on the condition that one's name will not be revealed to the public.

Whistle-blowing decisions are among the most difficult that professionals face. Typically the decisions center on the ethical dilemmas created by conflicting professional obligations, namely: (1) loyalty to one's employer and colleagues, including specific duties of confidentiality and team play, versus (2) duties to protect one's patients, one's future patients, and the wider public. Given the harsh repercussions for whistle-blowing, the dilemmas also involve weighing (3) rights to pursue one's career and responsibilities to oneself and to one's family. Professionals who report to their supervisors the misdeeds or inefficiencies that result in diminished safety or care might find management in their organization unresponsive, and in fact more eager to silence the objection than fix the problem. Indeed, as we noted, some argue that most whistle-blowing is a betrayal of one's organization and colleagues. These critics insist that organizations should be permitted to deal with their problems internally, without the damage to their reputation caused by whistle-blowers.

What guidance concerning whistle-blowing can be found in the APTA *Guide for Professional Conduct*? Principle 9 states: "A physical therapist shall protect the public and the profession from unethical, incompetent, and illegal acts." This principle is vague, but it seems to convey a spirit of support for responsible whistle-blowing aimed at protecting the public and the profession. Principle 9.1(c) apparently supports that interpretation: "A physical therapist shall report any conduct that appears to be unethical, incompetent, or illegal." Yet we are not told to whom the report may be made—to one's boss, to an appropriate government official, to a journalist, or to someone else? Critics opposed to whistle-blowing might interpret these statements as only requiring internal reporting—that is, reporting within the organization's approved channels, and not as supporting external whistle-blowing. Perhaps it is fair to say that currently the APTA guide does not provide explicit and strong support for whistle-blowing based on responsible professional judgment.

Some philosophers have attempted to state general rules about situations in which whistle-blowing is justified. Richard T. De George distinguishes two senses of "justified": permissible and obligatory. He suggests that whistle-blowing is morally permissible when (1) serious harm to the public is at stake, (2) one reports one's concerns to one's supervisor, and (3) one exhausts other channels for solving the problem within the organization—for example, by taking advantage of a company's open door policy. Whistle-blowing is justified as obligatory when two further conditions are met: (4) one has documented evidence that would convince reasonable parties that one's view of the situation is correct, and (5) there is good reason to believe that the whistle-blowing will lead to solving the problem.[32] De George adds the last two conditions because whistle-blowers typically suffer severe retaliation from their employers, a point to which we will return in a moment. In his view, it is fair to make whistle-blowing a requirement, rather than a permissible option, only when the two additional strong conditions (4 and 5) are met.

Gene G. James argues that De George's conditions are too stringent.[33] Regarding conditions (2) and (3), suppose that a therapist discovers that her immediate supervisor and/or other manager is committing major fraud by billing the government for services not actually provided to patients. In a case in New York, several post–acute brain injury treatment facilities were engaged in several kinds of fraud:

Rather than basing patient discharge on functional or clinical criteria . . . these facilities retained patients until third-party reimbursement was exhausted. Patients and their families further complained that the facilities under investigation not only failed to provide contracted services, but virtually imprisoned patients by staunchly refusing discharge requests made both by the patients themselves and by their families.[26(p31)]

Confronted with such a case of widespread fraud, a therapist who tells a supervisor or even a higher manager about the problem might merely enable them to take steps to cover up the wrongdoing. Again, conditions (4) and (5) seem too strong because often one cannot have such strong evidence supporting one's case, much less have strong assurance that one's act of whistle-blowing will solve the problem.

James does not attempt to provide an alternative set of rules for justified whistle-blowing. Instead, he offers a list of proposals that individuals should consider, including the following:

- Make sure the situation is sufficiently serious to involve great harm, specifically in the form of violating important rights.
- Examine your motives to make sure your judgment is not being distorted, as often it is in such situations.
- Verify and document information about the problem.
- In informing relevant authorities, state the facts clearly, effectively, and without making personal attacks.
- Determine who is the best individual or group to alert of the problem.
- Determine whether internal or external and open or anonymous whistle-blowing is likely to be most effective while causing the least amount of adverse side effects.
- Consult an attorney, to ascertain that you are not violating the law and also to protect against retaliation.
- Expect retaliation.

The personal consequences for "taking on" the organization are usually serious. Studies find that up to 90 percent of whistle-blowers experience some form of retaliation from their employers.[34] These retaliations might take the form of harassment, social ostracism, unsatisfactory job ratings, suspension, outright dismissal, and blacklisting by other similar organizations. Sometimes phone calls and mail are monitored, and not infrequently whistle-blowers are transferred to jobs they are not qualified to do, making them likely to fail so that employers can dismiss them for incompetence. In most cases, whistle-blowers face a drastic social and financial change for the worse, even when they make a valuable social contribution.

In recognition of both the benefits to society and the costs to the whistle-blower of speaking out, the federal False Claims Act rewards whistle-blowers with 10 percent to 30 percent of triple damages and fines for fraud uncovered in federally funded programs. Government employees are protected by the First and Fourteenth Amendments to the Constitution, the Civil Service Reform Act of 1978, the Whistle-blower Protection Act of 1989, and the 1994 amendments, along with over 28 other whistle-blower protection policies. In the private sector, however, there is no comprehensive federal law that offers this protection. At present, 42 states and the District of Columbia offer redress through civil action, which entitles whistle-blowers to a jury trial in an effort to collect compensatory and punitive damages for employer acts of retaliation.[34]

Marilyn Killane and Debra Krahel

One example of whistle-blowing in the health-care environment occurred at the University of California, Irvine (UCI). Marilyn Killane, the office manager at the Center for Reproductive Health, and Debra Krahel, the senior administrator, were forced from their jobs "because they believed in the most basic of moral precepts—honesty and integrity in the workplace."[35] Killane blew the whistle on doctors in the unit who were prescribing drugs that were not FDA-approved, as well as on billing irregularities. Earlier, when she refused to participate in the cover-up of wrongdoing, she immediately started receiving negative evaluations from her boss. (Later her boss and two others were sued by UCI for failing to report nearly one million dollars in diverted patient cash fees, some placed in envelopes and taken home by the doctors.) Killane had reported her findings to Krahel, who then refused her boss's demand that she dismiss Killane. Soon afterward, Krahel discovered what later the university would acknowledge: "Human eggs were harvested from about 40 patients, fertilized, and, without consent of the donors, transferred as embryos to other patients. At least four children were born."[35] Krahel and Killane were quickly targeted by UCI for retaliation that took the form of questioning their integrity, humiliating them in public, isolating them from their peers, and ultimately firing them.

At the time Krahel had reported the improprieties to internal auditors, she requested protection under state and federal whistle-blower laws, which would impose a $10,000 fine and up to a year in jail for retaliating offenders, in addition to civil awards of punitive damages. Ultimately Killane received $325,436 and Krahel $495,000, which, after attorney fees, were reduced to $90,000 and $220,000, respectively. Because of their court appearances and the reluctance of other employers to hire whistle-blowers, both women remained unemployed for an extended time, imposing severe hardship on their personal lives and professional careers. Often, whistle-blowers must change fields of work and location, and even then, regaining their lives and jobs "can take a half-dozen years."[35(p4)] ◈

If there is any consensus on whistle-blowing, it is that responsible steps should be taken to prevent the need for it. Within organizations, that means maintaining an ethical climate in which the highest professional standards are institutionalized and in which workers are free to express responsible professional judgment without threats of retaliation. It also means maintaining open-door policies in good faith and, at least within larger organizations, offering the availability of an ombudsperson to whom one can talk in confidence about a problem. Within professional societies, hotlines can be established to enable professionals to confidentially seek advice. As for the government sector, virtually all federal agencies have hotlines to which employees can report wrongdoing. Government hotlines do not always provide safety for whistle-blowers, however, and even among the best hotlines, only 20 percent of calls are investigated within one year.[34]

Finally, in trying to provide an honest portrayal of the risks to whistle-blowers, we do not want to leave the impression that we are against responsible whistle-blowing. On the contrary, we express our personal admiration and gratitude for whistle-blowers like Krahel and Killane, who act at great personal sacrifice on behalf of the public and the clients they serve. In our view, they are exemplars of moral integrity. Our concern is that professionals and others who identify serious wrongdoing should not be required, as a matter of duty, to engage in extraordinary self-sacrifice on a routine basis. Both professional societies and the wider society—each of us—need to meet our obligation to protect responsible whistle-blowers.

Discussion Questions

1. Brent has been a therapist with Professional Sports Medicine for approximately three years. Four weeks ago he was assigned to provide therapy to Emily, a 23-year-old sports enthusiast who had injured her anterior cruciate ligament while skiing. Her surgery had been performed by one of the leading orthopedists in the state, and because she had been in excellent physical health at the time of the accident and was highly motivated, she did extremely well in physical therapy. Even this early in her rehabilitation, she was functional, without pain, and eager to start preparing herself for the next season on the slopes. Brent proposed a step-down therapy schedule, giving the home program the major emphasis, with weekly and then semiweekly checkups at the clinic. Brent was certain, since Emily was paying privately, that this would be a welcome accommodation. Instead, Emily seemed hurt when Brent proposed the change in schedule. She explained that the money was not a problem and she would prefer a more rather than less rigorous schedule at the clinic. Somewhat conservative in his care, Brent suggested that she take some extra time to allow maximal healing before pushing on to the next level. At this point Emily stated that what she really wanted was to see more of him, whether it be in the clinic or out of the clinic. She told him that over the past month she had developed a strong emotional attachment to him and wanted to explore what the relationship might mean. Brent admitted to himself that he found her attractive also. What should he say next and why? (Both Brent and Emily are single.)

2. Drawing on your education, personal experience, and research, discuss whether alcoholism and drug abuse are best approached in therapeutic terms (as sicknesses), in moral terms (as wrongdoing for which individuals are morally responsible), or some combination thereof. In doing so, indicate the implications of your view for how you will respond to substance abuse and substance dependence by colleagues and by patients. Use a concrete example, such as the case of Stuart in the chapter.

3. (a) With regard to the case of Troy, explain how a character explanation and a social explanation might be used to (1) understand and (2) help prevent the wrongdoing involved. Are the explanations, as well as the strategies for prevention, complementary or incompatible alternatives? (b) Choose an example of one type of conflict of interest from Chapter 7 involving wrongdoing, and answer the same questions.

4. Have you witnessed any suspected fraud in the health-care environment, and, if it was discussed or explained, how was it justified—or rationalized?

5. Present and defend your view about when, if ever, whistle-blowing by physical therapists and other health professionals is (a) morally permissible and (b) morally obligatory. When it is obligatory, should whistle-blowers be given legal protection? Would you favor revising the APTA *Code of Ethics* to include support for responsible forms of whistle-blowing? What other forms of support might the APTA provide?

As you answer these questions, discuss several types of examples, including the UCI case study and also cases of disgruntled employees seeking revenge against their bosses. If you have time, research another example, such as that of Jeffrey Wigand, who blew the whistle on dishonesty within the tobacco industry and who was portrayed in the movie *The Insider*. In thinking about these cases, what matters most—the likely good to be achieved, meeting one's professional duties (whatever the consequences), or acting from desirable motives?

References

1. Altman A. Making sense of sexual harassment law. In: Shaw WH, Barry V, eds. *Moral Issues in Business*. 7th ed. Belmont, CA: Wadsworth; 1998:441-448. First published in *Philos Public Aff*. 1996;25.
2. Petrocelli W, Repa BK. *Sexual Harassment on the Job*. 3d ed. Berkeley, CA: Nolo Press; 1998:1/19-1/20.
3. Equal Employment Opportunity Commission. Guidelines on discrimination because of sex. *Federal Register*. 1980;45:74676-74677.
4. Connell DS. Effective sexual harassment policies: unexpected lessons from Jacksonville shipyards. *Employee Relat*. 1991;17(2):191-206.
5. Woody WD, Viney W, Bell PA, Bensko NL. Sexual harassment: the "reasonable person" vs. "reasonable woman" standards have not been resolved. *Psychol Rep*. 1996;78:329-330.
6. Winer RL, Hurt LE. How do people evaluate social sexual conduct at work? A psychological model. *J Appl Psychol*. 2000;85(1):75-85.
7. Orlov D, Roumell MT. *What Every Manager Needs to Know about Sexual Harassment*. New York, NY: American Management Association; 1999:28.
8. Lasater NE, McEvoy TJ. The Supreme Court opens the door wide for harassment claims. *Clin Lab Manage Rev*. July/August 1999:213-214.
9. Siegel PJ, Kaplan RS. Sexual harassment, liability and disability discrimination: new rules apply. *Caring*. 1998;17(10):48-50.
10. Worthington, K. Violence in the health-care workplace. *Am J Nurs*. 2000;100(11):69-70.
11. McComas J, Hebert C, Giacomin C, Kaplan D, Dulberg C. Experiences of student and practicing physical therapists with inappropriate patient sexual behavior. *Phys Ther*. 1993;73(11):762-770.
12. DeMayo RA. Patient sexual behavior and sexual harassment: a national survey of physical therapists. *Phys Ther*. 1997;77(7):739-743.
13. Scott R. Sexual harassment: a reminder for managers. *PT Magazine*. December 1995:19-21.
14. Coombs RH. *Drug-Impaired Professionals*. Cambridge, MA: Harvard University Press; 1997.
15. Mill JS. *On Liberty*. Indianapolis, IN: Hackett Publishing Company; 1978:9. First published in 1859.
16. DesJardins J, Duska R. Drug testing in employment. *Bus Prof Ethics J*. 1987;6:3-21.
17. American Psychiatric Association. *Diagnostic and Statistical Manual of Mental Disorders, IV-TR*. Washington, DC: American Psychiatric Association; 2000:197.

18. Fingarette H. *Heavy Drinking: The Myth of Alcoholism as a Disease*. Berkeley, CA: University of California Press; 1988.

19. Peele S. *Diseasing of America*. New York, NY: Lexington Books; 1995.

20. Martin MW. Alcoholism as sickness and wrongdoing. *J Theor Soc Behav*. 1999;29:109-131.

21. Purtilo RB. Habits of thought: an instrument of our own minds. *PT Magazine*. 1993(Feb.):76-78.

22. Scott R. *Professional Ethics: A Guide for Rehabilitation Professionals*. Boston, MA: Mosby; 1998:128.

23. Medicare Improper Payments: While Enhancements Hold Promise for Measuring Potential Fraud and Abuse, Challenges Remain. Available at: http://freedom.house.gov/wastewatch/documents/a800281.pdf. Accessed on February 5, 2001.

24. Swisher LL, Krueger-Brophy C. *Legal and Ethical Issues in Physical Therapy*. Boston, MA: Butterworth-Heinemann; 1998.

25. Kornblau BL, Starling SP. *Ethics in Rehabilitation*. Thorofare, NJ: Slack Inc.; 2000:25-26.

26. Banja JD. On fraud and the rehabilitation profession. *PT Magazine*. 1993 (March):31-32.

27. MacIntyre A. *After Virtue: A Study in Moral Theory*. 2d ed. Notre Dame, IN: University of Notre Dame Press; 1984:181-203.

28. Eliot G. *Middlemarch*. New York, NY: Penguin Books; 1994:589. First published 1871–1872.

29. Martin MW. *Meaningful Work: Rethinking Professional Ethics*. New York, NY: Oxford University Press; 2000:176-179.

30. Milo RD. *Immorality*. Princeton, NJ: Princeton University Press; 1984.

31. Martin MW. *Self-Deception and Morality*. Lawrence, KS: University Press of Kansas; 1986:15.

32. DeGeorge RT. *Business Ethics*. 3rd ed. New York, NY: Macmillan; 1990:208-212.

33. James GG. Whistle-blowing: its moral justification. In: Hoffman WM, Frederick RE, Schwartz, MS, eds. *Business Ethics*. 4th ed. New York, NY: McGraw-Hill; 2001:291-302.

34. Government Accountability Project. Survival tips for whistle-blowers. Available at: http://www.whistleblower.org/www/Tips.htm. Accessed on October 3, 2000.

35. McGraw, C, Strong, B. Truth and consequences: 3 found that principle can have a high price; whistle-blowing takes toll on lives, careers. *Orange County Register*. August 13, 1995:1.

Justice and Access to Health Care

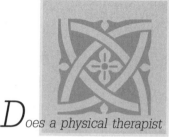

*D*oes a physical therapist
have a responsibility to provide equal treatment to
two patients with the same diagnosis but differing
insurance coverage?

Keywords

Microallocation

Macroallocation

Formal principle of distributive justice

Material principles of justice

Free-market system

Single-payer federal government plan

State-based managed competition

Theories of economic justice

Right to health care

Pro bono service

ealth care in the United States is in crisis, both financially and morally. The United States remains the only developed country without an effective health-care system for all its citizens. The exact cause of the financial crisis is in dispute, but clearly many factors are involved: expensive advances in health-care research, reliance on costly technology, public demand for the best care possible, high administrative costs in health-care organizations, and the dramatic extension of the average American life span, with its accompanying increase in medical intervention. Over 40 million Americans have no medical insurance, either because their companies do not provide it or because they cannot afford to pay for it. In addition, uncounted millions of people have only partial health-care coverage because of preexisting medical conditions or exclusion clauses in their policies. This, too, raises medical costs as public health facilities attempt to provide unreimbursed services.

The health-care crisis also presents a moral issue because of the enormous suffering caused when individuals lack proper medical coverage. This moral issue relates to distributive justice; in other words, given scarce (limited) resources, what is a just and fair way to make health-care services available? This question is germane to both **microallocation**—or determining what, for individuals and organizations, is the just or fair way to balance the competing claims of individuals for limited resources—and **macroallocation**, which is a determination of which resource allocation system for health care within a society is most in tune with principles of justice. In this chapter, we will note several main health-care options currently being debated in the United States. Then we will introduce some of the major ethical theories of justice that enter into assessing those options. We conclude with a discussion of the important, but often neglected, topic of *pro bono* services.

Microallocation: Balancing Patients' Needs

Microallocation deals with issues concerning justice in distributing resources to individuals and within health-care organizations. It involves balancing conflicting claims of patients and sometimes third parties, allocating the time spent by health professionals, and distributing other limited resources. For example, one type of conflict involves scheduling problems. When a clinical staff is overloaded on a given day because a therapist calls in sick, what is a fair way to allocate the time of other staff physical therapists? What if a patient arrives late for an important therapy session because of traffic delays beyond her control, necessitating postponement of the regularly scheduled care of a patient in less need? Does greater need override scheduled appointments? Another frequent problem concerns when to decrease or terminate treatment of a patient whose insurance coverage has ended.

Let us consider five cases in some detail.

Helen and Karen

Helen had been the chief physical therapist in Buena Vista Rehabilitation's physical therapy department for four years. She had made tremendous progress in raising the standard of care in the department by acquiring the funds from administration to hire the best available therapists. In doing so, she made a conscious effort to hire people educated at a variety of universities to enrich the professional peer interactions concerning patient care. Ironically, the resulting diversity of viewpoints was integral to the following dilemma.

Karen and Corey, two of Helen's staff therapists, expressed their frustration about the differential care of two patients. Each patient had the same diagnosis and was of the same age as the other, but each had different health insurance policies. Karen's patient was entitled to only 6 visits, exactly half of the 12 visits Corey's patient was allotted. Karen called the insurance company to explain the complexity of the diagnosis and her treatment proposal, but her request was refused. Karen and Corey were convinced there was an injustice, and Karen decided to give her patient six more sessions without reimbursement.

However, Helen had long ago implemented a policy of no courtesy treatments, because the department could not afford to lose the revenue that free treatments displaced. Helen told Karen that if she wanted to come back on her own time, she could use the department. But Helen would not change the policy because doing so would be unfair to the other therapists, who would also be damaged by any cuts in the revenue. Karen responded that it did not seem fair that she should have to give up her family time to solve the organization's problem.

Karen's desire to provide adequate treatment for her patient is compelling, but is it the duty of the department to administer justice between unequal plans? Helen is caught in a dilemma between her responsibilities to provide quality care to each patient, to be loyal to her staff, to be fiscally responsible by working within the restrictions of different insurance plans, and to maintain overall standards of excellence. She is aware that the APTA *Guide for Professional Conduct* states in Principle 10.1: "A physical therapist shall render pro bono publico (reduced or no fee) services to patients lacking the ability to pay for services, as each physical therapist's practice permits." However, it also says in Principle 7, "A physical therapist shall seek only such remuneration as is deserved and reasonable for physical therapy services." In Helen's department, "deserved and reasonable" means staying on budget or losing staff or equipment or both. ✖

Given such obstacles, how exactly does one go about determining the fair distribution of resources? A starting point is the **formal principle of distributive justice,** which says we should treat similar cases similarly. This purely logical principle provides important guidance by requiring consistency, but it says nothing about what makes cases "similar" in moral terms. That is, it says nothing about the substantive features of cases that should be taken into account, nor which features are most important in particular situations. Is medical need the only relevant feature in the cases at hand, or is the difference in health-care plans of most relevance?

Substantive considerations can be formulated as **material principles of justice.** Beauchamp and Childress identify six material principles:

To each person an equal share.

To each person according to need.

To each person according to effort.

To each person according to contribution.

To each person according to merit.

To each person according to free-market exchanges.[1]

It is possible to formulate a comprehensive theory of distributive justice that includes all six material principles, although typically a comprehensive theory emphasizes some of the principles, as we will illustrate later in this chapter.

In Helen's case, any of the six principles could be applied, but which should have priority? For example, should considerations of need lead Helen to modify her firm policy? Since the insurance for the fewer visits cannot be adjusted upward, should the patient with 12 authorized visits be cut to 6 so that patients with similar diseases are treated similarly? Considerations of justice also enter into how staff therapists are evaluated—a matter that bears on fair and effective allocation of care to patients. If Karen or Corey decides to engage in pro bono work on their own time, how should Helen acknowledge each of their efforts when it is time for staff evaluations? We leave further examination of these issues to the Discussion Questions section at the end of this chapter.

Helen and Stuart

Helen negotiated with management for money to cover the tuition costs and time with pay for the staff to take continuing education courses. The vice president in charge of the division explained that there was a precedent in another area to allow up to three days per year with pay for verified continuing education. She could not, however, create a new budget line item to pay for the courses without offering that same opportunity to nursing and all other health-care professionals, and there simply were not enough uncommitted funds to do that. So Helen requested use of the conference room and one treatment room for one night per week after 7:00 P.M. so that the department could provide continuing education courses and raise funds at the same time by charging a registration and attendance fee. The staff would teach the courses over a period of time. The funds raised could then be used for education courses for her therapists. The vice president agreed.

When Helen announced the plan, she stated that since all the therapists were professionals, they should all be treated as equals, and therefore they would share equally in the funds generated by the classes and would all have three paid days per year to use the money. Stuart, one of the senior therapists, objected, noting that not everyone on staff was capable of conducting a class. Even if they could all present programs of equal length, they would certainly not all have equal appeal and would therefore not deliver equal money to the general fund. As an example, he suggested that there would probably be high interest in his own area of joint mobilization, but he doubted that many would attend Mary's course, which would focus on her specialty of pediatric burn assessment, even though it was of equal value to the department. He questioned whether all rewards should be equal if contributions were going to be unequal.

Helen wanted the staff to be treated as equals in terms of the money because she wanted to maintain cohesion and unity in the department. But Stuart was correct in that the contributions, at least financially, would be different. After much discussion, Helen stated that market demands, while very real, should not be the basis for unequal treatment, because different expertise was needed in the department for it to remain a comprehensive physical therapy department. Unequal effort, however, was the greater difficulty, because some of the new therapists were recent graduates and could not be expected to produce an advanced program. In fact, they were in greater need of attending the continuing education courses than others. The compromise she proposed was that the newer therapists would not offer programs, but rather they would team up with the more experienced therapists who were presenting and be responsible for all handouts, announcements, and all other associated duties, leaving the presenters with only the preparation of the course content. She then stated that she wanted all the staff to attend all the presentations. ▨

Which of the principles did Helen use and which ones did she abandon? How would you have done it differently? We'll examine these questions further in the Discussion Questions section, after we have had the benefit of exploring other related topics in this chapter.

Jeff

Pacific Hospital was one of several long-term care facilities supported by the state of California. Pacific was unique in that it was dedicated solely to pediatric care. For the most part, the patient census was composed of children who were either too medically fragile to remain at home or had too many complex problems to be cared for by their parents. The parents had either voluntarily relinquished custody to the state or the courts had placed the children at the hospital after assuming custody because of either abuse or neglect. The hospital had a large campus and was efficiently managed by trained administrators and by a professional staff of physicians, nurses, physical therapists, occupational therapists, and other allied health professionals. Medical care was supplemented by a staff of volunteers from the community who played with the children, took them on walks, and in general were surrogate parents or grandparents to them.

Jeff had specialized in pediatric physical therapy early in his career and saw Pacific Hospital as an opportunity to help a segment of the pediatric population often overlooked. On his first day at the hospital, he was given his patient roster by the chief therapist, Rafael. The roster contained nearly 200 names. Jeff explained to Rafael that it was impossible to deliver care to all 200. Rafael agreed and said that it was not the expectation that he would, unless he wanted to use the "shotgun" approach and give a little care to each child, asking nurses and aides to assist him in carrying out assigned programs. Usually, Rafael explained, therapists selected approximately about 30 patients for more intensive therapy.

Later that day, during orientation, Jeff learned that Pacific Hospital was conducting a pilot program that would take the highest functioning children and place them in group homes located within the community and managed by paid custodial help. The children would return to the hospital for medical emergencies and physician appointments, but therapies would no longer be provided to them on an ongoing basis. The aim of this program was to place as many of the children as possible in a more normal community environment, making use of local community resources such as schools and clinics. Fiscally, the commitment was to reduce the census as much as possible to meet the demands of new admissions without having to expand the physical or professional resources of the hospital.

Over the next week, Jeff reviewed his charts and visited each of his 200 patients. They fell into two major groups. The first group, representing about one-third of his roster, was composed of patients who would probably be able to move into community homes. To do so they would need to acquire better skills in the activities of daily living and ambulate safely with or without assisting devices. Some children in this group needed to improve gross motor skills, such as throwing or kicking, so they could engage in play with other children. The second group, including patients with the most severe problems, would probably stay in the hospital. They would all benefit from therapy to relieve and prevent pain, specifically through better positioning, ROM, and varied postural activities. They could also acquire basic gross motor skills that would provide them with some control over themselves in their environment, such as rolling over to prevent skin breakdown. Others could benefit from activities to improve head control, allowing safer caretaker handling.

Jeff asked Rafael for advice about selecting patients for care, since nearly all could benefit. Rafael remarked that he was the professional and he would need to take responsibility for those choices. The other staff used varied criteria to make such choices, and he encouraged them to work out the triage system that made them feel comfortable with delivering care.

Who, then, should Jeff schedule for therapy? Applying the six material principles of distributive justice, we see that all the children have a need, but the principles of effort, contribution, merit, or free-market exchange do not seem to fit the situation. And adopting a "shotgun" approach by "giving to each person an equal share" would be a dubious way to help patients make a significant transition to other settings. Should Jeff spend more time and effort with the children in the first group so that they can move from the hospital to a community living environment, or should he focus on the others, who might acquire minimal motor milestones or benefit from help in the prevention of pain? ⊠

Many would argue that significant gains will require more intense therapy than the less than 10 minutes per week (in a 40-hour workweek) that equal distribution of time would allow for all 200 patients. As a consequence, we will have to sort through the variables to see which are most compelling. Is it fair to assume, for example, that community placement is in all cases such a highly desirable goal that it displaces consideration for those who must stay in the hospital? If a child in the second group, who most likely will stay in the hospital, had the capacity to address us, she might argue that she should not be blamed for her disabilities. She might even argue that the severity of her disabilities entitles her to more, not less, care.

On the other hand, perhaps it is the groupings themselves that distract us from a truly relevant variable. Perhaps, rather than determining whether community placement or increased control over the hospital environment is most important for any given child, we should try to judge which children are most likely to transition to a higher level of functioning with intervention. Similarly, should the administration's desire to move as many children out of the hospital be the deciding variable, or should we consider such additional variables as age, degree and type of abnormal motor tone, ability to appreciate acquired goals, and motivation, which are but a few of the relevant issues at the micro level of patient care? We might finally select children from both groups, although perhaps not proportionally.

Mark and Elizabeth

When Possibilities Unlimited, a private physical therapy practice, was purchased by Hartford Care, the staffing was left intact, as were the profitable methods for patient care delivery. The success of Possibilities Unlimited rested in part on patients who paid for their own therapy and whose programs were supervised by physical therapists but implemented by a staff of highly trained physical therapist assistants. Hartford Care brought with it a blend of patients financed by point-of-service, HMO, and Medicare insurance that by sheer volume reduced the clinic's ability to admit private-paying patients. The high volume of care necessitated that most of the care be delivered by assistants supervised by the physical therapists.

Mark had been with Possibilities Unlimited for three years before it was purchased, and he was confident in the quality of care delivered by the assistants. With Hartford's knowledge and consent, Mark, like all other therapists in the unit, would sign notes written by the assistants whenever third-party reimbursement honored only direct service by a therapist. Therapists would cosign all other care delivered by the assistants. The volume of patient care become so large that there were many patients for whom he signed that were known to him only through their initial evaluation. The increase in patient volume also brought a decrease in the time available for the therapists and assistants to case-conference, and the reviews became hurried and often incomplete.

When Elizabeth, a therapist, was hired, she immediately began to question the way in which care was delivered by the assistants. She refused to sign for the assistants and would cosign only when she had closely supervised the delivery of care. At the first staff meeting, she charged that the current policy of signing and cosigning was unethical and perhaps illegal. It had to be changed or she would be forced to report it to the relevant insurance companies. ▨

How do the material principles of justice apply in this case? The third-party payers have clearly defined the type of service, its amount, and by whom the services should be provided through their contracts and agreements. The free-market exchange principle entails compliance with a number of conditions, and to violate portions of an agreement without the consent of the contractor is to possibly commit fraud, as when the service is delivered by an assistant but signed (not cosigned) by the therapist to represent it as the therapist's care. And when patients selected their third-party payers, they were sometimes given the conditions and terms of the negotiated contracts; therefore, both the third-party payer and the patient have been deceived.

Lynn and Clara

Lynn, in her mid-thirties, had entered the physical therapy program at a respected university. Prior to entering the program she had been a paralegal with her father's law firm, but she decided she would rather help people in a more "hands on" profession. After graduating from the program, she focused her continuing education and work experience in the area of geriatrics. For the past two years she had been working at a skilled nursing facility contained within a retirement community. Her reputation as a therapist was unquestioned, and she had become known best for her patient advocacy. She almost always won her appeals with Medicare and the HMO when she felt a patient needed additional therapy, thanks in part to her paralegal background.

Clara Hopkins was a 82-year-old widow with mild dementia who had recently fallen and broken her hip. Lynn was particularly fond of Clara and had worked with her as intensely as with any patient she had encountered. The results, however, were less than one might reasonably expect. Clara, though clearly appreciating the attention and effort, was simply too weak and frail to carry out the traditional course of treatment to prepare her for ambulating. Clara's sedentary life style prior to the accident had in many ways contributed to her minimal muscle strength, range, and balance. Lynn decided that she would advocate a full rehabilitation program, five days per week, to bring Clara up to a level that would maximize her potential for ambulating once the fracture healed.

Although the course of treatment she proposed was virtually unheard of, Lynn felt confident that her understanding of the appeals process, with help from her father's firm, would result in the outcome she wanted for Clara. Two weeks after she submitted her written petition for additional treatment, which referenced her father's law firm, a representative from Medicare called to set up an appointment. At this meeting, the representative cited the history of extensions and additions granted to Lynn but stopped short of granting the full program requested for Clara. When Lynn protested, the Medicare representative looked at her and said, "I am just trying to decide if you are crossing the line between advocating for the patient's good and abusing the system. Because the resources are limited, someone else receives less each time we give your patients more." ⊠

Certainly Lynn has done nothing illegal, but are her actions ethical? She seems to be applying the material principle of justice "To each person according to need." One could argue that no one is harmed by Lynn's zealous advocacy for her patients, and some are indeed helped. Yet a closer investigation reveals hidden costs to the clinic beyond the therapist's time, such as administrative cost to review her numerous appeals. Has Lynn crossed the line?

Macroallocation: Priorities in Public Policy

Macroallocation addresses public policy issues related to distributing resources for health care within a society, whether at the federal, state, or local level. It might seem that macroallocation issues have little relevance to physical therapists in their daily work, but increasingly physical therapists are being called upon to be involved in public debates, in keeping with Principle 10 of the APTA *Code of Ethics*: "A physical therapist shall endeavor to address the health needs of society." Health-care reform is inevitable and currently in a state of flux. The extent to which physical therapy is a part of future standard care in the United States will largely depend upon on how well the profession justifies its interventions, mainly by documenting patient improvements scientifically, and on how convincingly the profession marshals persuasive arguments and presents them to the public and lawmakers. At some level, whether in the national forum of the APTA, at the state level through local APTA chapters, or in one-on-one campaigns for the profession with individual citizens, all physical therapists have a vested interest in seeing that decisions made about the inclusion of physical therapy in overall treatment are informed and fair.

Macroallocation issues might be sorted into three categories. The first concerns prioritizing health-care services and asks the question: Given limited funding for health care, which medical treatments should have priority? The second category concerns prioritizing health care among other societal "goods": Within the current system of health care, how should overall quantities of health-care resources be balanced against other social goods, such as education, environmental protection, and promotion of the arts? The third category focuses on establishing a viable system of health care within a society: Which system of health-care delivery best meets the requirements of justice? These are all large and complex issues, but we can briefly illustrate each.

1. Priorities Among Medical Treatments

As an example of prioritizing limited health care services, consider Oregon's experiment since 1988 in allocating health care for the poor. In its earliest version of the allocation process, Oregon developed a complex ranking of hundreds of medical procedures.[2] For example, it gave reproductive services—prenatal services, genetic counseling, amniocentesis, and others, but not including infertility counseling or treatment—the highest priority: 10 on a scale of 10. It set rehabilitation for improved function at level 7, and organ transplantation at 3. The specific rankings proved controversial, and Oregon revised them using opinion polls, interviews with residents, and commissioner votes. The list now includes a total of 688 medical services and procedures, with Oregon Medicaid paying for the top 568. Throughout the ongoing debate, the views of health professionals, as well as of the general public, are regularly solicited.

Individual physical therapists living in Oregon, as well as both the Oregon branch of the APTA and the national APTA, have had the opportunity to provide input. In this connection, Janet Coy asks us to consider the actions of a therapist who provides services for many patients with tendinitis, which was not covered under the original Oregon plan. The therapist was indignant and lobbied for a change in the policy, arguing that the therapy enabled patients to work and to function normally. Coy points out that, given the fixed allocation of medical resources under the plan, the single-minded lobbying for one service necessarily implies cutting back services in other areas. Hence, she argues, therapists need to adopt a community perspective in addition to their focus on the good of individual patients: "Justice may require some patient or professional interests to be less well-served to secure larger societal interests. It would be morally irresponsible to lobby for narrow patient or professional interests that are contrary to the interests of the commonwealth."[3]

Coy provides a valuable caution against using a blinkered approach when participating in public policy debates, acknowledging how one's own economic interests might distort judgment. At the same time, her conclusion leaves several questions unanswered: Is it inherently wrong to promote funding for one type of therapy that one sincerely believes is underfunded? It is, after all, standard practice for such one-issue advocacy to take place in funding programs. Should we think of lobbying at this level as partly a political act in which competing and partisan convictions are allowed to clash, with an outcome decided by legislators who are the ones most required to take a balanced view? Or is Coy correct in urging that professionals involved in the dispute themselves constantly seek to integrate their personal commitments with a vision of the wider public good? We tend to favor Coy's position, but we acknowledge that the passionate commitments of advocates for specific causes also play an important role, and those commitments are not always easily contained within an impartial perspective of the full good of the community.

2. Health Care versus Other Goods

The need to prioritize health-care services among other social goods routinely arises in debates about health-care funding at the national level. For example, should the federal government fund prescription drugs for Medicare recipients? The issue is an important one as prescription drug costs continue to increase rapidly and many retired persons living on fixed incomes are adversely affected. If the federal government assumes funding at a time when the public will not accept increased taxation, some other government programs have to be downsized.

3. Systems of Health Care

Which system of delivering health care within a society best satisfies the requirements of justice as well as the requirements of benevolence (compassion, decency)? There is no general answer to this, for health-care systems must be constructed in part to reflect the varied traditions of particular societies.

For example, when the nature of the Canadian medical system was being debated, the citizens made it quite clear that they wanted health care to be provided equally to all. The British system, however, has evolved into a two-tiered system in which the health care provided to all citizens can be supplemented at will with treatment by private practitioners, through use of either supplemental insurance or direct private payment. In each case, the system of delivery fits the predominant value of fairness in distribution in those countries. For Canadians, only the material principle of justice that states "to each person an equal share" was acceptable. The British system combined equal share with "free-market exchange" to allow those with the resources to acquire additional or different services. In each case the population is satisfied, on average, with the system in place. All health care systems are constantly in revision in order to best meet the changing needs of the population and the resources available to meet those needs.

In contrast, the majority of U.S. citizens are displeased with their current health-care system, which combines several traditions that pull in different directions: a strong sense of individualism and self-reliance that places responsibility for health on individuals; a free-market system that is open to profit-seeking in virtually all areas of health care; and, since the 1930s, a commitment to providing basic "goods," when they are available within the community, to individuals unable to secure them (welfare). Possibly as a result of powerful lobbying by physicians, the insurance industry, and pharmaceutical companies to preserve the entrepreneurial system of health-care delivery, health care in the United States has not been recognized as a right. Certainly it has not been recognized as a right backed by the obligatory duty of government to provide it, at least in the way police protection, fire protection, and public education are provided through local, state, and federal tax revenues.

In 1983, the President's Commission for the Study of Ethical Problems in Medicine and Biomedical and Behavioral Research argued that the federal government had a moral obligation to ensure that everyone has access to an adequate level of health care.[4] Acknowledging that the meaning of "adequate" is inevitably open to dispute, the commission used the term to indicate a medical and political middle ground, between the ideal maximum health service for everyone and minimal emergency care. The commission also underscored that maintaining health at some basic level should have a high social priority, given its centrality to the ability to pursue all other human activities.

The commission stopped short, however, of saying there is a human right to health care. Moreover, the commission drew a sharp distinction between placing responsibility with the federal government for ensuring *access* to basic health care (which was the commission's preference) and making the federal government the primary provider of health care (what is often called "socialized medicine"). The commission stipulated that the federal government must create a just health-care system, not that it should directly deliver health care. Critics found this conclusion unsatisfactory. They viewed it as a sad failure in the effort to ground the government's health-care obligation in the U.S. tradition of human rights, and it provided little guidance on how to implement the obligation it did ascribe to the government.

Clearly, Americans have had extreme difficulty reaching consensus on a fair and just health-care system. At present, the United States has a mixed system, combining for-profit managed-care corporations, nonprofit organizations, selected federal government programs, and various forms of oversight by state governments.

For its part, the APTA has outlined a "Position on Priorities in the Health Care System" in its *House of Delegate Standards, Policies, Positions and Guidelines* in HOD 06-97-07-20 (Program 19) that endorses universal coverage, exemption from restrictions based on preexisting conditions, and direct patient access to physical therapists.[5] The APTA document "Principles for Delivering Physical Therapy Within the Health Care System," states that "Patients or clients should have the option of selecting a physical therapist as their practitioner of choice [and] as their entry point into the health care system relative to the prevention, evaluation, and treatment of physical impairment, functional limitations, and disability due to musculoskeletal or neuromusculoskeletal disorders."[6] In its concise but comprehensive statement, APTA's "Position on Priorities in the Health Care System" addresses not only access-to-care issues but also the parameters of concern under "Quality of Care," "Prevention," "Benefits," "Cost Containment," and "State Autonomy."

While much of the impetus for change in the current U.S. system is argued from the justice point of view, there are additional concerns—humanitarian, practical, and national pride–related—that make change imperative. At one time, the common perception—fueled by nationalism and success in technology and research—was that the United States supplied the best health care in the world. While that may still be true in some regions of the country, high-quality care is generally accessible only to those with the financial resources to select among the best providers with access to the best facilities. At the current rates, only those in the highest income categories can afford unrestricted access to superlative care. When one reviews health outcomes for the aggregate of the U.S. population compared to those from other countries, the statistics are grim. Although the World Health Organization, in its "World Health Report 2000," ranks the United States first in per capita government health-care expenditure, the country is 37th in health-care performance. In the health-care performance category, based on disability-adjusted life expectancy, the United States was ranked number 72.[7]

If we look specifically at health outcomes rather than system delivery, the results are also unsatisfactory. In 1999, the National Institutes of Health ranked the United States last of the G-7 industrialized nations in life expectancy, placing it below France, Japan, the United Kingdom, Italy, Canada, and Germany, in that order.[8] Similarly, in other markers of health, such as infant mortality rates, the United States has not earned favorable averages.[9]

None of this would be quite so disquieting if the United States did not have the highest gross national product in the world.[10] Obviously, when comparing the United States with those countries having universal coverage, even minimal universal coverage will generate better averages. Nonetheless, the comparisons do speak to the health of the nation as a whole.

If health-care reform is imperative, what options do we have? Although no one at this point can foresee what will evolve even over the next decade, we will sketch here three proposals for alternative systems that are currently being debated: (1) **free market system**, (2) **single-payer federal government plan**, and (3) **state-based managed competition**.[2(pp805-830)]

A free market (a market operating by free competition), primarily managed-care, system would place full responsibility on individuals for the acquisition of their health care. They would have to acquire private insurance, enroll in the health coverage plan at their place of employment as part of a benefit package, or pay privately. As is currently done, most employers would negotiate annual contracts with health maintenance organizations (HMOs) that utilize a managed-care approach to control costs. (Essentially, managed care means reducing costs through a screening process that limits access to medical specialists and expensive technology and sets caps on costs for certain services. Beyond that, HMOs take various forms, including preferred provider operations (PPOs) that allow patients, for an added fee, to select their personal physician within an HMO.)

Libertarian ethicists favor this free-market approach. Alarm over escalating medical costs has also favored this general direction during the past two decades.

Defenders highlight the benefits of flexible options within HMOs, the emphasis on competition among health-care providers in the spirit of for-profit capitalism, the reduced costs to employers, and a minimum of government interference. In addition, individuals are encouraged to accept greater responsibility for their health, and HMOs have an incentive to provide better preventive care in order to minimize the onset of diseases and illnesses that require expensive treatment and intervention.

Critics of managed care argue that these systems give health-care professionals an incentive *not* to provide optimum care, primarily because of their profit motive and their short-term financial perspective. Critics also argue that the extensive profits once enjoyed by managed-care organizations have decreased over time, and lower profit margins often translate into decreased services. In addition, corporations with large numbers of employees who are disabled or who have special medical conditions have difficulty finding HMOs willing to negotiate fees for their services. And because of the high costs, small companies are often unable to offer health-care coverage as part of their benefit package, leaving many workers (often low-paid ones) without health-care insurance.

Critics also argue that preventive care coverage has been neglected by HMOs because often subscribers (employees) change jobs and/or insurance plans before the HMO profits from its prevention efforts by avoiding the more expensive treatment a major illness would require. And since contracts are usually negotiated yearly, the new contract can reflect any increase in the number of medically at-risk employees working at a corporation.

In contrast to the current U.S. system, a single-payer federal plan would have the strong advantage of ensuring automatic coverage to everyone, or almost everyone, at some level of adequate care. The drawbacks of the program would likely include higher taxes to fund the medical care and increased government involvement in the health-care environment at a time of concern about "big government." The actual cost and the amount of savings are difficult to project, but fiscal benefits could be realized from a reduction in administrative charges. Canada administers its national plan for less than one-half what the United States spends on its fragmented approach. Critics who object to "socialized medicine" believe it leads to long waiting lists for specialty care and low salaries for physicians, but advocates believe that some of its problems could be solved by allowing individuals to pay for supplemental coverage. Advocates also point out that under our current system, many still wait for care or are denied some care altogether, and those without insurance may never receive care. In any case, many doubt that Americans will ever embrace heavy federal government involvement in health-care delivery beyond the selective programs for the elderly (Medicare), for the poor (Medicaid), and for children (the 1997 Children's Health Insurance Program).

To some, state government involvement is more palatable than that of "big" (federal) government. State-based managed competition would organize the pool of health-care recipients as citizens of individual states (although, in one variation, small states might opt for more regional pools). The individual states would then negotiate each year (or so) with health-care providers to seek a combination of high-quality and low-cost care while making sure that the poor, the disabled, and other disadvantaged groups are included. The benefits of such a program are its universal coverage and the cost savings of managed care. The disadvantages, according to critics, combine the drawbacks of both of the previous systems: heavy government involvement (single-payer system) and pressures to withhold expensive treatments (managed-care system). When President Clinton proposed a version of state-based managed care in the mid 1990s, Congress rejected it. However, some states, most notably Oregon and Hawaii, are currently experimenting with various forms of state involvement.

Theories of Economic Justice

All the preceding issues, especially the alternative proposals for health-care delivery systems, can be approached within broader theories of economic justice. These theories attempt to identify and justify the basic moral principles that should govern the distribution of goods and services within societies, primarily at the national, or macro, level. Each of the ethical theories discussed in Chapter 2 provides its own principles of economic justice, and, as we emphasized, the detailed direction in which the theory is developed matters greatly. Consider three examples: rights ethics, utilitarianism, and duty ethics.

Rights Ethics

In libertarian versions of rights ethics, only liberty rights exist, and economic rights to seek and keep property (without taxation) are highlighted. Robert Nozick, for example, insisted that "the minimal state is the most extensive state that can be justified."[11] He suggested that justice consists of a simple, threefold principle of entitlement to the rights to (1) seek property, (2) exchange property without fraud or coercion, and (3) receive reparation when the first two rights are violated. His and others' libertarian views favor a free-market approach to health care with minimal government interference in the pursuit of profit.[12] If, for any number of reasons, individuals do not secure health-care coverage, libertarians believe that society cannot be expected to assume the costs for their care, although they leave room for voluntary philanthropic giving by individuals who freely choose to donate their money or time to help the disadvantaged.

In contrast to libertarians, most rights ethicists believe in positive rights to affordable health care, and that these rights call for universal health-care coverage at some level of care. After all, what is the point of declaring that individuals have rights to life and liberty if they are unable to pursue those rights because of severe disadvantages over which they have no control, such as genetic abnormalities or debilitating diseases that strike at random? This **right to health care**, however, does not mean a right to unlimited, optimum care. Although in public debates the idealistic notion of optimum care is sometimes encountered, medical ethicists who adopt a rights ethics approach argue for some "decent minimum" of health care assured for everyone, allowing individuals to pay more to receive additional benefits and insurance.[1(pp239-253)] Increasingly, they also add the need to impose additional insurance costs on individuals who smoke or in other ways irresponsibly threaten their own health.[13]

Utilitarian Ethics

Utilitarians focus on the maximization of total (aggregate) utility. Rule utilitarianism is the most widely used version of utilitarianism applied to public policy concerning health care. Yet there are different versions of rule utilitarianism, depending on the specific theory of good adopted, as well as different ways of interpreting how specific goods like health care contribute to individuals' overall well-being. Many rule utilitarians adopt a principle of equal access to some decent minimum level of health care, thus to that extent agreeing with most rights ethicists. This agreement arises because utilitarians appreciate the fundamental importance of health care in providing a basis for pursuing any other goods. The guarantee could be provided at the federal level or the state level, and the best system would be the one that maximizes the public well-being overall. However, in keeping with the utilitarian theme of maximizing total social good, many utilitarians are willing to restrict expensive forms of health care—to, for example, the elderly and very premature infants—in favor of providing preventive health care to the masses.

Duty Ethics

Duty ethics also has many versions. In one version, a duty of justice supports equal access to health care at some decent minimum. The most influential version of duty ethics, however, goes further, requiring a steady concern to raise the level of economic and social well-being of disadvantaged members of society. Such a version was set forth by John Rawls in 1971 in *A Theory of Justice*, a book widely regarded as the single most important work in 20th-century social and political philosophy. Rawls believes that two principles should govern economic systems, at least those of Western political democracies:

1. Each person is to have an equal right to the most extensive scheme of equal basic liberties compatible with a similar scheme of liberties for others.
2. Social and economic inequalities are to be arranged so that they are both (a) reasonably expected to be to everyone's advantage, and (b) attached to positions and offices open to all.[14]

In brief, the first principle prescribes maximum equal liberty for individuals. The second principle endorses differences in wealth and power if those differences benefit everyone, especially (as Rawls adds) the most disadvantaged members of society. Rawls also adds that the first principle has priority. It specifies that before we begin to discuss differences in money and authority, we must make sure that the most liberty possible is equally available to all members of society. This means establishing respect for basic political and legal rights, such as the right to vote, to assemble in voluntary groups, to exercise religious faith, and to be given due process in an effective system of law. After these basic liberties are ensured, the second principle then endorses the pursuit of wealth and power within a free market (capitalism), so long as this pursuit results in helping the least advantaged members of society. There are several ways this help can occur—for example, free markets create jobs, provide goods and services, and create wealth that sometimes is distributed through philanthropy. However, a graduated tax system (taxing the rich at a higher rate) is also considered to be essential in redistributing wealth with an intent to help the least advantaged.

Rawls's way of arguing for his two principles is as famous as the principles themselves. He asks, essentially, which moral principles would we, as rational and fair beings, agree to as governing the basic institutions and procedures in our society? This could be stated more fully as which principles would we agree to if we were to form a hypothetical agreement (social contract) with one another within a fair negotiating context in which none of us had a special negotiating advantage? As a heuristic device to ensure such fairness, Rawls has each of us imagine that we are in "an original [contracting] position" behind a "veil of ignorance" in which we do not know any specific details about ourselves that could bias our judgment.

To experience this scenario, right now imagine that we, as individuals, do not know if we are rich or poor, a member of any particular ethnic group or nation, living in this century or the last century, or even male or female—for each of these factors could bias the principles of justice we select. However, we do have general knowledge about psychology, economics, ethical theories, and so on. As rational beings, we are motivated to get as many "primary goods" as possible for ourselves and the people we care deeply about. Rational goods are desirable things that every reasonable person would want, such as liberty, opportunities, and self-respect. (Note: In saying we seek primary goods for ourselves, Rawls is not at all embracing ethical egoism, which says we should only care about ourselves. An ethical egoist would not be willing to get behind the veil of ignorance in the first place.)

In this fair-contracting situation, behind the veil of ignorance, Rawls argues that we would select his two principles to govern our society. We would select Principle 1 because it assures that whatever our position in society turns out to be we will have basic political and legal rights ensuring opportunities to participate in society and improve it—for example, by voting. We would select Principle 2 because it would ensure that even if we were to become disadvantaged, the differences in wealth and power within society would benefit us.

Rawls's principles are attractive because they seem to articulate many of the fundamentals of the American social, political, and legal system. That system is founded, first and foremost, on ensuring basic political rights (Principle 1). In addition, most Americans also endorse allowing individuals to keep large amounts of wealth and power when doing so tends to contribute to the well-being of the disadvantaged members of society (Principle 2). Moreover, Rawls's two principles combine some appealing aspects of both rights and duty ethics (Principle 1) and utilitarianism (partly reflected in Principle 2).

It might seem that Rawls's principles are too abstract to require any one health-care system. Nevertheless, Principle 2, which would steadily raise the well-being of the least-advantaged members of society, clearly supports concern for people who lack health-care insurance, or at least those who lack any realistic opportunity to afford it.

Although Rawls calls his approach "egalitarian," it is in fact a particular version of equality called "maximin," which means we should maximize (constantly increase) resources for people at the minimum level of well-being, even when doing so does not maximize the total good (contrary to what utilitarians favor).

This emphasis would be even more dramatic if health care were considered to be a primary good—a good that all rational beings would want—in developing the argument for the two principles. Rawls does not list health care as a primary good, but others have plausibly done so.[15] Without health, and hence health care, none of the other primary goods are possible, including the continued existence of life and the pursuit of all liberties. Indeed, some might view the opportunity to have affordable health care at some basic level as a basic liberty of the sort listed in Principle 1.

Nevertheless, despite Rawls's enormous influence, there is no consensus that he is correct. Critics challenge the plausibility of his veil of ignorance argument. Are we genuinely capable of imagining ourselves behind a veil of ignorance, not knowing our individual plans and interests, the circumstances in which we live, the communities in which we participate, or even our gender? But the difficulty is not only with the extent of our imagination. Morality seems to begin with our particular situation and identities in ways that require greater recognition in thinking about the principles we should live by. Also, Principle 2 requires constant attention to increasing benefits to the least advantaged, whereas some critics think it suffices to provide a basic safety that meets essential needs.

Defenders of each of the other major ethical theories have developed responses to Rawls. A familiar objection is that he makes unacceptable assumptions in specifying the original position (of fairness). For example, libertarians favor a spirit of greater risk taking. Utilitarians and most rights ethicists argue for only a minimum safety net rather than constantly raising the level of the least advantaged.

Where does this disagreement about justice leave us? As we concluded in Chapter 2, it is extremely unlikely that any ethical theory will ever prove convincing to all reasonable persons. Moreover, there is as much internal disagreement about the important details of a given type of ethical theory (say, libertarian versus other forms of rights ethics) as there is among defenders of different types of theories (say, rights ethics versus utilitarianism). Yet these results need not be a cause for despair. For there remain large and dramatic areas of overlapping agreement among the ethical theories when applied to specific situations. Above all, any sound ethical perspective will emphasize tolerance and reasonable compromise among different perspectives in working out shared health-care programs within democratic and pluralistic societies.[16]

Pro Bono Service

The APTA *Code of Ethics* states in Principle 10: "A physical therapist shall endeavor to address the health needs of society." The APTA *Guide for Professional Conduct* augments this principle by including pro bono service: "A physical therapist shall render pro bono publico (reduced or no fee) services to patients lacking the ability to pay for services, as each physical therapist's practice permits." It is noteworthy that the "shall" replaces the word "should," which was used in earlier versions of the code. As it is typically used in codes, "should" is a weaker term used to suggest "desirable, but not mandatory." "Shall" is a stronger term used to suggest a duty. Of course, "as each physical therapist's practice permits" seems to allow considerable latitude in interpreting the pro bono duty. Cynics would argue that it allows profit-driven organizations to essentially ignore any serious pro bono contributions.

Do physical therapists have a substantial responsibility to provide pro bono services, and what does that responsibility entail? Historically, medicine began with a strong tradition of pro bono service. In the 5th century B.C.E., Hippocrates urged physicians to offer such services:

> Sometimes give your services for nothing, calling to mind a previous benefaction or present satisfaction. And if there be an opportunity of serving one who is a stranger in financial straits, give full assistance to all such. For where there is love of man, there is also love of the art. For some patients, though conscious that their condition is perilous, recover their health simply through their contentment with the goodness of the physician. And it is well to superintend the sick to make them well, to care for the healthy to keep them well, also to care for one's own self, so as to observe what is seemly.[17]

In this passage, Hippocrates offers several reasons for what is now called pro bono service. He suggests that such services should be done in a spirit of gratitude, as a way to express thanks for one's good fortune—perhaps connected to the privilege of being able to work as a professional—as well as for having society's support in gaining an education to be a professional. He also suggests that a habit of providing pro bono service helps keep alive motives of caring ("goodness"). These motives promote the profession of physical therapy directly, by strengthening commitments to help, and indirectly, by contributing to a character that inspires trust and hope in patients.

Like other members of classical Greek society, Hippocrates thought in terms of virtues and moral ideals, such as caring (or goodness) and self-respect (or honor). He did not draw a sharp distinction, as we do today, between a mandatory duty and supererogatory acts—that is, acts that are morally desirable but also morally optional (beyond the call of duty). Debates concerning pro bono service often center on precisely this distinction. Is pro bono service a basic duty of each therapist, and if so, how much is required by that duty? Alternatively, is pro bono service a collective duty incumbent on the profession as a whole, but not necessarily a requirement for each therapist? Or, yet another possibility, is pro bono service a moral *ideal* that it is desirable to promulgate within a profession, in particular among physical therapists, but not a matter of basic duty at all?

These questions are critical because so many patients and members of the public are currently not receiving adequate services. The principle of benevolence straightforwardly seems to require filling this gap in access to services by widespread provision of pro bono service. In reply, libertarians state that mandatory pro bono service violates the rights of professionals, essentially functioning as an unfair tax on their labor and income. They say it also leads to shoddy work from individuals who feel resentment at being pressured to work without compensation. Other (nonlibertarian) critics contend that society should provide funding through taxation, rather than placing this special burden on professionals, a burden that results in sporadic help for individuals in need. These critics say it is simply unfair for society to allow a general health crisis to exist by failing to ensure adequate health insurance programs, and then to expect professionals struggling to earn a living to assume this responsibility.[18] Mandatory service also defeats the very spirit of voluntarism that is morally rewarding to professionals precisely because of the element of voluntary choice.

Defenders of a strong pro bono requirement argue that the public reasonably expects professions to help establish institutions and practices that foster public access to their services.[19] The public grants special recognition to a profession, essentially giving it a monopoly or quasi-monopoly in delivering a particular set of services. The public also provides financial support to universities and to students (in the form of scholarships, reduced-interest loans, and subsidized tuition), as well as to supportive related institutions such as licensing, regulation, and law. In return for such benefits and privileges, the public expects the profession to be responsive to the public interest in obtaining services. Some have argued that professions have a collective (shared) responsibility to foster pro bono service to help fill the gap between the rich and poor in obtaining services. Moreover, they argue, each individual should accept a portion of that shared responsibility, because it is unfair for only a few individuals to take on an excessive burden.

The legal profession has tried to strike a balance with a compromise position that states that attorneys should provide some pro bono services, but that this "should" does not state a mandatory requirement. In addition, the American Bar Association expands pro bono service to include not only services to patients at no fee or reduced fee, but also public service, service to charitable groups, service to one's professional organization, and making financial donations to organizations that provide pro bono services to clients. Critics view such statements as little more than window dressing—statements that make it sound to the public as if a serious duty exists ("should") while in fact requiring nothing. Defenders argue that this middle ground ("should" but not "ought") is a reasonable position in physical therapy and other professions: R. Scott states that, "Pro bono service should be an expectation (but never a requirement) of all professionals to whom the state has granted an exclusive license to practice a profession for profit."[20]

We leave resolution of this issue to the Discussion Questions section at the end of the chapter, but we conclude here by restating two issues discussed in this chapter—(1) what needs to be done to improve our current flawed system, and (2) the role of pro bono work within a system that is more just than our present one—and pointing out the benefits of pro bono service in addressing both. Recall that Hippocrates urged that physicians provide pro bono service in a spirit of generosity and gratitude. To help others was an "opportunity" and also a way to enliven the service commitments that drew one into medicine in the first place. The same argument can be made for physical therapists and other health-care professionals, even within systems of health care alone.

In addition to these profession-oriented reasons, some would argue that pro bono work is a desirable ideal, or even a civic duty, for all citizens who are able to engage in some form of philanthropy—that is, voluntary giving for public purposes.[21] Professionals often find pro bono service an especially fulfilling way to participate in philanthropy, although of course they might find other avenues of service equally fulfilling.

Discussion Questions

1. Referring to the two cases in the opening section of this chapter, which of the principles of microallocation did Helen use, and which ones did she abandon? What would you have done in her situation? Using which principles? Answer the same questions regarding the therapists in the other cases in the opening section.

2. Brenda, a physical therapist working in the outpatient department of a large medical center, is assigned two patients diagnosed with an anterior cruciate ligament (ACL) tear.[22] She has helped many patients with this knee injury using a treatment program of 16 to 24 visits over two months, the exact time varying according to the severity of the injury and individual differences in recovery progress. Patient X has traditional health insurance that reimburses for all warranted treatment. Patient Y has a managed-care plan that pays for only 12 visits for an ACL tear. Does Brenda face an ethical dilemma, or even two dilemmas, concerning (1) what to do for the course of treatment for the patient, and (2) whether to tell Patient Y about the drawbacks of her insurance program? If so, how should she respond to the dilemmas?

   Also, consider the following view expressed by the president of a physical therapy corporation in response to questions about this case requested by the editors of *PT Magazine*. Which view of justice seems to be in the background of the president's comments, and do you agree with his view?

> Brenda's dilemma is simple. (a) She is a staff physical therapist employed by (b) a medical center outpatient department. In accepting that employment, she has tacitly approved agreements that her employer may make with third-party payers. In short, as long as she is a staff physical therapist employed by this medical center, and as long as the medical center accepts the two "very different" health-care plans, she has an ethical obligation to provide the services as dictated by both payer and employer. . . . Should she tell patient Y about the difference in care? Only if Patient Y questions the care that he or she is receiving.[23]

3. Present and defend your view on whether pro bono service should be (a) mandatory for each therapist—and if so, how much should be required, (b) a collective duty of the profession as a whole, one that the profession is duty bound to find ways of implementing, but not necessarily a specific requirement of each practitioner, or (c) a desirable but supererogatory ideal for the profession as a whole but not a requirement of any kind for individuals. In presenting your answer, discuss how it would apply in the case of Helen and Karen. Also, discuss whether the current statement on pro bono service in the APTA *Guide for Professional Conduct* is satisfactory.

4. Japan has a health-care system that ranks in the top five in the world in health outcomes and delivery. Unlike the British or Canadian systems, Japan's government support is administered through insurance programs. No universal system in the world costs as much as the current system in the United States, either in per capita government expenditure or in percentage of gross national product. In administrative charges alone, list the expenses additional to actual care that you have witnessed (either as a patient or as a volunteer or paid staff in a hospital setting).

5. What elements would you want as a recipient of care in a health-care system if you could move behind Rawls's "veil of ignorance"? What elements would you want as a provider? Do you find Rawls's approach to justice promising, as a way to outline a fair system of health care in the United States? If not, what criticisms of his view would you raise?

6. During the middle and late 1980s, the British National Health Care Service launched a public education program about AIDS. It used prime-time television ads that were explicit and graphic in identifying the transmission routes and methods of protection. The education program also included posters and handouts targeted for bars and entertainment events, using language that was easily understood by the population. The transmission rate of AIDS in the United Kingdom has been approximately one-tenth the transmission rate in the United States. In the United Kingdom, the National Health Care Service is free to use whatever methods it deems necessary to curb epidemics and is immune from political censure or reprisal. AIDS education efforts in the United States, however, have been and continue to be heavily influenced by local, state, and national political mandates. When government funds health care, what areas should be protected from political interference and left solely to the medical community in order to ensure justice and compassion in health care? Should AIDS education be one of them?

References

1. Beauchamp TL, Childress JF. *Principles of Biomedical Ethics*. 5th ed. New York, NY: Oxford University Press; 2001:228.

2. Munson R. *Intervention and Reflection: Basic Issues in Medical Ethics.* 6th ed. Belmont, CA: Wadsworth; 2000:822-823.
3. Coy JA. Habits of thought: the community perspective. *PT Magazine.* July 1993:75.
4. President's Commission for the Study of Ethical Problems in Medicine and Biomedical and Behavioral Research. *Securing Access to Health Care: The Differences in Availability for Health Services.* Washington, DC: President's Commission; 1983.
5. American Physical Therapy Association. Position on priorities in the health care system. In: American Physical Therapy Association, *Ethics in Physical Therapy, Part 1.* Alexandria, VA: American Physical Therapy Association; 1998:71-73.
6. American Physical Therapy Association. Principles for delivering physical therapy within the health care system. In: American Physical Therapy Association. *Ethics in Physical Therapy, Part 1.* Alexandria, VA: American Physical Therapy Association; 1998:74.
7. World Health Organization. World Health Report 2000. Annex Table 1. Available at: http://www.who.int/whr/2000/en/report.htm. Accessed December 12, 2000.
8. National Institutes of Health. Life expectancy in G-7 industrialized nations may exceed past predictions, study suggests. Available at: http://www.nih.gov/nia/news/pr/2000/06-14.htm. Accessed December 13, 2000.
9. Euromonitor. International Marketing Data and Statistics 2000. 24th ed. London, England: Euromonitor PLC; 2000.
10. Kaul C, Tomaselli-Moschovitis V. *Statistical Handbook on Poverty in the Developing World.* Phoenix, AZ: Oryx Press; 1999:26.
11. Nozick R. *Anarchy, State, and Utopia.* New York, NY: Basic Books; 1974:149.
12. Nozick, we should note, has since modified his views. See Nozick R. *The Examined Life.* New York, NY: Simon & Schuster; 1989:286.
13. Callahan D., ed. *Promoting Healthy Behavior.* Washington, DC: Georgetown University Press; 2000.
14. Rawls J. *A Theory of Justice,* revised edition. Cambridge, MA: Harvard University Press; 1999:53.
15. Daniels N. *Just Health Care.* New York, NY: Cambridge University Press; 1985.
16. Benjamin M. *Splitting the Difference: Compromise and Integrity in Ethics and Politics.* Lawrence, KS: University Press of Kansas; 1990.
17. Hippocrates. *Precepts.* Jones, WHS, trans. Loeb Classical Library. Chapter 6.
18. Shapiro DL. The enigma of the lawyer's duty to serve. *N.Y.U.L. Rev.* 1980;55:735-792.
19. Luban D. *Lawyers and Justice: An Ethical Study.* Princeton, NJ: Princeton University Press; 1988:277-289.
20. Scott RW. For the public good. *PT Magazine.* January 1993:82-85.
21. Martin MW. *Virtuous Giving: Philanthropy, Voluntary Service, and Caring.* Bloomington, IN: Indiana University Press; 1994.
22. Purtilo RB. Allocation of care: readers respond. *PT Magazine.* February 1997:65-70. The case study was developed by Jim Dunleavy.
23. Glenn JE. Quoted by Purtilo RB. Allocation of care: readers respond. *PT Magazine.* February 1997:67-69.

Leadership and Administration

10

What duty do we have, if any, to shape the values expressed by the organizations that employ us?

Throughout their careers, physical therapists must work collegially with supervisors, managers, coworkers, and support staff. In doing so, therapists are well advised to understand ethical issues from the point of view of people in positions of authority, particularly because the therapist often oversees the activities of a variety of supportive personnel, thereby functioning as supervisors in the delivery of care, and because many therapists move into supervisory and management positions at some point during their careers. Under "Scope of Practice," the APTA *Guide to Physical Therapy Practice* specifies that an effective practice is one which includes the ability to "[i]nteract and practice in collaboration with a variety of professionals" and to "direct and supervise physical therapy services, including support personnel." For these reasons, this chapter discusses some of the ethical challenges of leadership.

In one sense, "leadership" is a descriptive term referring to the organizational roles of supervisors and managers. In another sense, the one explored here, **leadership** is a value—the value of influencing people in morally desirable ways. In this chapter, we will discuss several categories of duties in which leadership plays a role: decision making within different kinds of organizations, patient-related duties, personnel duties (including worker safety), and organizational duties.

Leadership in Promoting an Ethical Climate

Sara

Sara responded to an advertisement placed by Northeastern Health Care for the position of chief physical therapist at a local hospital not far from where she lived. She had decided to make the change from practicing physical therapist to supervising therapist because she hoped to improve the outcomes in health-care delivery. Aware that no system is ideal, she remained optimistic that the current system could be improved. The representative from Northeastern offered only a slightly higher salary than she had received as a practitioner, and the hours were going to be longer. Nevertheless, she saw the new job as a genuine opportunity. Northeastern immediately announced her appointment in the local paper.

At first, the job of supervising eight therapists and eight aides was overwhelming. In the first month she called a department meeting and asked the therapists and staff what they would like to see improved. To her surprise, their only concerns were to reduce the patient load and to increase the flexibility of work hours. She had fully expected to hear complaints about overdelegation of patient care to aides, lack of continuing education leaves, and the absence of certified specialists on staff. After the meeting, she set up an appointment with her boss, John Garcia, who was director of allied health. She expressed to John her surprise that the staff did not appear to be worried about the quality of care the patients were receiving or the absence of a dynamic professional exchange of ideas and expertise. She wondered about the feasibility of her plan to require weekly case conferences at which therapists could present difficult cases for input from other therapists. In fact, she was beginning to wonder whether any of her ideas for professional development would work.

John told her to relax; the hospital was happy with the way things were now. The department was producing a good profit, the employees performed their jobs, and few patients complained. He went on to say that anything she could do to increase productivity and profit would be welcomed, but any efforts, professional or not, that might detract from the current level of productivity would need to meet with his approval before they could be introduced to the staff. Sara began to realize that she was essentially being asked to function as an efficient manager, whereas she had changed jobs hoping to expand into more of a leadership role in the health-care environment.

What is the distinction between efficient managing and effective leadership? Was it impossible for Sara to express leadership skills given the constraints of her situation, or would a wider perspective reveal opportunities for furthering or at least maintaining an ethical climate within the organization? "Leadership" is different from "headship." Headship is simply being appointed to be in charge of a section, division, or larger unit within an organization or group. If an organization designates an individual as a supervisor, and assigns specific duties in accordance with the organizational chart and policy manual, then the individual is ipso facto a supervisor. But becoming a leader requires something more. Even some high-level managers who head an office are not leaders, and indeed some leaders do not hold official positions within organizations. What, then, is the difference?

The answer depends upon one's value perspective and the specific values one builds into the concept of "leadership." One view is that leadership is simply successful managing, influencing people to get things done. But while both leadership and successful managing certainly involve influencing people to achieve desired ends, what if the desired goals are immoral? This is sometimes called "the Hitler problem": Did Hitler exhibit leadership? He was enormously influential, but he is the epitome of an evil tyrant. Many theorists insist that leadership suggests the opposite of tyrannical control.

An enormous literature is devoted to defining leadership and to developing generic models for leadership as a value. As Joanne B. Ciulla argues, debates over models of leadership are invariably debates about moral values—specifically, about what it means to be a morally admirable leader, director, supervisor, or manager.[1] Such discussions focus on what moral values should guide the procedures of leaders (how they lead), their aims (purposes), and their effectiveness (morally desirable results). Thus, leadership means influencing people in morally desirable or at least morally permissible ways and directions. The centrality of moral values explains why the Hitler problem repeatedly arises in the search for a model for leadership.

For example, in his famous "transforming model" of leadership, James MacGregor Burns suggests that good leaders, "transforming leaders," seek to engage the full person, including the "higher needs."[2] Burns presents his view in contrast to the traditional concept of leaders as setting forth incentives in the form of self-interested gains, which include salary, medical insurance, and a pleasant work environment. Moral values enter this concept, but primarily as procedural constraints on the relationship between the leader and follower. These procedural values, such as fairness, trust, and honesty, are enormously important, but transforming leadership involves more. It is focused on end-result values, such as liberty and equality (especially in the political arena that Burns studied) and patient values (such as healing and respect for autonomy) in health-care professions. Clearly, Burns is not simply describing; instead, he is prescribing. He is attempting to portray a desirable form of leadership. In general, to present a model of good leadership is to present one's view of ethically desirable forms of leading.

Exactly what it means to show leadership needs to be determined contextually, but there are several tasks that leaders typically undertake: J. Gardner summarizes those tasks as follows: "[E]nvisioning goals, affirming values, motivating, managing, achieving a workable level of unity [within groups], explaining, serving as a symbol, representing the group externally [to other groups], and renewing [organizations]."[3] We will emphasize one umbrella role of leaders: promoting an ethical climate within organizations.

An ethical climate has several dimensions, including the following three features: moral responsibility, trust and trustworthiness, and effective conflict resolution or peacemaking. First, in the morally responsible organization, moral values in their full complexity are discussed and affirmed. Moral language, especially as set forth in the APTA *Code of Ethics and Guide for Professional Conduct*, is accepted as a legitimate part of the corporate dialogue. The moral dimensions of the organization are not allowed to be forgotten amidst a singular concern for profits or personal power. Of course, profits are essential in for-profit organizations, and even not-for-profit organizations must maintain a healthy "bottom line." But within morally responsible organizations, the moral goals embedded in the enterprise are promoted rather than eclipsed.

One example of the eclipse of moral values was described by Robert Jackall in his study of corporations in which ethics meant nothing more than obeying orders. One employee summed it up this way: "What is right in the corporation is what the guy above you wants from you. That's what morality is in the corporation."[4] Jackall's study focused on several large chemical and textile companies that were going through enormous upheavals during the 1980s climate of corporate takeovers. Professional standards, as well as the values of hard work, were consistently eroded. Interestingly, the force behind the erosion was not solely or even primarily profit maximization. Instead, it was the preoccupation of individual managers with their own survival and power in a tumultuous world of layoffs and hostile corporate takeovers.

At another extreme, we might add, corporations fail because of insufficient adjustments to changing realities. Leadership in the form of nurturing support of professionals is not to be confused with the "touchy-feely" acceptance of incompetent or substandard performance. Nor is it to be confused with obstinate refusals to respond to the ever-shifting challenges at the workplace. Instead, leadership is a dynamic process of defining goals and shaping responses with integrity.

A second important feature of an ethical climate within organizations is its strong sense of mutual trust, based in turn on a conviction of the trustworthiness of professionals. In such an environment, employees are allowed, invited, and encouraged to participate in the organization beyond their narrowly assigned duties. In particular, they have a role in developing the policies and procedures of the organization. Leadership, in order to achieve envisioned goals, must generate a unity that is also committed to those goals.

A third feature of an ethical organizational climate is effective and fair conflict resolution. Conflicts arise in all organizations, and they take many forms, such as disagreements over schedules, prioritizing projects, making resources available, technical issues about appropriate therapies, administrative procedures, cost and billing procedures, and personality clashes. Often several types of conflicts combine. For example, it can be difficult to see whether personality conflicts or professional judgment are at stake in how best to help a particular patient.

John and Tim

John and Tim often debated the merits of proprioceptive neuromuscular facilitation (PNF) and neuro-develomental treatment (NDT) for patients undergoing rehabilitation after a stroke. At the last staff meeting, a heated argument broke out between them about which approach would best fit a new patient. In desperation, the chair of the meeting assigned the patient to another therapist, with the instruction that she should use whatever techniques she felt were appropriate without feeling obliged to either Tim or John. In fact, the chair knew that the two men often disagreed and to some extent their personal conflicts affected the willingness of the staff to address difficult subjects. The chair set up an appointment with both men to start a program of conflict management whose ultimate goal was to help Tim and John develop cordial and professional work behaviors and skills without letting personal feelings escalate differences to the point of creating a hostile work environment.

It is worth noting that leadership is a widely applicable value rather than the sole province of managers. Ruth Purtilo, herself an enormously creative leader in the study of physical therapy ethics, argues for the need to go beyond two familiar models of leadership: captains and shepherds. The captain model, used in the military and in sports, places the focus on one key individual who has primary responsibility and authority. The shepherd model emphasizes the leader as a benevolent nurturer of employees. Both models capture elements of truth about what is needed, but both models are limited by their focus on encouraging leadership in only a few individuals. Instead, Purtilo calls for development of leadership as a quality in all individuals: "*Each member* of APTA must assume a central role in advancing the moral life of the profession: Each member must nourish a seed of self-governance, assume ultimate responsibility for his or her own actions, and be sensitive and responsive to those committed to his or her care."[5]

We will keep Purtilo's insight in mind as we proceed, for although we will focus on the leadership supervisors and managers exhibit in maintaining an ethical organizational climate, leadership is a virtue that all physical therapists can develop and exhibit. At the same time, we recognize that certain organizational settings present considerable obstacles to putting the concept into practice. Our primary concern is with individual decision makers, but we note that health-care organizations often have designated methods for solving organizational ethical problems. For example, Institutional Review Boards (IRBs) are responsible for protecting both human and animal subjects in research and are discussed in Chapter 11. A second type of organizational ethical monitoring system is the Institutional Ethics Committee (IEC). There might be two committees, one to address administrative ethical decisions, including resource allocation and cost control, and a second to govern patient concerns, such as decision making when the patient is incompetent and has no identified surrogate decision maker. Within hospitals, these committees are typically interdisciplinary and consist of physicians, attorneys, nurses, therapists, clergymen, and community members. There might be additional committees such as the Infant Care Review Committee that is encouraged by the Department of Health and Human Services to attend to the specialized ethical concerns originating in neonatal care units. Some large hospitals employ ethicists for consultation or provide consulting services through a team of ethicists and trained clinicians who work as a unit.

By having formal structures to respond to ethical concerns, organizations enforce expectations that ethical behavior will permeate the entire cultural climate. In an ethical cultural climate, it is far easier for division and department chairs to engage staff in decision-making strategies that emphasize "the right thing to do" instead of what is most expedient or what is solely in the best interest of the department.

Decision Making and Organizational Models

Most of us have experienced the frustration caused by organizational barriers that prevent us from achieving a fair and desirable outcome. Fortunately, bumbling bureaucracies are the exception, and we need only recall Habitat for Humanity, Ben and Jerry's Ice Cream, and a host of other organizations for examples of pioneering value-based changes made both inside and outside the organization. To better understand the capacity of organizational values to influence employees, we will first review three types of structures within organizations: (1) formal hierarchies, (2) informal hierarchies, and (3) professional hierarchies.

Formal Hierarchies

The formal chain of command in a typical business acknowledges the tasks and duties of key players, but, more important, it outlines the distribution of decision-making authority inherent in each position. Organizational theorists propose multiple structural models, which Gareth Morgan has clustered into four main types of formal hierarchies, using the metaphors of machine, organism, brain, and culture.[6] Each of these formal structures has the potential to influence the quality of the ethical decisions made by employees.

Machine models refer to organizations that have bureaucratic structures with numerous strata of highly specialized staff, each with clear demarcations in authority. These structures work well in protected environments such as surgical suites, mailrooms, or businesses such as McDonalds, in which the market is reasonably secure, the product standardized, and efficiency is most important. To achieve this efficiency, priority is placed on obedience to rules and uniform ways of performing tasks. This ensures equal and impartial treatment to the consumer base. However, machine models can also emphasize dominance and control that translate into an oppressive work environment devoid of creativity, one in which decisions follow the rules even when the rules do not offer the best solution in a particular situation. When corruption is uncovered in organizations using this machine model, it is not uncommon for the participants to excuse their behavior with "I was just following orders."[7]

Organism models stress participative decision making, a reduced hierarchy, and psychological incentives largely achieved through "family" groups. These models work well in organizations integrating multiple professions, but they tend to be self-insulating, leading to consensus at the cost of innovation and tolerance of dissent. Where organizations put groups in competition for resources without oversight, the common excuse for corruption is the belief that "everyone does it."[8]

Brain models blend elements from the machine and organism models. They are best exemplified by the stratum theory, which divides any organization into six strata based on the attention span needed for a task completion. These attention spans range from up to three months in stratum one to thirty years and beyond in stratum six. In the top strata—the outer cortex—the CEO is expected to make decisions based on a vision that projects up to or even beyond 30 years into the future. At the bottom strata, the tasks are essentially maintenance, much like the workings of the brain stem. Without the addition of collaborative decision making and excellent communication between strata, short-term goals and long-term goals do not match, and ethical decisions tend to be uninformed by a cross-strata perspective. These decisions are thus inadequate to address the plurality of concerns that exist in every organization.

Culture models are based largely on the concept that each organization is like a separate culture with its own set of beliefs and values. Within the organization there are mini-cultures that define themselves. As an example, for many years the U.S. Atomic Energy Commission consciously created shields to protect its internal culture of secrecy and expansiveness. One of these shields, used to protect the agency from public criticism and political accountability, was a diversification program in which the commission was decentralized, with contracts given to outside companies to perform research and development. Although the agency was well aware of the environmental hazards secondary to the research, and aware of the public's concern about those hazards, it made no effort to hold the outside contractors responsible for the contamination. When criticism was expressed about the increased environmental hazards being generated, the Atomic Energy Commission stated that each diversified location was separately responsible. As a result, the commission avoided holding itself or its contractors accountable for wrongdoing.[8(p177)]

Although organizational structures can greatly damage the quality of ethical decisions, they can also enhance them. Terry Cooper distinguishes between two important avenues for improving formal hierarchies with an eye to enhancing ethical conduct: external controls and internal controls.[9]

External controls include any attempt outside the individual to shape or prescribe the conduct of the individuals in the organization. Codes of ethics for the organization and even for the department are examples of external controls. R. Ford and W. Richardson report that the research shows that "[t]he existence of corporate codes of conduct will positively increase an individual's ethical beliefs and decision behavior."[7(p216)] It appears that organizational, including departmental-specific, statements are of even greater value to employees than professional codes of ethics. The likely reason is that they are more personalized to the particular environment and directly linked to organizational expectations, thereby potentially affecting promotion and pay.

Internal controls consist of the internalized values of employees that guide the individual, especially in the absence of external controls. An example of a way these internal values are expressed and nurtured is the regular effort by employees and employers to identify and discuss ethical concerns. For example, the identification process might involve creating ways for employees to report suspicious behavior or wrongdoing while offering protection and confidentiality to the informant.[10,11] The discussion of ethical concerns probably is best accomplished when ethics training courses are introduced as one would introduce any other continuing education course. The discussion meetings that follow should be held on a regular basis, focused on the identification and solution of current problems, and conducted using a Socratic method of dialogue.

There are at least three additional strategies that, when added to a hierarchical organization, further promote ethical conduct but that neatly fit neither the internal nor external control definition. One is the publication of clear lines of accountability at each level of the organization that specify the limits of authority. The second is to create a "constitutional bureaucracy" in which each level of the organization has an advisory board made up of elected employee representatives who participate in policy formation and conflict resolution.[10(p178-183)] The third is the use of ad hoc committees. Such committees can resolve an immediate problem and then be dissolved, thus avoiding the power struggles that often occur in fixed committees. They carry the added flexibility that managers can quickly alter the blend of personnel composing them.

Informal Hierarchies

Although the formal hierarchy can have a profound influence on the ethical decision making in an organization, the informal hierarchy is also very influential. The informal hierarchy encompasses the politics of the organization and access to key decision makers. For example, the formal organizational chart will probably not list administrative assistants and secretaries prominently, but in the informal structure they are the ones who have crucial access to key decision makers and to classified information, and who often control the timing of disclosure of information. Informal groups are also in this invisible hierarchy and have much to do with defining the values of the organization.

The informal hierarchy exists within the larger context of the organizational culture. As G. Morgan states, "Organizations are mini-societies that have their own distinctive patterns of culture and subculture. Such patterns of belief or shared meaning, fragmented or integrated, and supported by various operating norms and rituals, can exert a decisive influence on the overall ability of the organization to deal with the challenges that it faces."[6(p121)]

Unfortunately, the informal culture sometimes encourages unethical dealings. An example of this occurred when the informal hierarchy of the Rampart Division of the Los Angeles Police Department encouraged unethical dealings by encouraging officers to manufacture evidence to convict perceived gang members, creating an underground of drug dealing, drug consumption by officers, and alleged murder. It discouraged ethical conduct through the legendary "code of silence" that permeates many police departments, in which group loyalty forbids turning in a fellow officer even for serious violations of law and organizational policy.

Formal and informal structures of organizations constantly influence each other. The ethical conduct sanctioned by the informal culture has a dramatic impact on the formal operations of the organization, and in turn the formal operations influence the ethical climate of the organizational culture. As an example, the actions of a metropolitan university president in refusing to approve an underqualified candidate for tenure sent an important message of fairness to the rest of the university community. The university had just recently experienced financial cutbacks, and many of the faculty believed that one of the professors up for tenure would be welcomed, despite a less than impressive academic performance, because of strong ties with a wealthy foundation. There were rumors that the chairman of the foundation had recently given the university an unsolicited award and that the implicit message was that more support would come if the candidate received tenure. The president of the university vetoed the tenure application. Although no one wished harm to the candidate, there was a renewed sense of the importance of fairness based on merit and an increase in the respect for the president among those who knew the extenuating circumstances.

The reverse can also be true. One chairperson of an academic department, whose management style was best described as "urban guerrilla fighter," blamed higher administration for her own errors. She manufactured convincing stories that portrayed senior administrators as ruthless and unethical opportunists who were using the department to fund unrelated pet projects on campus. To claim her just compensation, she co-taught courses in which she did minimal work while claiming full teaching credit, and awarded unearned administrative units to friends who also complained of being overworked. As a result, the faculty in the department had low morale and similarly assisted other faculty to claim unearned teaching units. When senior administrators finally uncovered the source of a faculty-to-student ratio twice that of the rest of the campus, she was removed from the chair position. The new chair forged a better relationship with senior administrators and asked them to explain their decisions to the department faculty. They did so, and slowly the faculty better understood the context of administrative decisions and in general agreed with the policies. As the senior administrators were perceived to be ethical in their behaviors, the faculty voluntarily reorganized themselves around ethical standards and honest accounting of their labor.

Professional Hierarchies

The professional hierarchy, operating as a distinct structure that also overlaps other structures, is usually built on the traditional roles of domination in health-care decision making: physicians at the top, followed by nursing, physical therapy, occupational therapy, respiratory therapy, and so on. The historical dominance of physicians within the domains of nursing and physical therapy is linked in part to the role of the physician as the case manager. It is also historically linked to sexism, given the predominance of physicians who are male and physical therapists and nurses who are female. P. Decker states that, within health care, "formally, administrators are in charge. But informally, clinical expertise holds much of the power. For many physicians, that power often does not require accountability to administration or to other staff."[12] In a study of purchases of high-technology equipment, most of which was already available at other private or shared locations, it was discovered that physicians, not hospital administrators, were primarily responsible for the purchases, in part to maintain status among other physicians.[13]

All three internal hierarchies—formal, informal, and professional—are concerned with power. Having power means having the ability to cause change, directly or indirectly, and thus power is a necessary component of leadership. However, unlike leadership, which is a virtue, power can be used for evil as well as good. Thus we too often stereotype powerful people using negative examples, such as Hitler or Mussolini. We tend to forget that Jesus, Mohammad, Confucius, Eleanor Roosevelt, Jimmy Carter, and the current "Teacher of the Year" are/were also enormously powerful individuals.

Typically people acquire power by being perceived as having special knowledge or skills, access to information, and control over resources affecting the actions of the group. The powerful could not, however, maintain their influence without the conformity of others.

Several major research projects have studied the power of conformity within groups. The best known is the Milgram study.[14] In this experiment, the subjects were told that they were part of a study to understand the effect of punishment on memory. However, the true purpose of the study was to examine obedience and conformity to authority within the study group. They were told that the person just out of their view, but whom they could hear, was the "learner," and that whenever the "learner" made a mistake, they were to administer an electrical shock. There were 30 lever switches labeled as ranging from 15 volts to 450 volts, with adjacent labels ranging from "Slight Shock" to "Danger: Severe Shock." As the shocks became stronger, the "learner" (who was not truly receiving a shock) would shout and exclaim that he had a weak heart and at 300 volts he would kick the wall. After 300 volts he made no noise at all. Nearly 65 percent of the subjects continued to deliver the shocks at the instruction of the researcher all the way to the 450-volt level.

A few of the other studies that support these findings, while augmenting them with attention to "groupthink," follow. In the Sherif experiment in 1936, a group of subjects were put in a room in which there was only one light hanging in an otherwise dark room.[15] The group developed a common way of viewing the light and actually identified a pattern of the light's movement. When the subjects were put back into the room singly, they each reported seeing the same pattern defined by the group. The light in fact was stationary.

Solomon Asch conducted a series of experiments in which groups of individuals were assembled and asked questions to which the answers were obvious.

However, all members of each group except one, who was the subject of the experiment, had been coached to give the same incorrect answer. Over 74 percent of the experimental subjects conformed to their group even though their conformed answers were obviously incorrect.[16]

Conformity to authority was also demonstrated in the Stanford Prison Study, conducted by Phillip Zimbardo in 1971. Student volunteers from Stanford University were brought to a simulated jail where they drew lots to determine if they would be the prisoner or the guard. Although all were informed that they could leave at any time, they became completely immersed in their roles. The project had to be cancelled on the sixth day because of the unconscionable physical and psychological brutality that occurred.[17]

 ## Patient-Related Duties

Having discussed general theory and related overarching problems, we next turn to the responsibilities of a generic physical therapy department manager (chair, supervisor) who is given opportunities for moral leadership as well as risks of failed leadership. These responsibilities are multiple and include duties to the patients seen in the department, to professional and staff employees, to the organization, and to themselves to find solutions that do not compromise their own moral integrity.

It would be a mistake to think that the role of managers, such as department chairs, is to deal primarily with staff rather than patients. Department chairs are commonly asked to make decisions that have rather profound effects on patients, as illustrated in the following case adapted from Gervais and colleagues.[18]

Marcia Lewis

Complete Care Health Systems is an integrated nonprofit health-care delivery system with the advertising slogan of "Quality health-care services across the continuum of care." Because of severe financial losses in the prior year, all divisions in the company are given the directive to cut costs. Marcia Lewis is a physical therapist who manages the division called Peerless Home Therapy Care, which delivers physical therapy to the full continuum of patients covered by Complete Health Care Systems.

One of the subdivisions is a program called the Pediatric High-Intensity Home Care Program, which provides therapy in home care to medically compromised children with complex health-care needs. It differs from other subdivisions, even from another pediatric home health-care subdivision, in its increased frequency and duration of treatments. Nearly all the patients in this program are funded by Medicaid, which has failed to increase its payments proportionally to the increase in the costs of the services. The costs include continuous in-service training needed by therapists to interact with the high-tech equipment and special needs of these children. As a consequence, each year the program has operated at an escalating loss of profit. In the past the losses had seemed justified because the unit saved other divisions the cost of providing for these children at rates that would have been even higher in a hospital. Yet, when costs were analyzed, each unit was segregated from the whole. Unless it could stand on its own, something had to change.

Other providers in the area had already withdrawn from this type of service because of the cost, and so it seemed apparent to Marcia Lewis that this program would have to close or change drastically. It could be closed by simply not taking on any new patients. Another option was to limit access to the program, and yet another was to take on new patients but do it in a time-limited contractual manner. Marcia felt that the best solution, consistent with the "continuum of care" commitment, was to provide services for only six months and in that time help families find other services or make other arrangements. Marcia requested the help of Peerless Home Care's ethics committee, which, along with her staff, developed a respectful way to announce this new policy to the current patients.

The committee called the patients' parents the day that certified letters were sent out, to give them advance notice. The letters contained an announcement that service would be discontinued in six months, a list of home-care providers, the name of a staff person at Peerless who would assist them in the transition, and the name of a management person they could contact with questions. Physicians, social workers, and departments that would be affected were also notified. Despite these efforts, one parent contacted a reporter who, following an investigation, made it a high-profile story. The story generated so much bad publicity that ultimately a high-level administrator reversed Marcia's decision and made the public announcement that Complete Care Health System would not abandon its patients.

The primary difficulty in this case was that Marcia Lewis accepted, or was forced to accept, a level of decision making that was beyond the scope of her job description and training. In doing so, she squandered an opportunity to provide leadership within the organization that would have maintained the trust of the public and perhaps even improved the care given. Anytime a course of action is in opposition to the mission statement of an organization, or requires balancing the business interests of the organization with its responsibility to deliver care, the decision should be made further up the organizational hierarchy, ultimately by the board of directors. Had Marcia recognized the limits of her authority and presented the problem to the board, the board could have notified all patients of their concerns with the program and asked for a joint meeting to gather information and share possible solutions. The board would retain the formal decision-making powers, but the texture and depth of information that board members would then possess would make a just decision more likely. The decision would also be more satisfying to the public if the board informed them of how they weighted the relevant variables. Regardless of the decision, trust would not have been eroded so seriously.

We now highlight some managerial duties, beginning with patient-related responsibilities. Productivity and efficiency of staff should be key expectations of department chairs, in the eyes of the organization and patients alike. While managers usually cannot correct inequities between patients' health plans, managers do have a responsibility to oversee the fair allocation of the primary assets of the profession—in particular, treatment time and treatment effectiveness. Organizations see this as a supervisory function to ensure revenue, but patients regard it as an accountability issue for their treatment expectations. Staff therapists, however, do not always see it from either perspective; rather, they view it from a position of how it impacts their jobs.

As part of their duty to patients, supervisors must be diligent in detecting bias in treatment by staff because it affects treatment time and efficacy. In the past, bias has on occasion been expressed as a refusal to treat, but more frequently it disguises itself as the "professional judgment" that some patients will not benefit from an intervention. Such patterns of professional judgment need to be tracked by a supervisor to detect either a conscious or an unconscious bias influencing the allocation of care. Consider the following example.

Renee and Sue

Renee (a supervisor) noticed that Sue consistently focused on ambulation for the elderly male patients who were being rehabilitated after a stroke and on ADL for the female patients with the same diagnosis. When Renee questioned this pattern, Sue was obviously embarrassed and admitted that she just assumed, without asking, that these would be the patients' priorities. Sue volunteered that her selections of goals could easily be considered sexist and promised to document the patient priorities for treatment goals.

While efficiency of the staff is a manager's duty to patients, effectiveness is an equally important duty. A department supervisor is morally responsible for ensuring that the therapists hired are effective and competent. Thus, during the hiring process, the supervisor confirms graduation from an accredited program, checks licensure to assure it is current, seeks recommendations from prior employers, and makes inquiries about felony convictions. The duty is to hire people who will not harm patients or staff, or be so disruptive that the department is damaged. There are, however, limits to diligence in making inquiries about prospective employees. For example, a supervisor is not permitted to make any inquiry into conduct outside the employment setting, both because it violates privacy laws and because it fails to demonstrate respect for the autonomy of the applicant. The fact that a therapist is a staunch environmental activist, for example, has nothing to do with whether that therapist is fit to practice. Although no one person can judge with certainty the competence of another in a single interview, potential employees should be interviewed by other therapists in the unit. Interviewers can use case studies to evaluate the candidate's proposed treatment strategies and then meet with the chair to synthesize their impressions and arrive at a recommendation.

After the new therapist is employed, the supervisor can help ensure efficiency and efficacy in patient care by providing opportunities for continuing education, including reviewing issues of cultural sensitivity and diversity. Many health-care organizations working within managed-care limitations do not provide funds or time for formal continuing education, but a supervisor can provide the leadership to initiate a group effort to critically review current research through a journal club held after work or on weekends. At the very least, the manager should not be an obstacle to efforts to ensure current competency. When therapists wish to attend conferences relevant to enhancing their skills, managers should work with them to provide a flexible workweek or other strategy so that time missed can be accrued through additional patient treatment time.

Assignment of patients, often tedious and time consuming, brings with it a host of considerations. The patient expects to receive the best care available. Therapists expect to be treated fairly and equally. However, all therapists are not equally skilled in all areas of practice. The profession is simply too expansive for everyone to hold equal expertise in pediatrics, geriatrics, sports medicine, acute care, and other specialized areas. Even within any one of these areas, it is doubtful that all will be equally skilled in all facets of that specialty. It is the responsibility of the manager to know the staff's skills, strengths, and weaknesses, and assign patients appropriately. If a therapist has a deficit that causes patient assignment to be unequal (either in complexity of care or in number of patients), the manager has the responsibility of providing opportunities for the therapist to develop the essential skills. If the therapist refuses or simply is unable to acquire the needed competencies, and the deficiencies are significant, the manager must dismiss that therapist and find a replacement.

Personnel Duties

Ron

Ron has been practicing clinically for fourteen years. Six years ago he returned to school, where he earned a master's degree in health-care administration. He accepted the position of chair of the physical therapy department at Mercy Hospital two years ago. Immediately he made needed changes in the methods used to assign patients to therapists, instituted flexible work schedules, and established a weekly case review time that was more like continuing education than peer review. He is generally perceived as a strong leader by the therapy staff, which is made up of 12 full-time therapists and 3 physical therapist assistants.

Mercy Hospital had been on the brink of bankruptcy for years. It has managed to survive through the efforts of a highly competent CEO who could generate donations and assistance when times were difficult. Nevertheless, the board of directors sold the hospital to Partners in Health Care, Inc., one of the larger publicly traded national managed–health-care organizations. Ron met with his new supervisor, Harold, the vice president of rehabilitation, who alerted him that the therapy department was losing money. The losses were not great and certainly did not constitute a threat to the organization as a whole, but the problem had to be solved so that the department would make at least a 10 percent profit. This was the margin of profit essential to support other services, such as the prevention and immunization programs, that could not be expected to be self-supporting. If this profit goal could not be reached, the organization would abolish the physical therapy department as it was currently structured and retain Ron as chair to manage per diem therapists. Harold explained that the cost savings of such a change would be significant because per diem therapists were paid only for their hours of patient contact and received no benefits, which totaled over 35 percent of the salaries of the current staff. Harold said that he would give Ron one week to develop and implement a plan that was equal, or nearly equal, to the per diem strategy.

Based on his experience, Ron reasoned that a full per diem staff was simply not acceptable. Patients would lose the continuity that was essential to good care, and there was no way he could assure competency in specialized areas for complex patient needs. His solution was a proposal that left the current team intact but imposed a 10 percent reduction in pay across the board. The proposal would also end overtime pay, and it would impose unpaid "voluntary" time for the case reviews that had proved professionally valuable. In addition, he requested that each therapist donate one weekend day every six weeks without pay.

According to Ron's calculations, which were confirmed by the accounting staff, this proposed solution would slightly improve the return that a per diem staff would generate for the organization. He called a departmental meeting and explained his reasoning for the proposal. Initially the staff seemed accepting. He felt confident that, after giving them a couple of days to think it over, they would rally behind his ideas.

At the end of the second day he called another departmental meeting and opened with this item of business. Sharon, one of the therapists, said that the staff had met without Ron to assess their options and the group had asked her to speak for them. She expressed her thanks to him for proposing what he clearly believed was the best alternative. The group had decided, however, to take another course of action, which was also currently being considered by the nursing staff in response to cuts in their area. They had contacted the labor union to ask it to represent them in their dealings with management.

The therapists had in theory endorsed a job action that would leave patients without any therapy, and they believed that management would quickly realize that they could not afford such an action, in terms of either patient liability or bad publicity. The group saw no reason why they should lose salary or personal time. They were all prepared to take this job action for a duration of up to three weeks, and some would continue even longer. ▨

Ron thought he was providing responsible leadership when he made his proposal to the staff. Was he? He could probably have reached a much better decision about "the right thing to do" if he had had more information. For example, he might have tried to hear from the therapists on an individual basis how they weighed such issues as patient abandonment, future long-term goods versus the short-term harm, or perhaps their perspective on how good a leader they perceived him to be. Because more information tends to generate better decisions, we wisely seek a "thick" rather than a "thin" case description. Nevertheless, whether in textbook cases or in real life, there is always a limit on what can be known before having to make a decision.

One of the most important findings about organizational life was the discovery that administrative units make decisions in what is called a "bounded rationality."[19,20] That is, organizations typically come up with decisions that are good enough (satisfactory) but usually not ideal because of very real constraints on time and information. The time constraints exist especially in businesses operating in volatile markets where agile, quick responses are needed to survive. In turn, the time constraints limit the information managers can gather and analyze. The time and information deficits force decisions that will "suffice"—that is, solve problems—even though better solutions could be found under more ideal conditions.

Personnel duties are particularly sensitive to issues of justice and fair dealings and are also usually under tight time constraints. Under such constraints, there is a tendency to treat everyone equally. But is that fair, and does that mean that the support staff (secretaries, administrative assistants, aides) should be managed in the same way as the professional staff? Probably not, because of one major difference: the professional's job is defined primarily by the profession. The manager of a professional team monitors for incompetence but does not define or teach competency; this is handled through the professionals' training and schooling. Staff, on the other hand, must be given specific expectations about what their job entails and taught the process by which to achieve those expectations. That does not mean that their autonomy is not just as worthy of respect as that of the professionals, but in work behaviors, they do in fact have fewer opportunities for making autonomous decisions.

The key to fair treatment of personnel starts with an honest, detailed job description that includes both the skills and values that are required from the organizational point of view. The job description, in essence, defines the contractual agreement between the employee and the employer. Obviously, the skills possessed by the employee must match the needs of the organization. Less obviously, the basic organizational values must also match those of, or at least be acceptable to, the employee.

For example, let us say that hospital Z has an interdisciplinary team approach to patient care, a corporate culture that values diversity, and a commitment to put quality of care on equal footing with profitability. A potential employee who prefers to work autonomously with a homogeneous population, and who feels that only quality of care should be addressed in the professional setting, is clearly a poor risk. Thus, the best time to address a match in values is during the employment interview prior to candidate selection. Employers must be honest and straightforward about the values of the organization and stress that if there is not a match, the candidate would be better served by employment elsewhere.

As stated earlier, the job description is the single most important element in hiring. Advertising must accurately reflect the job content, and the job description must be posted in a public area accessible to all potential candidates. The candidate's resume must be validated, but the degree to which this can be accomplished is affected by state laws concerning the right to privacy that should be consulted prior to inquiry. If possible, it is best to inform applicants on the job application form itself that the application information will be verified by calling former employers, law enforcement agencies, and schools. Steingold recommends having the applicant sign a consent form to authorize this investigation and thereby reduce the risk for the employer.[21] This procedure also fairly informs potential employees that truthfulness is of value in the organization. Employers must then verify the dates and responsibilities provided by the prospect, as well as any comments or written communication they are willing to share concerning past job performance. These steps are critical; unfortunately, in business, more than a few individuals inflate and even lie about job responsibilities in previous employment. Truthfulness is an essential component in employment, for if it is lacking, the manager will have to either set up a surveillance system to check the accuracy of any statement made by that employee or disregard their input. Neither is a reasonable option.

Once the applicant pool is defined, the format and content of the application and interview process must treat all candidates equally. The initial application process will probably be managed by human resource personnel who usually have the assistance of legal advisors, but the department chair usually conducts the interview and may request other staff members to also interview candidates. Each interviewer should have a written list of questions so that all candidates are treated equally. Since the landmark case of *Griggs v. Duke Power Company* in 1971, only items proven to be reasonably relevant to the job task(s) can be asked in the process of selecting employees. In that particular case, heard before the U.S. Supreme Court, Mr. Griggs was refused employment as a manual laborer because Duke Power Company required that employees in that job function have a high school diploma. Since the company could show no relevancy of a high school diploma to laying telephone lines (the job Mr. Griggs had applied for), it lost the court case.

Because managers purchase the skills and talents that fit a specific job description, there is no need to ask irrelevant questions, such as "Are you married?" or "Where were you born?" or "When did you graduate from high school?"—all of which imply a selection bias that is irrelevant and may be illegal.[21] Questions that reveal an applicant's age (especially if over 40), such as the question about high school graduation, or that pertain to race, religious beliefs, physical disability, financial status, birthplace, or ethnicity are illegal, in addition to many others, which vary by state and often include references to marital status and sexual orientation.[21]

A manager must be completely honest with prospective employees and be especially careful not to promise or imply a job security that is unrealistic. The 1877 U.S. document "Horace Wood's Treatise on Master and Servant" officially endorsed the tradition of "at-will" employment in the United States, which means that an employee can leave a job at any time and an employer can dismiss an employee at any time for any reason, and even for no reason.[22] Since that time, the courts and Congress have limited the employer's legal reasons for dismissal, but the employee remains free to come and go at will.

In truth, there is no job security unless a contract employment is created. This can happen when an administrator informs a prospective employee that "if you do a good job, you need not worry about your employment."[23] Statements such as this create a contract that is additional to the "at will" employment tradition and leaves the organization subject to charges of wrongful termination if employment is terminated. In fact, the three most common bases for lawsuits include wrongful termination based on stated or implied conditions of work, discrimination based on legally protected classifications, and retaliation that violates rights granted under state or federal law.[22(p205)]

Workers' Safety

One category of an organization's personnel duties warrants separate mention here: duties to maintain a safe workplace. Employees have the expectation that their employer will act in their behalf to make their work environment as safe as possible. That expectation became a legal right under the Occupational Safety and Health Act (OSHA) passed by Congress in 1970.

The intent of the act was to reduce workplace hazards by requiring employers to meet specified health and safety standards. The act contained a provision for a new agency, called the Occupational Safety and Health Administration (also called OSHA), to be housed in the U. S. Department of Labor for the purpose of establishing additional health and safety standards. In Section 18 of the act, states were encouraged to set up their own job safety and health programs, which OSHA would then approve and monitor. Presently, 23 states have their own programs, many of which are more stringent than the federal OSHA standards.[24]

Both state and federal programs cover all health service organizations, with the exception of self-employed professionals with no employees. In addition to maintaining a safe environment, organizations are required to keep records of accidents requiring more than simple first aid. They are also required to provide safety training.

Workers were given two basic legal rights by OSHA. First, workers have a right to register a complaint with OSHA, and they cannot be harmed by the employer for doing so. Second, if workers sincerely believe that a serious injury or death might occur because the work area is unsafe, they can refuse to work and employers may not retaliate. OSHA does have the right to issue citations and can enforce fines and even prison sentences, although these harsher consequences usually occur only in extreme cases and after repeated warnings. Because each state program has unique properties, we will discuss only the broad categories of recommendations outlined by OSHA for health-care settings.

Hospital and other health-care settings are particularly vulnerable to hazards because of the complex nature of the services delivered and the speed at which they must often be administered. Unlike employees in most businesses, hospital employees are often near explosive gases and liquids, do heavy lifting, and often encounter wet floors. Examples of the types of common hazards and injuries that OSHA addresses are hernias, back injuries, fires (patient rooms, storage areas, and equipment are most frequently involved), compressed gases, flammable/combustible liquids/vapors/gases, and electrical equipment. In 1991, OSHA issued its Blood-borne Pathogens Standards, which provide essential protection for health-care workers who might be at risk for blood-borne diseases such as hepatitis and HIV infection. Detailed recommendations can be referenced at OSHA's Website.[25]

The two risks of greatest concern to physical therapists are addressed in OSHA's long-standing recommendations for preventing back injuries and the more recent OSHA standards for preventing violence in the health-care setting. Proper lifting techniques and strategies for managing the physical demands of the profession are solidly embedded in the preparatory educational programs, but violence in the workplace is often overlooked, even though therapists are specifically mentioned among those health-care workers who are covered by the guidelines. Assaults are more common in the health-care and social services than in any other setting, according to 1993 figures from the Bureau of Labor Statistics. The incidence is probably seriously underreported because for too long many have felt that the risk of assault and violence came with the territory. Unfortunately, health-care workers and administrators too often believe that when violence occurs, it is probably the result of a health-care professional who did not properly respond, thereby signaling a type of professional incompetence.[26]

Many factors contribute to violent responses in the health-care workplace, not the least of which is the level of violence in the nation itself and the general population's easy access to handguns. In a 1989 report by J. Wasserberger, G. Orlog, and M. Kolodny, et al., 25 percent of patients in emergency rooms treated for major trauma carried weapons.[27] In addition, there are increasing numbers of mentally ill patients carrying guns who are released from hospitals with no follow-up care. In 1991, 17.3 percent of patients with psychiatric disorders carried weapons.[28] The more salient reason, however, for the prevalence of assault in health care probably has to do with the stress of patients' life-altering injuries, including loss of income and disruption of social and emotional support.

In response to violence in health-care settings, OSHA has recommended the use of metal detectors, closed-circuit video recordings, and bullet-resistant and shatter-proof glass in reception, admitting, and client service rooms. In addition, OSHA recommends that alarm systems that are not dependent on telephone lines be installed throughout the facility, including panic buttons in hallways and stairwells supplemented with handheld alarm devices and hardwired reporting devices in the admissions area, nursing stations, and emergency rooms. Furniture should be affixed to the floor, and other items that could be used as weapons, such as vases and pictures, should be properly secured.

There are a host of other recommendations for reducing violence in the workplace, including employee training in assault management, but at this time the recommendations are not required standards unless mandated by state OSHA regulations.

Organizational Duties

In addition to patient- and personnel-related duties, managers have a cluster of duties concerning the general well-being of the organization. These duties include risk management, fair allocation of resources, sustaining teamwork within the organization, and a host of additional duties at the level of upper management.

Risk Management

Managers typically function as departmental risk managers. Most large hospitals have full-time risk managers whose job includes monitoring compliance with local, state, and accrediting agency regulations. These managers will also create systems to monitor all departments for safety and patient violations, and they are called upon to respond immediately to any patient who has been injured by hospital personnel. At the departmental level, the manager is expected to ensure compliance in the following five directions, among others.

1. All employees in the department are expected to adhere to hospital/organizational policies. We relinquish much of our personal freedom in the employment setting in exchange for the resources we are unable to procure on our own. However, a good manager, and certainly an effective leader, knows that managing is far more than compliance to the letter of each rule. It is rare that a general rule will correctly fit each situation. As a consequence, the manager is constantly deciding how much compliance with selected policies is needed and when policies need revision to better fit the current work environment. Although staff expect to be treated equally, frequently supervisors have to decide when decreased productivity is valid. In order to maintain the trust of the staff, management must avoid even the appearance of wrongdoing or favoritism by communicating the rationale for different standards of productivity where it will not break a rule of confidentiality such as an illness that the employee does not want revealed. In general, the manager should take care in open communications to respect the confidentiality and personal information of all employees.

2. All equipment should be maintained according to manufacturer instructions and inspected on a regular basis to assure that it is safe for patient treatments. When new equipment is purchased, it should be tested prior to patient use to ensure it is properly calibrated and safe.

3. In the event of a patient or employee injury in the department, there must be an immediate and medically appropriate response that is professional, sympathetic, and followed by a written incident report. Most departments have well-established policies and procedures that prescribe the format of this response.

4. Staff must understand that it is essential to respect patients' informed consent, and that it is important to inform patients about treatment and the methods that will be used, where and why touching of the patient is required, and expected outcomes. Any procedure, including evaluations, that involves touching the patient in areas that might be interpreted as sexual should be explained in advance and must be documented.[29]

5. Supervision must be available for all staff while patients are treated in the department. Managers are the organization's representatives, as well as

representatives of the staff, hence they are expected to be available as needed. Thus they must keep the receptionist or some other staff member informed about their daily activities and how they can be reached.

Fair Allocation of Resources

One of the most important functions of any manager is the fair allocation of resources to employees. Traditionally, the higher the manager is in the hierarchy, the greater the resources at hand to distribute. Because of the perceived power that goes with the allocation of resources, managers must be keenly aware that even the appearance of wrongdoing or unfairness, no matter how unfounded, will damage the trust employees have in them.

Because managers work in a fiduciary role when it comes to allocation, it is usually best if all concerned parties are involved in the decision making about resource allocation. Often, staff are involved as advisors, with final decision resting with the manager. This is because, while employees have a vested interest in their own rewards and maintenance, the manager has the responsibility of managing both present and future goals for the entire department. Thus, rather than distributing the resources to the individual members of the department, the manager might make better use of those resources by investing them in long-term department development. In that event, managers should explain to their staffs the principles that guided their thinking and the potential tradeoffs between benefits and burdens.

Unfortunately, there are times when information cannot be shared with staff, perhaps because it is proprietary or because it violates the privacy rights of another employee. For example, if managers are aware of confidential negotiations for a merger with another company, they are not free to reveal that information, even if it is the reason for a sudden staffing "freeze." As another example, funds might have to be spent to secure a 30-inch computer monitor to give reasonable accommodation as a part of ADA compliance to a new receptionist with a vision disability. And although it would be clear that a disability is involved, that information cannot be released to the staff without the employee's permission. Even so, managers are best advised to explain that there are reasons they cannot express at the time, but that as soon as possible they will explain their reasoning.

Maintaining Teamwork

The manager's responsibility to promote and ensure teamwork is an organizational duty that overlaps with personnel duties and that also affects patient-related duties. There are three basic types of teams in health-care rehabilitation: multidisciplinary, interdisciplinary, and transdisciplinary, as were already defined in Chapter 7.

All teamwork raises ethical concerns. Teamwork creates the obvious gain of peer interaction through participation in team decision making, but teamwork also brings the equally obvious loss of professional autonomy in making requisite compromises. Individuals are no longer completely free to intervene as they see fit, because decisions are now joint ventures and interventions are tailored and scheduled around the team's resources. Moreover, it seems that in all groups there is the somewhat troublesome problem of "free riders"—those who produce just enough to get by and who do not contribute as equal members. Fairness is a powerful force in the workplace. When it is perceived as absent, morale in the entire group is affected. Peer pressure might be effective in changing the free-loading behavior when the person actually values the opinions and wishes of the other team members. However, as long as the person is meeting minimum expectations, the manager might lack the leverage to implement change.

The more troublesome aspect of team membership is its fracturing of the individual provider's sense of responsibility for the patient. When the team is the accountable unit, sometimes, in spite of ethical responsibilities, none of the members feel individually accountable for the outcomes. This phenomenon is reminiscent of the by-stander effect brought to national attention in 1964 when New Yorker Kitty Genovese was murdered near her home following a half-hour attack. More than 38 neighbors heard her screams but no one came to her defense and no one called police. A large number of studies were initiated following this event that produced multiple findings to explain it, including the natural tendency to assume that someone else will respond to a problem. The studies tended to agree that the diffusion of responsibility is proportional to the number of people involved.[30]

Upper Management Duties

As one moves up the hierarchy, decision making becomes increasingly complex. In part this is because the decisions that cannot be comfortably made at a lower level must be taken to the next level. Also, the increasing number of variables needing consideration increases. Decisions that have a global effect on the organizational culture or fiscal stability of the organization are typically made by the top managers along with the chief executive officer (CEO) and the board of trustees. A decision that might be made at this level is whether to establish a voluntary affirmative action program.

Top managers must juggle and integrate numerous competing interests. The CEO of a hospital is typically responsible to the board of directors or trustees not only for the decisions which she makes but also for all the decisions made by her vice presidents and their managers. The CEO must communicate with the Joint Commission on Hospital Accreditation and other accrediting agencies, as well as negotiate with labor unions that represent employees of the hospital. The CEO must assure that the hospital complies with city, county, and state laws as they relate to patient care, building codes, and various other regulations. Fund-raising in the form of attracting charitable donations and submitting grant applications is part of the CEO's responsibilities, as well as developing long-range strategic plans for the hospital. At each successive move up the hierarchy, the manager has greater contact with the external environment of the organization. Most of these responsibilities rest on making fair distribution of existing and future resources. While the primary focus of the hospital should be the patients it serves, the hospital also has a role as an employer with broader social and legal obligations.

Discussion Questions

1. Outline what you envision as the key ethical values, both procedural and result-oriented, that define leadership. Then apply this normative concept of leadership to Sara's situation in the case early in this chapter. What avenues for effective leadership might she have available in her situation?

2. What variables do you hope Ron's staff considered before deciding to join the union and embark on a job action? How would you weigh the variables and options, and what course of action would you have taken if you had been a therapist in Ron's unit?

3. As a cost-saving measure, a managed-care organization announced that it would do away with the chairs of each department and ask each department to run itself. Members of the physical therapy department were to leave any unmanageable problems to the division chief, who would handle performance appraisals and strategic planning for the division and thus for each department. What are some strategies you could use to keep the operations of the department fair for the department employees? Be sure to address patient scheduling, conflict management, and resource allocation for such things as continuing education and patient supplies.

4. The CEO of a health-care organization announces, through the division chief, that staff therapists will have to reduce the time currently spent with patients so the organization can meet the time allowance that the third-party payers are willing to fund. In the past, therapists were scheduled in 30-minute blocks of time, both for ease of scheduling and because most therapists needed that amount of time to prepare for, assess, treat, and educate each patient. Now, some cases will receive only 20 minutes. The reason seems clear: the hospital is trying to make more money. You are concerned that the patients will receive less care than is desirable. What options might you pursue?

5. You are the chief physical therapist at a small private hospital, in a department with four additional therapists. The chief occupational therapist at the hospital has quit after a long dispute with management, and the vice president in charge of rehabilitation announces that the two departments will be combined under your leadership. How will you assuage the fears of the occupational therapists concerning your ability to fairly and credibly evaluate their patient care?

6. The therapist in charge of the whirlpool area reports to you that the Hubbard tub sample sent for a bacteria reading has come back positive for *E. coli.* Since the unit has a full roster of patients from the burn unit to be treated each day, either a new Hubbard tank will have to be found, whether purchased or rented, or the patients will have to be sent to another hospital. New admissions will also have to be rerouted until the tank is sterilized and key components are disassembled and sterilized. Even with a crew working around the clock, it will be days before a tank will be ready for patient use. You take the matter to the division chair. Instead of authorizing transfers for treatment, the chair says to fill the old tank with as much disinfectant as available, add alcohol and anything else that might kill the bacteria, run it, rinse it, and readmit patients. What should you do?

7. As chief therapist in the rehab unit, you are initially impressed with Susan's efficiency. Although a new graduate, she treated more patients in her first month than some of the senior therapists on staff. Early in the third month, Steve, one of the physical therapist assistants, approaches you in your office. Steve has been in the department for 15 years and is generally considered the best assistant on staff. He comments that while he thinks Susan is very competent, he is concerned that she has instructed him to do full patient evaluations parallel to her while she evaluates other patients. In addition, she has asked

him to propose treatment plans, which up until now she has approved without question. Steve adds that he considers himself competent to do what is requested, but he questions if this is entirely permissible. What would be your response, and what would be your course of action?

References

1. Ciulla JB. Leadership ethics: mapping the territory. In: Ciulla JB, ed. *Ethics: The Heart of Leadership*. Westport, CT: Praeger; 1998:3-25.
2. Burns JM. *Leadership*. New York, NY: Harper; 1978.
3. Gardner JW. The tasks of leadership. In: Rosenbach WE, Taylor RL, eds. *Contemporary Issues in Leadership*. 2d ed. Boulder, CO: Westview Press; 1989:24.
4. Jackall R. *Moral Mazes: The World of Corporate Managers*. New York, NY: Oxford University Press; 1988:6.
5. Purtilo RB. Habits of thought: beyond captains and shepherds. *PT Magazine*. June 1993:76-77.
6. Morgan G. *Images of Organizations*. Beverly Hills, CA: Sage Publications; 1986.
7. Ford RC, Richardson WE. Ethical decision making: a review of the empirical literature. *J Bus Ethics*. 1994;13:205-221.
8. Denhardt KG. Organizational structure as a context for administrative ethics. In: Cooper TL, ed. *Handbook of Administrative Ethics*. New York, NY: Marcel Dekker; 1994:179.
9. Cooper TL. *The Responsible Administrator*, 4th ed. San Francisco, CA: Jossey-Bass; 1998:140–153.
10. Bowman JS, Elliston FA, Lockhart P. *Professional Dissent: An Annotated Bibliography and Resource Guide*. New York, NY: Garland; 1984.
11. Elliston F, Kennan J, Lockhart P, Van Schaick J. *Whistleblowing: Managing Dissent in the Workplace*. New York, NY: Praeger; 1985.
12. Decker PJ. Sexual harassment in health care: a major productivity problem. *Health Care Superv*. 1997;16(1):2.
13. Friedman LH, Goes JB. The timing of medical technologies acquisitions: strategic decision making in turbulent environments. *J Healthc Manag*. 2000;45(5):317-331.
14. Milgram S. *Obedience to Authority*. New York, NY: Harper & Row; 1974.
15. Sherif M. A study of some social factors in perception. *Arch Psychol*. 1936:187.
16. Asch SE. *Social Psychology*. Englewood Cliffs, NJ: Prentice-Hall; 1952.
17. Zimbardo PG, Haney C, Banks WC, Jaffe D. The psychology of imprisonment: privation, power, and pathology. In: Rubin Z, ed. *Doing Unto Others*. Englewood Cliffs, NJ: Prentice-Hall; 1974:61-73.
18. Gervais KG, Priester R, Vawter DE, Otte KK, Solberg MM, eds. *Ethical Challenges in Managed Care: A Casebook*. Washington, DC: Georgetown University Press; 1999:303-320.
19. Simon HA. *Administrative Behavior: A Study of Decision Making Processes in Administrative Organizations*. 2d ed. New York, NY: Collier/Macmillan; 1957.
20. Burrell G, Morgan G. *Sociological Paradigms and Organizational Analysis*. Portsmouth, NH: Heinemann; 1985:150-156.
21. Steingold FS. *The Employer's Legal Handbook*. 4th ed. Berkeley, CA: Nolo; 2000.
22. Walsh J. *Mastering Diversity: Managing for Success Under ADA and Other Anti-Discrimination Laws*. Santa Monica, CA: Merritt Publishing; 1995:1.
23. Steingold FS. *The Employer's Legal Handbook*, 3d ed. Berkeley, CA: Nolo; 1999:1/7.
24. Occupational Safety and Health Administration. State Occupational Safety and Health Plans. Available at: http://www.osha-slc.gov/fso/osp. Accessed on November 20, 2000.
25. National Institute for Occupational Safety and Health Guidelines for Protecting the Safety and Health of Health Care Workers. Available at: http://www.ced.gov/niosh/hcwold3.html. Accessed on November 20, 2000.

26. OSHA Preambles: Bloodborne Pathogens. Summary and explanation of the standard. Available at: http://www.osha-slc.gov/Preamble/Blood_data/BLOOD9.html. Accessed on November 20, 2000.

27. Wasserberger J, Ordog GJ, Kolodny M, Allen K. Violence in a community emergency room. *Arch Emer Med.* 1989;6:266-269.

28. Goetz RR, Bloom JD, Chenell SL, Moorhead JC. Weapons possessed by patients in a university emergency department. *Ann Emerg Med.* 1981;20(1):8-10.

29. Swisher LL, Krueger-Brophy C. *Legal and Ethical Issues in Physical Therapy.* Boston, MA: Butterworth-Heinemann; 1998:146.

30. Atkinson RL, Atkinson RC, Smith EE, Bem DJ. *Introduction to Psychology.* 10th ed. San Diego, CA: Harcourt Brace Jovanovich; 1990.

Scientific Integrity and Experimentation

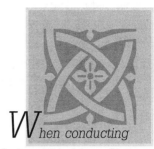

*W*hen conducting

research, is it acceptable to withhold conflicting

data to gain financing?

Keywords

Scientific integrity	Competence
Exploiting the vulnerable	Substituted judgment
Tuskegee Syphilis Study	Best-interest standard
Willowbrook experiments	Imagination principle
Respect for autonomy	Animal-rights proponents
Voluntary consent	Animal-welfare proponents
Informed consent	Authorship credit

Scott Conway

For years, Scott Conway has resented teaching at a less prestigious school, and he also feels overdue for a promotion to full professor. To improve his chances for both a promotion and a better teaching position at a more prominent university, he insists on being the first author listed in articles he developed with the graduate students he supervised. His curriculum vitae, which no one at his school has checked closely, contains misleading entries designed to make his contributions to several research projects appear significantly greater than they were, although he has never engaged in outright fabrication.

Currently he is desperate to renew a substantial grant from a school district for research he hopes will show that participation in a school band is equivalent in exercise value to the state-mandated physical education program. This particular school district has an exceptional football team and is intent on promoting the athletic program in every possible way, including its half-time entertainment. To do this, the district wants to use Conway's research to exempt band members from state-mandated physical education units. Scott is confident the project has promise, but the results have been inconclusive so far, and he doubts that the school district will continue to fund his research unless significant results are likely. He knows there is a way to massage the data by highlighting the promising results and not reporting some conflicting data. He also knows it is unlikely that anyone will be caught. Convinced he is doing no serious harm to anyone, he quickly makes the changes and mails the grant proposal.[1]

The validity and usefulness of scientific studies depend on whether research-ers proceed with **scientific integrity**. As the APTA document "Integrity in Physical Therapy Research" states, "A concern for integrity in research follows quite naturally from the dual commitment to research and professional ethics."[2] In everyday life, moral integrity is a complex virtue that implies respect for others, honesty, fairness, decency, and moral consistency (*integritas* means "wholeness" in Latin). The same complexity comprises scientific integrity, a virtue that combines and extends several key values studied in earlier chapters: (1) respect for autonomy, shown by securing informed consent of persons who participate in research projects; (2) justice, shown by a concern about who benefits from scien-tific experimentation; (3) humaneness, shown by acting with beneficence toward both humans and (research) animals; and (4) honesty, shown by, for example, providing full disclosure of research findings, as well as giving proper credit to authors of publications. In Chapter 8 we discussed fraud—which is what Scott Conway engaged in—but the ethics of research involves many additional facets, a sampling of which we explore in this chapter.

Exploiting the Vulnerable

By their very nature, the sciences seek new knowledge that can be validated objectively, and nowhere is that more important than in the health sciences.[3,4] Beliefs based on clinical experience alone, passed from generation to generation without question, will not suffice. Scientific validation of treatment techniques is increasingly required for reimbursement by government and health-care facili-ties,[4] but more than money is at stake.

In the past, the charge has been made that much of the practice of physical therapy is inadequately supported by objective research.[5,6] But this situation is changing, and for good reason. First, respect for patients requires that we be able to discuss with them the likelihood of success of a particular intervention, and that information can only come from outcomes research. Patients cannot make informed decisions without relevant information.

Second, what is right for the patient in physical therapy care should be within the domain of the profession, not the third-party payer. Yet, as long as we say that we do not know if an intervention will work, or at least know the likelihood that it will work, the payer will make those decisions, and there will be little hope of a successful challenge by the professional or the patient.

Third, and most important, the worthiness of physical therapy as a profes-sion depends on its ability to scientifically back its claims that it promotes better health, avoids harm, and is worthy of the public's investment of money, time, trust, and emotional energy. In the words of the editor of the journal *Physical Therapy*, "Scientifically collected data allow us to look beyond our biases at the reality of our patients, their lives, and their resources and at how they bene-fit from our interventions. These data allow us to lay claim to treatments that work, to shed those that do not work, and to modify those that need improve-ment."[7]

Thus, scientific experimentation is essential in extending human knowledge, but it also has an alarming history of abuse. We begin by highlighting a few episodes from that history to show why increasingly strict regulation of research has become necessary.

In the early 18th century, when immunizations were first being developed, it was common for physician-researchers to use their own children, servants, and slaves as subjects.[8] Smallpox vaccination was just one of the immunizations initially tested on children. By the late 19th century, medical journals carried reports of experimentation with gonorrheal cultures by applying them to the eyes of sick children to document the progression of the disease. In 1914, Alfred Hess, who was medical director at the Hebrew Infant Asylum in New York City, said that institutionalized children offered those conducting experiments the distinct advantage of living in "conditions which are insisted on in considering the course of experimental infection among laboratory animals, but which can rarely be controlled in a study of infection in man."[8(p6)]

In Nazi Germany, human experimentation reached a previously unimagined level of horror. Jews, homosexuals, gypsies, and other oppressed minorities were used freely by the medical schools in Germany for experimentation. Additional atrocities were committed by physicians in the service of the German state in hopes of acquiring university appointments through their scientific publications.[9] Experiments included the "High-Altitude Experiments," in which prisoners were locked in airtight compartments and exposed to rapid pressure changes that caused tremendous pain, with death occurring during dissection of the living "subject." In the "Freezing Experiments," prisoners were left in the cold with no clothing between 9 and 14 hours as measurements were taken to record each phase of death. The numerous failed experiments to change homosexuality included castration and the surgical insertion of hormone briquettes, which resulted in horrible deaths.[10,11]

Although the Nazi atrocities are unparalleled in their viciousness, barbaric experiments were not limited to wartime. Deeply disturbing experiments took place in the United States during peacetime, even after dissemination of numerous international treaties on research ethics. The Tuskegee and Willowbrook experiments are among the most infamous.[12]

The **Tuskegee Syphilis Study**, a longitudinal study conducted by the U.S. Department of Public Health between 1932 and 1969, followed 400 black men infected with syphilis to confirm existing research on the long-term effects of untreated syphilis. Those effects included blindness and death for at least 40 of the participants. Long after penicillin was discovered to be an effective treatment for syphilis (in the 1940s), the men were given only aspirin or other ineffective treatments to prevent them from acquiring effective treatment. They were also promised a $50 bonus for funeral expenses if they lived 25 years and agreed to an autopsy at time of death.

Major breeches of medical ethics in this study included the following:[13]

1. The experiment was redundant and scientifically pointless.
2. The research design was so flawed that meaningful results could not have been detected.
3. The participants were deceived and coerced.
4. A socially deprived and financially vulnerable population was exploited.
5. Participants were knowingly allowed to die even though life-saving treatment was available.
6. The participants were not compensated for injuries.

Almost 25 years after the initiation of the Tuskegee studies, Saul Krugman and Joan P. Giles, through the New York University School of Medicine, began the **Willowbrook experiments**. This research, like the Tuskegee Syphilis Study, was designed to follow the natural progression of a disease—in this case, viral hepatitis. It also was designed to test the effectiveness of a known treatment, gamma globulin. Gamma globulin was already known to be effective in the treatment of this disease, yet it was withheld from half of the experimental group so that the natural progression of the disease could be observed. The research was conducted on mentally disabled children residing at the Willowbrook School on Staten Island, New York; the children were intentionally infected with the virus and then studied during the progression of the disease.

A particularly disturbing aspect of the Willowbrook research was that it was reviewed and approved by the New York State Department of Mental Hygiene, the New York State Department of Mental Health, the Armed Forces Epidemiological Board, and the New York University School of Medicine, in addition to the Willowbrook School. Although parental consent was given for each child, the consent was based upon the school's declaration that there was room for new students at the school only in the experimental unit. Initially the study was even supported by the *Journal of the American Medical Association,* but it was judged indefensible by the *British Journal of Hospital Medicine*. At the core of the objections was the principle that children should not be used in research unless the children themselves stand to gain by the research, a concept enforced in British law at the time.

Serious attempts to protect participants in research began after World War II, on December 9, 1946, at the Palace of Justice in Nuremberg.[14] There, twenty-three physicians were tried for war crimes and crimes against humanity. The judges relied on 10 rules for ethical experimentation on humans, which became known as the Nuremberg Code, a document that has exerted unparalleled influence in the scientific community. In March 1960, Henry K. Beecher recommended a general code be developed to guide physicians, comparable to the Nuremberg Code. The World Medical Association's Committee on Medical Ethics had developed a document that was ratified at the 18th World Medical Assembly in Helsinki in 1964. This Declaration of Helsinki was revised in 1975, 1983, and, most recently, in 1989.

Additional guidelines were developed by professional groups, including the American Medical Association and the American Academy of Pediatrics. On May 30, 1974, the U.S. Department of Health, Education and Welfare, now known as the Department of Health and Human Services, published specific guidelines for adults, and a 1977 appendix addressed the unique problems regarding children. Over the years, many revisions and competing models were offered, and in 1991 the "Federal Policy for the Protection of Human Subjects" was published and endorsed by government departments and agencies.[15]

These guidelines are quite specific and mandate an Internal Review Board (IRB) located at every institution that engages in human research and receives federal funds.[16] The IRB must have at least five members, including one who represents nonscientific interests, such as an ethicist, attorney, or member of the clergy.[17] Typically, the IRB reviews each full research proposal before the project begins. Depending on the risk level of the project, the IRB will characterize it as (1) exempt from review, (2) for expedited review, or (3) for full review. Projects typically exempt from review include surveys that are anonymous and do not deal with sensitive topics. Expedited reviews—projects reviewed by the chairperson of the IRB and at least one other member of the IRB rather than the entire committee—may be granted to research in the clinic setting that is noninvasive and to studies of normally occurring events. Full review covers all other experiments and especially those using invasive procedures.

 ## Respect for Autonomy

Respect for autonomy is at the heart of scientific integrity in research on humans. Each major ethical theory affirms respect for autonomy as an important value. For example, rights ethics emphasizes respect for the human right of self-determination. Utilitarianism points to the good consequences of allowing people to exercise autonomy and sometimes counts autonomy as an intrinsic good. Unquestionably, the greatest emphasis on respect for autonomy was articulated by Kant: Treat persons as autonomous rational beings who have their own purpose, and never as mere means to reaching your own purposes. The "mere" here is important. In one sense, we constantly use other persons in order to gain benefits, just as they use us. This reciprocity is essential to our lives as social creatures. Kant's point is that we must not treat them as if they were only our instruments—as if they were things whose value consists solely in what we can get from them. All persons have an inherent moral dignity rooted in their capacity (or potential) to govern their own lives. To ignore, undermine, or assault that autonomy is to degrade persons.

In one sense, to experiment on humans is to make them objects—namely, objects of scientific study (even though they are usually called "experimental subjects"). The danger comes when researchers shift to a view of people as mere objects—as mere means to achieving the aims of an experiment. Making that shift is a constant danger, because the goals of research are to maximize good consequences by discovering new knowledge, not to promote the welfare of individual participants. Respect for autonomy means that these benefits to others must never be won by sacrificing the autonomy of individuals who participate in experiments.

As noted in Chapter 3, respect for autonomy requires obtaining the voluntary informed consent of competent persons. (See Fig. 1.) Following is a review of three (overlapping) types of consent—voluntary, informed, and competent—as they apply to research.

Voluntary Consent

Respect for autonomy means acknowledging that participation in research must be voluntary. Mere assent, whether verbal or behavioral, is not necessarily **voluntary consent**. For example, handing over money in response to the threat, "Your money or your life," is hardly a fully voluntary act. Voluntary means there is no coercion in the form of threats, physical force, or other objectionable pressures. This includes subtle pressures that come in the form of undue influence—that is, offering positive benefits rather than threatening harm.

Minor tokens of appreciation may be given, but they must not be substantial or "irresistible." Also, assembling prospective participants in a group to request their participation and to inform them of their rights might allow peer pressure to shadow their judgments. In cases in which the researcher and care provider are one and the same, every effort must be made to separate the therapist-patient

Figure 1: A SAMPLE INFORMED CONSENT DOCUMENT

Subject	Comments
Title of Study	The title should give a brief, accurate statement about the study.
Location	Include the complete mailing address.
Investigators	List all members of the research team, including faculty sponsor.
Purpose of Study	The purpose should be clearly and briefly written so that the intent is known.
Participant Selection	Prospective participants are frequently unwilling to engage in the study unless they know how they were selected.
Institutional Review Board Disposition	All research conducted through an educational institution must have the university IRB approval and the approval of other participating institutions.
Methods	The methods should be as detailed as possible while still holding the reader's interest.
Risks	Social, legal, psychological, or economic risk must be made explicit. The reasonableness standard compares the risk of research participation with the normal risk of daily living without participation in the study. If the research risks are greater, then they must be expressed.
Benefits	Name the specific benefits, such as frequent medical exams, or, if there are no benefits, state that no benefits are anticipated.
Confidentiality	State specifically how confidentiality will be protected, noting that the designates of the Food and Drug Administration and the Department of Health and Human Services may inspect the records. Note that if the study plan is changed or the information is to be used in ways not explained to the subject, the subject will be informed and a separate consent will be required.
Financial Concerns	Financial concerns include both the direct effect on the participants and a disclosure of funding for the research project itself.
Questions	Tell the research subjects how they can have their questions answered personally, either by phone or in person.
Injury	In the event of injury, tell the subjects exactly what they should do and who will pay for the treatment or diagnosis.
Withdrawal and Discontinuation of Study	Subjects MUST be assured that they can withdraw from the study at any time with no negative consequences to them.
Questions Concerning Rights and Consent	Tell the subjects who they should call or see if they have questions specific to their rights or their consent.

(continued)

Figure 1: A SAMPLE INFORMED CONSENT DOCUMENT
(*continued*)

Subject	Comments
Study Design Changes	In the event that, during or after the study is completed, there is a design change that will result in the information being used in a new or different manner, the subjects must be assured that a new consent from them will be requested.
Concluding Statement	Review briefly the intent of the study.
Funding Sources	All sources of funding must be disclosed to the research participants.
Signatures	Signatures cannot be on a separate sheet. They must clearly be a part of the document.

relationship from the researcher-subject relationship, including having someone else request patient participation in research. This is important because patients often feel a sense of dependency on their physical therapists, and they might feel that to preserve that relationship they must agree to the therapist's suggestion to participate in the research.

Informed Consent

Two bodies of information are essential for patients to give their **informed consent**. First, to exercise our rights we must know them, and participants in experiments must be made aware of their right to give informed consent or to refuse. They must also be made explicitly aware of: their right to withdraw from the research at any time without suffering negative consequences; their right to confidentiality; and additional rights, all formalized in a patient's "Bill of Rights."

Second, participants must know specifically what they are agreeing to do in the particular experiment. Lying to participants, providing them false data, and withholding needed information are morally equivalent in this context. Most important, individuals must be provided with a detailed account of the risks—or potential harms greater than those experienced in daily life—involved in the study. Five basic types of risk are possible and, if foreseeable, should be assessed and expressed.[18] (See table.)

Type of Risk	Examples
1. Physical	Muscle soreness, adverse reaction to drugs
2. Psychological	Depression, confusion
3. Social	Loss of privacy
4. Legal	Revocation of parole, prosecution
5. Economic	Loss of employment

Risk assessment is an ongoing part of research, and new risks discovered in the course of experiments must be revealed to the participants immediately. If physical risks are involved, available medical care must be documented in the consent form.

The language of consent documents needs to be at the level of comprehension of the target population. If technical words, such as goniometer and isokinetic, are used, their meaning must be explained. In addition, it is essential that prospective participants have a way to speak personally with the researcher or someone informed about the research. Wanting to preserve the appearance of being knowledgeable, many people will be reluctant to ask questions unless it can be done privately. To assure both voluntariness and understanding, persons must be allowed time to weigh and consider the choices and risk inherent in participation in research.

Competent to Consent

So far we have assumed that the persons asked to participate in research are competent to make autonomous decisions. Voluntary informed consent implies this **competence,** but we will provide a separate discussion of it.

In most cases in which the sample of participants is drawn from the general population, competence is rarely a critical issue. Typically, persons are considered competent if they can demonstrate that they understand the research methods, have weighed the benefits and risks, and can express a decision. However, the burden of proof of competency increases proportionally to the risks involved. When risk is low, as in measuring the active range of motion at the knee, then a simple assessment of the participant's understanding of the methods, combined with an explicit decision upon considering the risks and benefits, is sufficient. When the risks are severe and the population studied is at risk for incompetence, it may be appropriate to have a psychiatrist or psychologist render a judgment using objective measurement tools. Between these extremes are other special circumstances warranting attention.

Competence is on a wide continuum and should be assessed in the specific context of the research with respect to each individual. Just because persons are incompetent in one area, such as world banking issues, does not mean they are incompetent in another area, such as personal finances or making a decision to participate in a research project. Moreover, it is not uncommon to witness intermittent competence. That occurs, for example, when a patient or someone with whom they have a significant relationship is given diagnostic information that either overwhelms them or causes grief. For a brief period of time, that patient may be incompetent to make a decision.

Some research topics, such as Alzheimer's disease, require populations in which incompetence is a common occurrence. Obviously, valid research for such populations must involve its members, even though autonomous consent is not possible. If the experimental subjects are in an institutional setting, the institution's IRB will assess a request to use their patients in research. The institution must also acquire the consent of the family member or guardian who acts as the patient's surrogate decision maker. In noninstitutional settings, such as home care, courts will typically appoint a legal guardian authorized to make such decisions for the patient.

Depending on the state, surrogate decisions will be made using either a "**substituted judgment standard**" or a "**best-interest standard.**"[19] According to the substituted judgment standard, someone appointed by the court—typically someone who knew the patient well when they were competent—is instructed to make a decision as the patient would have made if they were competent. In contrast, according to the "best-interest standard," the surrogate decision maker must weigh all possibilities and decide on a course of action that would give the highest benefit to the now incompetent person. They may consider former preferences of the patient as they help interpret quality of life issues, but the judgment is based on what will best serve the patient now.

Children are another special population legally defined as not competent. The states define legal competency by age, although surely we have known persons at age 14 who were considerably more mature than others at age 22. Nevertheless, even with some legal exceptions such as the "emancipated minor," who is awarded a decision-making right by the court, even a mature 14-year-old will need his or her parent's or guardian's consent to participate in a research project. If the risk of the research is minimal, usually only one parent's signature is necessary, but if moderate to great risk is involved, both parents must consent. (Exceptions occur when one parent has been given sole legal guardianship rights or when one parent is absent from the home and unavailable.)

When children are wards of the state—for example, abused and abandoned children living in shelters—then the relevant agency must provide institutional consent. Also, since 1983 the U.S. Department of Health and Human Services has recommended that children give assent in addition to the parent's consent. The form and content of assent are determined by IRBs and take into account the developmental level of children and their ability to understand. At the very least, the assent should be based on a simple description of the study and the procedures that will occur, together with some explanation of the risks involved and assurances of confidentiality. If the child refuses permission, the refusal must be honored. The one exception is when the parent overrides the child specifically because the child will personally profit from the research in ways greater than the risk or inconvenience.

Who Benefits?

Voluntary informed consent is the most important ethical consideration in experimentation on humans, but there are other important ones as well. A cluster of issues concern justice and fairness regarding who benefits from the research. These issues include the selection of participants for experiments, research topics, and control groups.

Experiment Participants

The selection of participants can determine the population that reaps the primary rewards of the research. Generalizations from one population to another require knowledge of all the variables that might affect a particular disease process and the proposed intervention. Typically, not all the important variables can be anticipated, and hence it is important to have an adequate representation of all groups that might be affected by the topic of the research. Because white adult males are frequently the only group sampled, they are the only population to which the results from those studies can be generalized with statistical confidence. As a result, there is a growing effort to find more equitable ways to share the benefits and burdens of scientific research with women, children, and minorities.

Having highlighted some of the abuses visited upon children in experiments, we nevertheless emphasize that it would be unfair to exclude them altogether.

Children are not "little adults." Physiologically, biochemically, metabolically, and psychologically, children are very dissimilar to adults.[20] They even experience different kinds of diseases, some unique to them. Medications suitable for adults can have paradoxical effects in children, resulting in exact opposite reactions to those in adults. Even when drugs have similar effects, the appropriate dosages are not always predicted by body weight.

Women are the most notable group not treated equitably in research designs, even though they constitute half the population.[21,22] For example, clinical drug trials are frequently performed with only male subjects. One often cited justification is the fear of unknown effects on a fetus should one of the female subjects become pregnant. A second frequently used justification is that if women are included, thereby adding extra variables, the sample size would have to be larger in order to achieve the same level of statistical significance that can be achieved with one sex only. In general, the physiological differences between men and women make it problematic to generalize from all-male studies to women. The additional cost and inconvenience are warranted by the far greater danger of giving women drugs that lack proven safety and efficacy for them.

Minorities have also been denied inclusion in many research designs. Nearly 63 percent of health-related studies excluded nonwhite subjects between 1921 and 1990.[23] Worse, the use of nonwhite subjects in clinical field trial studies has actually been decreasing. As discussed in Chapter 5, advocating the inclusion of minorities in research designs does not imply the falsehood that "races" are genetically or physiologically unique. Rather, it allows us to investigate socioeconomic and sociocultural factors that might not be adequately present in a white male sample.

Selecting Research Topics

Achieving justice in the distribution of benefits from research hinges greatly on the selection of topics. Throughout much of the history of science, there was a consensus that knowledge is morally neutral and that data could be used for either good or evil, with the burden of right action resting on the user rather than the discoverer of information. Since then, however, researchers have witnessed a history of horrible consequences that can evolve from the misuse of scientific findings.

In 1976, Callahan introduced the concept of what he called the **Imagination Principle**, which states that researchers have a responsibility to imagine the evil as well as the good ways in which findings might be used. In brief, if the research would produce more evil than good, as may be the case in biological warfare research, then the research should be stopped. If the results would likely be a mixture of good and evil, then the project should be structured so that the good would be maximized and the harmful results minimized. If the results would produce equal amounts of good and evil, then professional groups should be consulted, and if consensus cannot be reached at that level, the project should be presented for public scrutiny.[24]

Callahan's approach, if broadly implemented, would bring dramatic change. Researchers have additional duties, just as anyone in a position of power has further duties, to ensure right decisions. Moreover, we do not exempt other competent persons from responsibility for their products, and we hold them accountable for negligence if unintended consequences are the result of their failure to exercise reasonable foresight. If anything, the expectations outlined by Callahan would merely equalize the playing field so that researchers would have the same responsibilities as anyone else in a similar situation, rather than enjoy an extraordinary exemption.

In any case, researchers are responsible for the selection of research topics. Given finite resources, researchers must establish priorities and pursue questions most likely to produce beneficial results. But beneficial studies should not be equated with studies grand in scope. Out of a sincere desire to bring needed change to the profession, therapists sometimes assume that research must approach global concerns in order to be valuable. However, an incremental approach to solving large problems offers many strategic advantages.[25] For example, decisions about the need for physical therapy are frequently based on range-of-motion findings compared to standards. Unfortunately, in all known cases, these standards were established using adults and do not reflect averages in childhood. But, rather than have one study attempt to establish standards for all joints in children of all ages, an incremental approach through a series of studies would be far more manageable, and beneficial.

Finally, the researcher has a responsibility to acquire the skills and knowledge to select and implement studies with effective research designs. This expectation is justified from the perspective of the patients who will receive the experimental treatment, of those who will be influenced by the findings of the study, and also of the institution which invests resources in the process.

Control Groups

Frequently, the only appropriate study design requires a control group that receives no treatment or a placebo, so that the experimental treatment can be evaluated for effectiveness. The control group may come to a clinic for the same number of visits as the experimental group but participate in activities known to have no effect on the topic under investigation. In drug tests in particular, control groups might even be given medications that will produce some degree of harm—namely, the same side effects as the experimental group, such as dizziness, nausea, and other symptoms.

Many physical therapists are reluctant to use the control-group design, believing that it would be wrong to withhold treatment.[26] In some cases the problem can be resolved by comparing one treatment to another existing treatment, but often we do not know that either treatment is truly effective compared to the results that would occur over time alone. Researchers must decide if greater harm will occur when treatment is withheld from a small control group or when an ineffective treatment is perpetuated in large numbers of patients in the future. Of course, the individuals participating in the research should be considered. One of several ways to minimize damage, when it cannot be eliminated, is to conduct continuous data analysis, preferably by someone unaware of the group designations, and to call the experiment to a halt as soon as statistical significance is achieved. The control group can then immediately be given the experimental treatment.

The potential clash between the dual responsibilities of the researcher—to current research subjects and to future beneficiaries of experiments—became salient during the AIDS epidemic. Activists argued that when an illness is terminal, when options are limited, and when there is reason to believe that an experimental treatment could offer some benefit, the victims of a disease had primary authority to make therapy decisions and to receive drugs still in the experimental stages of development. The final judgment about what is an "acceptable" risk of nonefficacy or of negative side effects rested with those who might benefit. In support of this argument, guidelines by the U.S. Food and Drug Administration have been significantly streamlined to allow patients with terminal illnesses to make selections not available in less life-threatening situations.

Animal Research

Physical therapists, like scientists in other areas of health science, use animals in much of their research and therefore must confront the moral questions about animal research that have become prominent in our society. Since the publication of *Animal Liberation* by Peter Singer in 1975, the assumption that humans have unqualified dominion over animals has been widely challenged. Since the late 1970s, two groups in the United States have argued for including animals in the "moral community" and have strongly opposed abuses in animal experimentation—animal-rights proponents and animal-welfare proponents.[27] Both groups emphasize that human beings are themselves animals and that excluding other animals from moral consideration is a form of bigotry, which they refer to as "speciesism," a term paralleling "racism" and "sexism."

Animal-rights proponents extend rights ethics to apply to nonhuman sentient (conscious) animals, and use that moral framework to oppose most, if not all, animal experimentation. They draw attention to the striking parallels between human agency and the capacities of mammals to act as "subjects of experiences." Not only are sentient animals able to feel pain and pleasure, but they have beliefs, desires, intentions, memories, and in general the capacity to act purposefully based on their preferences. Even though they lack moral autonomy, many species are capable of elaborate social interaction and display remarkably human-like forms of caring for each other, especially within their kin groups.

Animal-welfare proponents extend utilitarian theories to animals. They see moral significance in all creatures capable of feeling pleasure and pain. They remind us that even Charles Darwin, the person who developed the theory that justified many generalizations from animals to humans, was convinced there is an "emotional continuum" in animal life and was troubled by the suffering he knew experimentation would likely cause.[28] Some animal-welfarists, like Peter Singer, argue that relatively few animal experiments are justified. Other animal-welfarists, perhaps placing greater value on the benefits humans have received from animal research, stipulate that animals must be treated in a humane way so as to minimize suffering.

Opponents of these movements typically build on an exclusively human-centered moral perspective which emphasizes obligations to humanity. Discoveries of the causes of diseases, of vaccines to prevent disease, and of life-saving surgical techniques have all been made possible by animal research.[29] In addition, they observe that throughout the life chain, species prey upon other species, and we do not consider this a moral wrong.[30] That is not to say they countenance wanton cruelty to animals, but the reasons given refer back to humanity. As Kant suggested, cruelty to animals degrades perpetrators of the cruelty, making them callous and sadistic in ways likely to foster cruelty toward human beings. Interestingly, these defenders of the status quo sometimes point to the benefits to animals (including endangered species) of experimentation, because they often profit from research-based advances in veterinary medicine, thereby implying that animals deserve some consideration as recipients of research benefits.

Substantial arguments are offered on both sides of this difficult issue. Here we highlight several points that offer hope for some compromise by identifying a middle ground of accepting animal experimentation with strict safeguards. First, there is an intricate web of interdependence in nature such that all living things contribute to the whole that supports individual species and lives. As we have collectively learned from our environmental mistakes, changes in a single unit can have a ripple effect over the entire fabric. For example, the ozone changes have affected amphibian life, which in turn can unbalance entire ecosystems.

Second, respect for nature does not demand identical treatment of all categories of animals. The boundaries between species, including those between plants and animals, are at times ambiguous even to experts. Nevertheless, in a general way humans tend to divide the continuum of life into at least four major categories: human, vertebrate, invertebrate, and plant. Our basic emotional responses signal differences in appropriate treatment of these groups even before we are able to give reasons justifying those responses. We might feel regret when neighbors neglect their plants to the point of death, but we feel much more strongly when they neglect their pets, and worse yet if they abuse their children—at which point we feel an obligation to call authorities.

Third, two general principles are widely affirmed on all sides of the debate and are now embedded in legislation. The minimal harm principle says that when harm is done, it must be justified with a good reason. The Principle of Proportionality calls for the least amount of harm to achieve the desired good.[31] Although these principles seem relatively simple, they have significant implications. Because suffering includes anxiety as well as the presence of pain, reducing harm means reducing anxiety, both for individual participants and for the sum of participants.

Suffering occurs at two levels for laboratory animals. The first level is composed of the husbandry conditions in which animals live on a day-to-day basis; some suffering is imposed simply by the removal or absence of an environment normal for that animal.[32] Reasonable animal husbandry will by necessity require the expertise of persons trained to recognize suffering and to appreciate species-specific conditions to reduce suffering. This staff must be held accountable through supervision by qualified and experienced staff.

The second level of suffering is posed by the scientific procedures themselves. In keeping with the Principle of Proportionality, scientists must select species from the lowest level of the animal hierarchy that meets the research requirements. They must also use the best statistical procedures to assure that the fewest numbers of animals are used. With regard to those animals used, every effort must be made to minimize pain and suffering. Before the experiment begins, end points must be established so that the process is not unnecessarily prolonged. Appropriate sedation, anesthesia, and ultimately painless euthanasia are used if chronic pain cannot be relieved.

The translation of these principles into specific laws and recommendations has for the United States been somewhat limited and prolonged compared to the process in Europe, Canada, Australia, and New Zealand. Over the past 15 years, in their efforts to find alternative models for animal usage in research, Germany has spent about $6 million annually, the Netherlands $2 million, and the European Center for the Validation of Alternative Methods (established in 1992) $9 million.[28] In comparison, the United States has contributed $1.5 million per year for three years. Since 1985 every scientist using animals in experimentation in the Netherlands has been required to take a three-week course in correct anesthesia and techniques in animal handling and management. In general, use of animals in experimentation in Europe has slowly declined, although comparisons with the United States are difficult because U.S. legislation and accounting exempt mice, birds, and rats, which make up roughly 90 percent of animal research subjects.

Nevertheless, numerous steps have been taken in the United States at the federal, state, and local levels to protect animals. Additional regulations also are specified by private foundations for projects they fund. The landmark federal legislation was the Animal Welfare Act (AWR) of 1966, which was revised in 1970, 1976, and 1985. More stringent standards are established by individual federal agencies, such as the 1996 Public Health Services Policy on Humane Care and Use of Laboratory Animals, for projects they fund. Because they receive federal research funding, most universities are required to have an Institutional Animal Care and Use Committee (IACUC), which functions in a manner similar to the IRB for human subjects. The IACUC members include a veterinarian who has specific training or experience in the proper management of laboratory animals, a scientist with experience in animal research, and a person representing the general community. Veterinary medicine must be made available as needed. For details, we recommend purchasing the *Guide for the Care and Use of Laboratory Animals* from the National Academy Press (see References for contact information).[33]

Authorship

In scientific literature, **authorship credit**—the listing, in order, of authors of published articles or books—is taken seriously because it acknowledges the intellectual contributions and assigns credit for the findings and outcomes of the study. As stated by Pool, "Publication is the coin of the realm, and authorship is analogous to patents for inventions and copyright for creative works of literature, art, music, and computer software."[34] Decisions related to tenure, promotion, and hiring are frequently contingent on authorship and order of authorship. The perceived value of authorship itself depends on the prestige—as determined by its review process, rejection rate, and readership—of the journal that publishes the study.

Authorship would appear easy to determine, but in fact it has become increasingly difficult given the movement toward multiple authors, a movement reflecting the increased specialization of talents used in generating knowledge. Complicating matters, different journals adopt different standards. We recommend the Medical Journal Editors' "Uniform Requirements for Manuscripts Submitted to Biomedical Journals," which states that:

> Authorship credit should be based only on substantial contributions to
> (a) conception and design, or analysis and interpretation of data; and to
> (b) drafting the article or revising it critically for important intellectual
> content; and on (c) final approval of the version to be published. Conditions
> (a), (b), and (c) must all be met.[35]

We note that this is essentially the same standard used by the journal *Physical Therapy*, expressed in its "Information for Authors."[36]

All scientific journals agree that minor or routine contributions such as editing, data tabulations, inputting data, or typing should be acknowledged (typically in footnotes), but they do not qualify a person for authorship.[37] Nor should personal qualities of the researchers, such as institutional position (department chair), status, or seniority be considered. Furthermore, "acquisition of funding, collection of data, or general supervision of the research group by itself would not justify a claim of authorship."[38] The wage status of the researcher is not a relevant variable in assigning authorship, and consultants should not be disqualified as authors merely because they are paid to assist in projects, for there is no significant difference between their pay and the pay that faculty receive from universities or grants while participating. Finally, time invested in the project is not an adequate gauge for either authorship or order.[39]

Even though these guidelines are relatively clear, some key ambiguities remain. Most journals stipulate that authorship requires "professional" or "significant" contributions to the creative and intellectual components of the project, such as the research design, assessment tools, interpretation of data, integration of existing theory, and development of new conceptual models. Yet the performance of just one of these areas might not in itself qualify a researcher for authorship. At the very least, following the guidelines from the Medical Journal Editors, one must have contributed to the design of the study or interpretation of the data, contributed to intellectual content to the article, and given final approval of the draft to be published. The precise requirements are not always clear, but the presumption is that every effort at honesty and fairness is required by scientific integrity.

Recognition of authorship brings with it a duty. The Council on Biology Editors argues that each author must be prepared to assume public responsibility for the content of the paper.[34] The American Physical Therapy Association states that by being authors, researchers "certify that they have participated sufficiently to take public responsibility for the work."[36] At the same time, fairness requires that researchers in the study have equal opportunity to contribute in the specified areas. Denying authorship because opportunities for contribution were denied is cause for an authorship dispute and appropriate appeal.

Although authorship is itself a mark of distinction, the order of authorship can be equally important. Some universities only consider first-author publications in determining promotion, tenure, and pay. Unfortunately, the intuitive descending scale of significance in terms of contribution to the research project is not universal. In some fields (physics) and in some journals, authors are listed alphabetically. In most cases, however, as is usually true in physical therapy, order of authorship is in descending order based on level of contribution, with the most significant contributions having been made by the first author. Because of the way in which articles are referenced, frequently the first author is the only author listed, followed by "et al."

Student-faculty research efforts are especially vulnerable to injustices in authorship distribution. The faculty member comes to the project with a disproportionate amount of knowledge about the process and significantly more power. There is a general tendency by both students and faculty to give undue credit to faculty for their contributions.[40] Ironically, senior faculty also tend to give more credit to students than they truly deserve. Just as students should be protected from unfair treatment by faculty, faculty have a responsibility to accurately report student authorship. Giving students more credit than they deserve falsely represents students' scholarship, gives them an unfair professional advantage compared to other students, and places them at risk for subsequent assignments that are beyond their competence.[41]

The dissertation process is qualitatively and quantitatively unlike other student-faculty research collaborations. In recognition of the difficulties in this area, the American Psychological Association Ethics Committee adopted the position that:

(a) dissertation supervisors may be *only* second authors;

(b) second authorship is obligatory if the supervisor designates the primary variables, makes *major* interpretive contributions, or provides the database;

(c) second authorship may be extended as a courtesy if the supervisor is *substantially* involved in developing the research design or measurement techniques/data collection or if the supervisor substantially contributes to the writing of the publication; and

(d) authorship is not acceptable if the supervisor only gives or provides encouragement, facilities, financial support, critiques, or editorial assistance.[39]

In all cases, it is recommended that everyone meet to discuss authorship early in the development of the research project. Those most informed on the subject should share relevant articles, and the terms for authorship and order of authorship should be discussed and outlined. The agreement might have to be renegotiated at a later time, given that research projects often take unexpected turns. Even with all precautions taken, there is still the possibility that disagreements will arise. Therefore, the first meeting of the research parties should arrive at a consensus that if disputes cannot be settled amiably, arbitration will be binding on all parties. Appropriate arbitration groups vary with the committee structures in each university, but typically they include IRBs, ethics committees, or ad hoc committees composed of faculty and students not involved in the dispute.[42]

In conclusion, we have touched on only a few areas of scientific integrity, albeit important ones. The literature on research ethics is currently undergoing rapid expansion, due in part to increasing public demand for scientific integrity as well as awareness of how increasing pressures to achieve financial gain and career development encourage wrongdoing. As we noted in Chapter 1, professionals are motivated by a combination of compensation motives (money, prestige), craft motives (excellence and creativity), and moral concern (caring, integrity). Integrity can quickly fade when self-interested compensation motives become dominant. Both character and societal-organizational factors enter into understanding wrongdoing, as we noted in Chapter 8. Exactly the same can be said of understanding the morally responsible conduct of professionals. At the levels of both individual character and social structures, ethics is the heart of professionalism.

Discussion Questions

1. Discuss the case of Scott Conway, introduced at the beginning of this chapter. What is morally troublesome about his conduct and his character, and why? Does the seriousness of misrepresenting and tampering with data turn solely on its likely consequences in the particular situation? Are there any changes in scientific or organizational practices you can recommend to discourage his type of behavior and to encourage scientific integrity in individual researchers?

2. Some critics complain that informed consent is impossible or worthless, since no one knows all the risk inherent in a project. Moreover, they say, experimental subjects lack the advanced education to fully grasp the risks that are understood by researchers. Finally, in some cases of patient care it is permissible to engage in mild paternalism—withholding some information for a short time because immediate release would likely cause more harm. By analogy, should not the same considerations apply in research? How would you reply to these critics?

3. At present, prisoners are banned from participating in medical experiments. Present and defend your view on whether the ban should continue, taking into account arguments on both sides. Those favoring the ban point to past abuses in which prisoners were not given full information about experiments and in which the hope for early parole served as undue influence. Indeed, since 1952, the House of Delegates of the AMA has insisted that prisoners not be allowed to participate because their coercive environment disqualifies them from giving full voluntary consent. Opponents argue that with proper safeguards prisoners should be allowed to participate in research because it reduces boredom, increases a sense of self worth, and allows them to act as moral agents.

4. Identify and discuss the ethical issues raised by the following case. Helen Mather is junior faculty member in a highly research-oriented physical therapy department of a large university.[43] For several years she has worked closely and published articles with her mentor, Henry Goldberg, but she has begun to feel her recognition is being overshadowed by his far greater reputation. Using techniques they had developed together, but based on an experiment she had designed by herself, she writes an article invited for an international conference. The galley proofs for the article, which is to be published in the proceedings of the conference, are given to the secretary to be mailed. Goldberg happens to see the galleys and adds his name as a coauthor. When Mather confronts Goldberg, he apologizes for not telling her what he had done, but explains that he regards the research as sufficiently belonging to him to warrant status as coauthor.

5. Present and defend your view on whether ethics should be entirely human-centered or widened to recognize moral worth in other mammals and animals. Do you see merit in the animal rights or animal welfare viewpoints? Also, assess the differences between the latter two viewpoints. In doing so, take into account that utilitarianism and rights ethics can have many variations (as discussed in Chapter 2), depending on the specific theory of good and rights, respectively, that is endorsed.

6. Feminists and others have pointed out that the language we use shapes as well as reflects our basic opinions and values. Assess the terms commonly used in experimentation, such as research "subject," and discuss how the pursuit of objectivity can easily reduce humans to objects, something Kant would find particularly objectionable. What terms might you suggest as alternative or more appropriate terms in research?

7. At a well-known university, the physical therapy students, in groups of three, are required to complete a research project with the assistance of a faculty sponsor and a second faculty member as an advisor. During one particularly difficult but meaningful research project, the second faculty member offered valuable editorial comments but did so in a manner that was condescending and insulting to all other members of the team, including the primary faculty

sponsor. The students approached the faculty sponsor about the behavior of the second faculty member and he agreed to speak privately to the person. Unfortunately, the situation only grew worse and the second faculty person refused to sign off on the project because a spacing error was discovered after the deadline in one cell of one table (although it did not affect the values). The primary sponsor overrode the second and passed the students. After graduation, the students prepared the manuscript for publication. They worked closely with the primary sponsor but refused to submit manuscripts to the second advisor. When it came time to submit the article to the journal, the students refused to sign the release if the second advisor's name was to be listed as fourth author, as had been customary in the division. When the second faculty advisor discovered that the article was to be submitted without her name, she threatened to engage an attorney to force her inclusion as an author, and if that failed, she stated that she would contact the editor and block publication. What are the merits of the demand by the second faculty member for inclusion in authorship credits? What merits support the students' position? How might this conflict have been avoided? How can it best be resolved?

References

1. This example is a composite of real events. For other examples, see Broad W, Wade N. *Betrayers of the Truth: Fraud and Deceit in the Halls of Science.* New York, NY: Simon and Schuster; 1982.
2. American Physical Therapy Association. Integrity in physical therapy research. Available at: https://www.apta.org/pdfs/governance/bod1_3_oo.pdf. Accessed March 25, 2001.
3. Atkinson HW. Head in the clouds, feet on the ground. *Physiotherapy.* 1988;74: 542-547.
4. Jette AM. Outcomes research: shifting the dominant research paradigm in physical therapy. *Phys Ther.* 1995;75(11):965-970.
5. Mooney V. The impact of managed care on musculoskeletal physical treatment. *Orthopedics.* 1995;18(11):1063-1064.
6. Robertson VJ. A quantitative analysis of research in physical therapy. *Phys Ther.* 1995;75(4):313-321.
7. Rothstein JM. Editor's note: outcomes and survival. *Phys Ther.* 1996;76(2):126.
8. Lederer SE, Grodin MA. Historical overview: pediatric experimentation. In: Grodin MA, Glantz LH, eds. *Children as Research Subjects: Science, Ethics & Law.* New York, NY: Oxford University Press; 1994.
9. Annas GJ, Grodin MA, eds. *The Nazi Doctors and the Nuremberg Code.* New York, NY: Oxford University Press; 1992.
10. Grau G. *Hidden Holocaust?* London, England: Cassell; 1993.
11. Plant R. *The Pink Triangle.* New York, NY: Henry Holt and Company; 1986.
12. For helpful readings, on which our discussion is based, see the articles on medical experimentation in Arras JD, Steinbock B, eds., *Ethical Issues in Modern Medicine*, 4th ed. Mountain View, CA: Mayfield Publishing; 1995. And Munson R, ed., *Intervention and Reflection*, 6th ed. Belmont, CA: Wadsworth Publishing; 2000.
13. Arras JD, Steinbock, B. Experimentation on human subjects. In: Arras JD, Steinbock B, eds., *Ethical Issues in Modern Medicine*, 4th ed. Mountain View, CA: Mayfield Publishing Company; 1995.
14. Taylor T. Opening statement of the prosecution, December 9, 1946. In: Annas GJ, Grodin MA. *The Nazi Doctors and the Nuremberg Code.* New York, NY: Oxford University Press; 1992.

15. Available through http://ohrp.osophs.dhhs.gov/humansubjects/guidance/ 45cfr46.htm.
16. For a detailed review of current regulations sponsored by the Department of Health and Human Services, see http://www.access.gpo.gov/nara/cfr/waisidx99/45cfr46 99.html.
17. Portney LG, Watkins MP. *Foundations of Clinical Research*. Norwalk, CT: Appleton & Lange; 1993.
18. Prentice ED, Purtilo RB. The use and protection of human and animal subjects. In: Bork CE, ed. *Research in Physical Therapy*. Philadelphia, PA: J.B. Lippincott Company; 1993:37-56.
19. Beauchamp TL, Childress JF. *Principles of Biomedical Ethics*, 5th ed. New York, NY: Oxford University Press; 2001.
20. Munson R. *Intervention and Reflection*, 6th ed. Belmont, CA: Wadsworth Publishing; 2000:480.
21. Fausto-Sterling A. *Myths of Gender: Biological Theories about Women and Men*, 2d ed. New York: Basic Books; 1992.
22. Dresser RS. Wanted: single, white male for medical research. *Hastings Cent Rep*. January-February, 1992:24-29.
23. Jones CP, LaVeist TA, Lillie-Blanton, M. 'Race' in the epidemiologic literature: an examination of the *American Journal of Epidemiology*, 1921-1990. *Am J Epidemiol*. 1991(134):1079-1084.
24. Callahan D. Ethical responsibility in science in the face of uncertain consequences. *Ann NY Acad Sci*. 1976;265(10).
25. Weick KE. Small wins: redefining the scale of social problems. *Am Psychol*. 1984;39(1):40-49.
26. Moffroid MT, Hofkosh JM. Development of a research section. *Phys Ther*. 1969;49(11):1208-1212.
27. Peter Singer, who is an act utilitarian, represents animal-welfarists. Although he occasionally used rights language in the first edition of his book, he has made it clear that his concern is with suffering. See *Animal Liberation*, rev. ed. New York, NY: Avon Books; 1990. Tom Regan is a leading animal rights ethicist: *The Case for Animal Rights*. Berkeley, CA: University of California Press; 1983. An insightful moderate position is set forth by Mary Midgley, *Animals and Why They Matter*. Athens, GA: University of Georgia Press; 1984.
28. Mukerjee M. Trends in animal research. *Sci Am*. 1997(Feb.):86-93
29. Botting JH, Morrison AR. Animal research is vital to medicine. *Sci Am*. 1997(Feb.):83-85.
30. Elliott D, Brown M. Animal experimentation and ethics. In: Elliott D, Stern J, eds., *Research Ethics: A Reader*. Hanover, NH: University Press of New England; 1997.
31. Donnelley S. Introduction, the troubled middle: in medias res. *Hastings Cent Rep*. 1990(May/June):2-4.
32. Russow LM. Ethical theory and the moral status of animals. *Hastings Cent Rep*. 1990(May/June):4-8.
33. *Guide for the Care and Use of Laboratory Animals*. National Academy Press (2101 Constitution Avenue, NW, Lockbox 285, Washington, DC 20055).
34. Pool R. More squabbling over unbelievable results. In: Elliott D, Stern J, eds., *Research Ethics: A Reader*. Hanover, NH: University Press of New England; 1997:127.
35. International Committee of Medical Journal Editors. Uniform requirements for manuscripts submitted to biomedical journals. *JAMA*. 1993;269(17):2283.
36. American Physical Therapy Association. Information for authors. Available at: http://www.ptjournal.org/aut_info.html. Accessed March 25, 2001.
37. Fine MA, Kurdek LA. Reflections on determining authorship credit and authorship order on faculty-student collaborations. *Am Psychol*. 1993;48(11):1141-1147.

Costa MM, Gatz M. Determination of authorship credit in published dissertations. *Psychol Sci.* 1992;3(6):354-357.

38. American Physical Therapy Association. Information for authors. *Phys Ther.* 1996;76(10):1156-1157.

39. Winston, RB. A suggested procedure for determining order of authorship in research publications. *J Couns Dev.* 1985;63:515-518.

40. Costa MM, Gatz M. Determination of authorship credit in published dissertations. *Psychol Sci.* 1992;3(6):354-357.

41. Fine MA, Kurdek LA. Reflections on determining authorship credit and authorship order on faculty-student collaborations. *Am Psychol.* 1993;48(11):1141-1147.

42. Goodyear RK, Crego CA, Johnston, MW. Ethical issues in the supervision of student research: a study of critical incidents. *Prof Psychol-Res Pr.* 1992;23(3):203-210.

43. Based on a case by Deni Elliott and Judy E. Stern (and earlier by C.K. Gunsalus), in *Research Ethics: A Reader.* Hanover, NH: University Press of New England; 1997:91.

Appendix

I APTA Code of Ethics

HOD 06-00-12-23

(Program 17) [Amended HOD 06-91-05-05; HOD 06-87-11-17; HOD 06-81-06-18; HOD 06-78-06-08; HOD 06-78-06-07; HOD 06-77-18-30; HOD 06-77-17-27; Initial HOD 06-73-13-24]

PREAMBLE

This Code of Ethics of the American Physical Therapy Association sets forth principles for the ethical practice of physical therapy. All physical therapists are responsible for maintaining and promoting ethical practice. To this end, the physical therapist shall act in the best interest of the patient/client. This Code of Ethics shall be binding on all physical therapists.

PRINCIPLE 1

A physical therapist shall respect the rights and dignity of all individuals and shall provide compassionate care.

PRINCIPLE 2

A physical therapist shall act in a trustworthy manner towards patients/clients, and in all other aspects of physical therapy practice.

PRINCIPLE 3

A physical therapist shall comply with laws and regulations governing physical therapy and shall strive to effect changes that benefit patients/clients.

PRINCIPLE 4

A physical therapist shall exercise sound professional judgment.

PRINCIPLE 5

A physical therapist shall achieve and maintain professional competence.

PRINCIPLE 6

A physical therapist shall maintain and promote high standards for physical therapy practice, education, and research.

PRINCIPLE 7

A physical therapist shall seek only such remuneration as is deserved and reasonable for physical therapy services.

PRINCIPLE 8

A physical therapist shall provide and make available accurate and relevant information to patients/clients about their care and to the public about physical therapy services.

PRINCIPLE 9

A physical therapist shall protect the public and the profession from unethical, incompetent, and illegal acts.

PRINCIPLE 10

A physical therapist shall endeavor to address the health needs of society.

PRINCIPLE 11

A physical therapist shall respect the rights, knowledge, and skills of colleagues and other health care professionals.

Appendix

II APTA Guide for Professional Conduct

Purpose

This *Guide for Professional Conduct* (Guide) is intended to serve physical therapists in interpreting the *Code of Ethics* (Code) of the American Physical Therapy Association (Association), in matters of professional conduct. The Guide provides guidelines by which physical therapists may determine the propriety of their conduct. It is also intended to guide the professional development of physical therapist students. The Code and the Guide apply to all physical therapists. These guidelines are subject to changes as the dynamics of the profession change and as new patterns of health care delivery are developed and accepted by the professional community and the public. This Guide is subject to monitoring and timely revision by the Ethics and Judicial Committee of the Association.

Interpreting Ethical Principles

The interpretations expressed in this Guide reflect the opinions, decisions, and advice of the Ethics and Judicial Committee. These interpretations are intended to assist a physical therapist in applying general ethical principles to specific situations. They should not be considered inclusive of all situations that could evolve.

PRINCIPLE 1

A physical therapist shall respect the rights and dignity of all individuals and shall provide compassionate care.

> ### 1.1 Attitudes of a Physical Therapist
> A. A physical therapist shall recognize individual differences and shall respect and be responsive to those differences.
> B. A physical therapist shall be guided by concern for the physical, psychological, and socioeconomic welfare of patients/clients.
> C. A physical therapist shall not harass, abuse, or discriminate against others.
> D. A physical therapist shall be aware of the patient's health-related needs and act in a manner that facilitates meeting those needs.

PRINCIPLE 2

A physical therapist shall act in a trustworthy manner towards patients/clients, and in all other aspects of physical therapy practice.

> ### 2.1 Patient/Physical Therapist Relationship
> A. To act in a trustworthy manner the physical therapist shall act in the patient's/client's best interest. Working in the patient's/client's best interest requires knowledge of the patient's/client's needs from the patient's/client's perspective. Patients/clients often come to the physical therapist in a vulnerable state and normally will rely on the physical therapist's advice, which they perceive to be based on superior knowledge, skill, and experience. The trustworthy physical therapist acts to ameliorate the patient's/client's vulnerability, not to exploit it.
> B. A physical therapist shall not exploit any aspect of the physical therapist/patient relationship.
> C. A physical therapist shall not engage in any sexual relationship or activity, whether consensual or nonconsensual, with any patient while a physical therapist/patient relationship exists.

    D. The physical therapist shall create an environment that encourages an open dialogue with the patient/client.

    E. In the event the physical therapist or patient terminates the physical therapist/patient relationship while the patient continues to need physical therapy services, the physical therapist should take steps to transfer the care of the patient to another provider.

2.2 Truthfulness

A physical therapist shall not make statements that he/she knows or should know are false, deceptive, fraudulent, or unfair. See Section 8.2.D.

2.3 Confidential Information

    A. Information relating to the physical therapist/patient relationship is confidential and may not be communicated to a third party not involved in that patient's care without the prior consent of the patient, subject to applicable law.

    B. Information derived from peer review shall be held confidential.by the reviewer unless the physical therapist who was reviewed consents to the release of the information.

    C. A physical therapist may disclose information to appropriate authorities when it is necessary to protect the welfare of an individual or the community or when required by law. Such disclosure shall be in accordance with applicable law.

2.4 Patient Autonomy and Consent

    A. A physical therapist shall not restrict patients' freedom to select their provider of physical therapy.

    B. A physical therapist shall communicate to the patient/client the findings of his/her examination, evaluation, diagnosis, and prognosis.

    C. A physical therapist shall collaborate with the patient/client to establish the goals of treatment and the plan of care.

    D. A physical therapist shall use sound professionalism judgment in informing the patient/client of any substantial risks of the recommended examination and intervention.

    E. A physical therapist shall respect the patient's/client's right to make decisions regarding the recommended plan of care, including consent, modification, or refusal.

PRINCIPLE 3

A physical therapist shall comply with laws and regulations governing physical therapy and shall strive to effect changes that benefit patients/clients.

3.1 Professional Practice

A physical therapist shall provide examination, evaluation, diagnosis, prognosis, and intervention. A physical therapist shall not engage in any unlawful activity that substantially relates to the qualifications, functions, or duties of a physical therapist.

3.2 Just Laws and Regulations

A physical therapist shall advocate the adoption of laws, regulations, and policies by providers, employers, third party payers, legislatures, and regulatory agencies to provide and improve access to necessary health care services for all individuals.

3.3 Unjust Laws and Regulations

A physical therapist shall endeavor to change unjust laws, regulations, and policies that govern the practice of physical therapy. See Section 10.2.

PRINCIPLE 4

A physical therapist shall exercise sound professional judgment.

4.1 Professional Responsibility

    A. A physical therapist shall make professional judgments that are in the patient/client's best interests.

    B. Regardless of practice setting, a physical therapist has primary responsibility for the physical therapy care of a patient and shall make independent judgments regarding that care consistent with accepted professional standards. See Section 2.4.

    C. A physical therapist shall not provide physical therapy services to a patient/client while his/her ability to do so safely is impaired.

D. A physical therapist shall exercise sound professional judgment based upon his/her knowledge, skill, education, training, and experience.

E. Upon accepting a patient/client for physical therapy services, a physical therapist shall be responsible for: the examination, evaluation, and diagnosis of that individual; the prognosis and intervention; re-examination and modification of the plan of care; and the maintenance of adequate records, including progress reports. A physical therapist shall establish the plan of care and shall provide and/or supervise and direct the appropriate interventions. See Section 2.4.

F. If the diagnostic process reveals findings that are outside the scope of the physical therapist's knowledge, experience, or expertise, the physical therapist shall so inform the patient/client and refer to an appropriate practitioner.

G. When the patient has been referred from another practitioner, the physical therapist shall communicate the findings of the examination and evaluation, the diagnosis, the proposed intervention, and re-examination findings (as indicated) to the referring practitioner.

H. A physical therapist shall determine when a patient/client will no longer benefit from physical therapy services.

4.2 Direction and Supervision

A. The supervising physical therapist has primary responsibility for the physical therapy care rendered to a patient/client.

B. A physical therapist shall not delegate to a less qualified person any activity that requires the unique skill, knowledge, and judgment of the physical therapist.

4.3 Practice Arrangements

A. Participation in a business, partnership, corporation, or other entity does not exempt physical therapists, whether employers, partners, or stockholders, either individually or collectively, from the obligation to promote, maintain, and comply with the ethical principles of the Association.

B. A physical therapist shall advise his/her employer(s) of any employer practice that causes a physical therapist to be in conflict with the ethical principles of the Association. A physical therapist shall seek to eliminate aspects of his/her employment that are in conflict with the ethical principles of the Association.

4.4 Gifts and Other Considerations

A physical therapist shall not accept or offer gifts or other considerations that affect or give an appearance of affecting his/her professional judgment.

PRINCIPLE 5

A physical therapist shall achieve and maintain professional competence.

5.1 Scope of Competence

A physical therapist shall practice within the scope of his/her competence and commensurate with his/her level of education, training, and experience.

5.2 Self-assessment

A physical therapist shall engage in self-assessment, which is a lifelong professional responsibility for maintaining competence.

5.3 Professional Development

A physical therapist shall participate in educational activities that enhance his/her basic knowledge and skills.

PRINCIPLE 6

A physical therapist shall maintain and promote high standards for physical therapy practice, education, and research.

6.1 Professional Standards

A physical therapist shall know the accepted professional standards when engaging in physical therapy practice, education, and/or research. A physical therapist shall continuously engage in assessment activities to determine compliance with these standards. If a physical therapist is not in compliance with these standards, he/she shall engage in activities designed to reach compliance with the standards. When a physical therapist is in compliance with these standards, he/she shall engage in activities designed to maintain such compliance.

6.2 Practice
A. A physical therapist shall achieve and maintain professional competence. See Section 5.
B. A physical therapist shall demonstrate his/her commitment to quality improvement by engaging in peer and utilization review and other self-assessment activities.

6.3 Professional Education
A. A physical therapist shall support high-quality education in academic and clinical settings.
B. A physical therapist participating in the educational process is responsible to the students, the academic institutions, and the clinical settings for promoting ethical conduct. A physical therapist shall model ethical behavior and provide the student with information about the Code of Ethics, opportunities to discuss ethical conflicts, and procedures for reporting unresolved ethical conflicts. See Section 9.

6.4 Continuing Education
A. A physical therapist providing continuing education must be competent in the content area.
B. When a physical therapist provides continuing education, he/she shall ensure that course content, objectives, faculty credentials, and responsibilities of the instructional staff are accurately stated in the promotional and instructional course materials.
C. A physical therapist shall evaluate the efficacy and effectiveness of information and techniques presented in continuing education programs before integrating them into his or her practice.

6.5 Research
A. A physical therapist shall support research activities that contribute knowledge for improved patient care.
B. A physical therapist shall report to appropriate authorities any acts in the conduct or presentation of research that appear unethical or illegal. See Section 9.

PRINCIPLE 7
A physical therapist shall seek only such remuneration as is deserved and reasonable for physical therapy services.

7.1 Business and Employment Practices
A. A physical therapist's business/employment practices shall be consistent with the ethical principles of the Association.
B. A physical therapist shall never place her/his own financial interest above the welfare of individuals under his/her care.
C. A physical therapist shall recognize that third-party payer contracts may limit, in one form or another, the provision of physical therapy services. Third-party limitations do not absolve the physical therapist from making sound professional judgments that are in the patient's best interest. A physical therapist shall avoid underutilization of physical therapy services.
D. When a physical therapist's judgment is that a patient will receive negligible benefit from physical therapy services, the physical therapist shall not provide or continue to provide such services if the primary reason for doing so is to further the financial self-interest of the physical therapist or his/her employer. A physical therapist shall avoid overutilization of physical therapy services.
E. Fees for physical therapy services should be reasonable for the service performed, considering the setting in which it is provided, practice costs in the geographic area, judgment of other organizations, and other relevant factors.
F. A physical therapist shall not directly or indirectly request, receive, or participate in the dividing, transferring, assigning, or rebating of an unearned fee.

G. A physical therapist shall not profit by means of a credit or other valuable consideration, such as an unearned commission, discount, or gratuity, in connection with the furnishing of physical therapy services.

H. Unless laws impose restrictions to the contrary, physical therapists who provide physical therapy services within a business entity may pool fees and monies received. Physical therapists may divide or apportion these fees and monies in accordance with the business agreement.

I. A physical therapist may enter into agreements with organizations to provide physical therapy services if such agreements do not violate the ethical principles of the Association or applicable laws.

7.2 Endorsement of Products or Services

A. A physical therapist shall not exert influence on individuals under his/her care or their families to use products or services based on the direct or indirect financial interest of the physical therapist in such products or services. Realizing that these individuals will normally rely on the physical therapist's advice, their best interest must always be maintained, as must their right of free choice relating to the use of any product or service. Although it cannot be considered unethical for physical therapists to own or have a financial interest in the production, sale, or distribution of products/services, they must act in accordance with law and make full disclosure of their interest whenever individuals under their care use such products/services.

B. A physical therapist may receive remuneration for endorsement or advertisement of products or services to the public, physical therapists, or other health professionals provided he/she discloses any financial interest in the production, sale, or distribution of said products or services.

C. When endorsing or advertising products or services, a physical therapist shall use sound professional judgment and shall not give the appearance of Association endorsement unless the Association has formally endorsed the products or services.

7.3 Disclosure

A physical therapist shall disclose to the patient if the referring practitioner derives compensation from the provision of physical therapy.

PRINCIPLE 8

A physical therapist shall provide and make available accurate and relevant information to patients/clients about their care and to the public about physical therapy services.

8.1 Accurate and Relevant Information to the Patient

A. A physical therapist shall provide the patient/client information about his/her condition and plan of care. See Section 2.4.

B. Upon the request of the patient, the physical therapist shall provide, or make available, the medical record to the patient or a patient-designated third party.

C. A physical therapist shall inform patients of any known financial limitations that may affect their care.

D. A physical therapist shall inform the patient when, in his/her judgment, the patient will receive negligible benefit from further care. See Section 7.1.C.

8.2 Accurate and Relevant Information to the Public

A. A physical therapist shall inform the public about the societal benefits of the profession and who is qualified to provide physical therapy services.

B. Information given to the public shall emphasize that individual problems cannot be treated without individualized examination and plans/programs of care.

C. A physical therapist may advertise his/her services to the public.

D. A physical therapist shall not use, or participate in the use of, any form of communication containing a false, plagiarized, fraudulent, deceptive, unfair, or sensational statement or claim.

E. A physical therapist who places a paid advertisement shall identify it as such unless it is apparent from the context that it is a paid advertisement.

PRINCIPLE 9

A physical therapist shall protect the public and the profession from unethical, incompetent, and illegal acts.

9.1 Consumer Protection

    A. A physical therapist shall provide care that is within the scope of practice as defined by the state practice act.

    B. A physical therapist shall not engage in any conduct that is unethical, incompetent, or illegal.

    C. A physical therapist shall report any conduct that appears to be unethical, incompetent, or illegal.

    D. A physical therapist may not participate in any arrangements in which patients are exploited due to the referring sources' enhancing their personal incomes as a result of referring for, prescribing, or recommending physical therapy. See Section 5.

PRINCIPLE 10

A physical therapist shall endeavor to address the health needs of society.

10.1 Pro Bono Service

A physical therapist shall render pro bono publico (reduced or no fee) services to patients lacking the ability to pay for services, as each physical therapist's practice permits.

10.2 Community Health

A physical therapist shall endeavor to support activities that benefit the health status of the community. See Section 3.

PRINCIPLE 11

A physical therapist shall respect the rights, knowledge, and skills of colleagues and other health care professionals.

11.1 Consultation

A physical therapist shall seek consultation whenever the welfare of the patient will be safeguarded or advanced by consulting those who have special skills, knowledge, and experience.

11.2 Patient/Provider Relationships

A physical therapist shall not undermine the relationship(s) between his/her patient and other health care professionals.

11.3 Disparagement

Physical therapists shall not disparage colleagues and other health care professionals. See Section 9 and Section 2.4.A.

Issued by Ethics and Judicial Committee
American Physical Therapy Association
October 1981
Last Amended November 2002

APTA Standards of Ethical Conduct for the Physical Therapist Assistant

HOD 06-00-13-24

(Program 17) [Amended HOD 06-91-06-07; Initial HOD 06-82-04-08]

Preamble

This document of the American Physical Therapy Association sets forth standards for the ethical conduct of the physical therapist assistant. All physical therapist assistants are responsible for maintaining high standards of conduct while assisting physical therapists. The physical therapist assistant shall act in the best interest of the patient/client. These standards of conduct shall be binding on all physical therapist assistants.

Standard 1

A physical therapist assistant shall respect the rights and dignity of all individuals and shall provide compassionate care.

Standard 2

A physical therapist assistant shall act in a trustworthy manner towards patients/clients.

Standard 3

A physical therapist assistant shall provide selected physical therapy interventions only under the supervision and direction of a physical therapist.

Standard 4

A physical therapist assistant shall comply with laws and regulations governing physical therapy.

Standard 5

A physical therapist assistant shall achieve and maintain competence in the provision of selected physical therapy interventions.

Standard 6

A physical therapist assistant shall make judgments that are commensurate with their educational and legal qualifications as a physical therapist assistant.

Standard 7

A physical therapist assistant shall protect the public and the profession from unethical, incompetent, and illegal acts.

Guide for Conduct of the Physical Therapist Assistant

This *Guide for Conduct of the Physical Therapist Assistant* (Guide) is intended to serve physical therapist assistants in interpreting the *Standards of Ethical Conduct for the Physical Therapist Assistant* (Standards) of the American Physical Therapy Association (APTA). The Guide provides guidelines by which physical therapist assistants may determine the propriety of their conduct. It is also intended to guide the development of physical therapist assistant students. The Standards and Guide apply to all physical therapist assistants. These guidelines are subject to change as the dynamics of the profession change and as new patterns of health care delivery are developed and accepted by the professional community and the public. This Guide is subject to monitoring and timely revision by the Ethics and Judicial Committee of the Association.

Interpreting Standards

The interpretations expressed in this Guide reflect the opinions, decisions, and advice of the Ethics and Judicial Committee. These interpretations are intended to guide a physical therapist assistant in applying general ethical principles to specific situations. They should not be considered inclusive of all situations that could evolve.

STANDARD 1

A physical therapist assistant shall respect the rights and dignity of all individuals and shall provide compassionate care.

1.1 **Attitude of a physical therapist assistant**
  A. A physical therapist assistant shall demonstrate sensitivity to individual and cultural differences.
  B. A physical therapist assistant shall be guided at all times by concern for the physical and psychological welfare of patients/clients.
  C. A physical therapist assistant shall not harass, abuse, or discriminate against others.

STANDARD 2

A physical therapist assistant shall act in a trustworthy manner towards patients/clients.

2.1 **Trustworthiness**
  A. To act in a trustworthy manner a physical therapist assistant shall act in the patient's/client's best interest. Working in the patient's/client's best interest requires sensitivity to the patient's/client's vulnerability and an effective working relationship between the physical therapist and the physical therapist assistant.
  B. A physical therapist assistant shall act to ameliorate the patient's/client's vulnerability, not to exploit it.
  C. A physical therapist assistant shall clearly identify him/herself as a physical therapist assistant to patients/clients.
  D. A physical therapist assistant shall conduct him/herself in a manner that supports the physical therapist/patient relationship.
  E. A physical therapist assistant shall not engage in any sexual relationship or activity, whether consensual or nonconsensual, with any patient entrusted to his/her care.
  F. A physical therapist assistant shall not invite, accept, or offer gifts or other considerations that affect or give an appearance of affecting his/her provision of physical therapy interventions.

2.2 Exploitation of Patients
A physical therapist assistant shall not participate in any arrangements in which patients/clients are exploited. Such arrangements include situations where referring sources enhance their personal incomes as a result of referring for, delegating, prescribing, or recommending physical therapy services.

2.3 Truthfulness
A. A physical therapist assistant shall not make statements that he/she knows or should know are false, deceptive, fraudulent, or unfair.

B. Although it cannot be considered unethical for a physical therapist assistant to own or have a financial interest in the production, sale, or distribution of products/services, he/she must act in accordance with law and make full disclosure of his/her interest to patients/clients.

2.4 Confidential Information
A. Information relating to the patient/client is confidential and may not be communicated to a third party not involved in that patient's care without the prior consent of the patient, subject to applicable law.

B. A physical therapist assistant shall refer all requests for release of confidential information to the supervising physical therapist.

STANDARD 3
A physical therapist assistant shall provide selected physical therapy interventions only under the supervision and direction of a physical therapist.

3.1 Supervisory Relationship
A. A physical therapist assistant shall provide services only under the supervision and direction of a physical therapist.

B. A physical therapist assistant shall provide only those physical therapy interventions that have been selected by the physical therapist.

C. A physical therapist assistant shall not carry out any selected physical therapy interventions that are outside his/her education, training, experience, or skill and shall notify the physical therapist.

D. A physical therapist assistant may adjust specific interventions within the plan of care established by the physical therapist in response to changes in the patient's/client's status.

E. A physical therapist assistant shall not perform examinations or evaluations, interpret data, determine diagnosis or prognosis, or establish or alter a plan of care.

F. Consistent with the physical therapist assistant's education, training, knowledge, and experience, he/she may respond to the patient's/client's inquiries regarding interventions that are within the established plan of care.

G. A physical therapist assistant shall have regular and ongoing communication with the physical therapist regarding the patient's/client's status.

STANDARD 4
A physical therapist assistant shall comply with laws and regulations governing physical therapy.

4.1 Supervision
A physical therapist assistant shall know and comply with applicable law. Regardless of the content of any law, a physical therapist assistant shall provide services only under the supervision and direction of a physical therapist.

4.2 Representation
A physical therapist assistant shall not hold him/herself out as a physical therapist.

STANDARD 5
A physical therapist assistant shall achieve and maintain competence in the provision of selected physical therapy interventions.

5.1 Competence

A physical therapist assistant shall provide interventions consistent with his/her level of education, training, experience, and skill.

5.2 Self-assessment

A physical therapist assistant shall engage in self-assessment in order to maintain competence.

5.3 Development

A physical therapist assistant shall participate in educational activities that enhance his/her basic knowledge and skills.

STANDARD 6

A physical therapist assistant shall make judgments that are commensurate with their educational and legal qualifications as a physical therapist assistant.

6.1 Patient Safety

A. A physical therapist assistant shall discontinue immediately any components of interventions that, in his/her judgment, appear to be harmful to the patient and shall discuss his/her concerns with the physical therapist.

B. A physical therapist assistant shall not carry out any selected physical therapy interventions that are outside his/her education, training, experience, or skill and shall notify the physical therapist.

C. A physical therapist assistant shall not perform interventions while his/her ability to do so safely is impaired.

6.2 Patient Status Judgments

A physical therapist assistant participates in patient status judgments by reporting changes to the physical therapist and requesting patient re-examination or revision of the plan of care. See Section 3.1.

6.3 Gifts and Other Considerations

A physical therapist assistant shall not invite, accept, or offer gifts or other considerations that affect or give the appearance of affecting his/her provision of physical therapy interventions or that exploit the patient in any way. See Section 2.1(B).

STANDARD 7

A physical therapist assistant shall protect the public and the profession from unethical, incompetent, and illegal acts.

7.1 Consumer Protection

A physical therapist assistant shall report any conduct that appears to be unethical or illegal.

7.2 Organizational Employment

A. A physical therapist assistant shall inform his/her employer(s) and/or appropriate physical therapist of any employer practice that causes him or her to be in conflict with the Standards of Ethical Conduct for the Physical Therapist Assistant.

B. A physical therapist assistant shall not engage in any activity that puts him or her in conflict with the Standards of Ethical Conduct for the Physical Therapist Assistant, regardless of directives from a physical therapist or employer.

Issued by Ethics and Judicial Committee
American Physical Therapy Association
October 1981
Last Amended July 2001

Index